T0139849

METHODS IN MOLECULAR BIOLOGY

Series Editor
John M. Walker
School of Life and Medical Sciences
University of Hertfordshire
Hatfield, Hertfordshire, AL10 9AB, UK

Lentiviral Vectors and Exosomes as Gene and Protein Delivery Tools

Edited by

Maurizio Federico

National AIDS Center, Istituto Superiore di Sanità, Rome, Italy

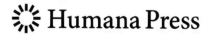 Humana Press

Editor
Maurizio Federico
Istituto Superiore di Sanità
National AIDS Center
Rome, Italy

ISSN 1064-3745   ISSN 1940-6029   (electronic)
Methods in Molecular Biology
ISBN 978-1-4939-8129-8   ISBN 978-1-4939-3753-0   (eBook)
DOI 10.1007/978-1-4939-3753-0

© Springer Science+Business Media New York 2016
Softcover reprint of the hardcover 1st edition 2016
This work is subject to copyright. All rights are reserved by the Publisher, whether the whole or part of the material is concerned, specifically the rights of translation, reprinting, reuse of illustrations, recitation, broadcasting, reproduction on microfilms or in any other physical way, and transmission or information storage and retrieval, electronic adaptation, computer software, or by similar or dissimilar methodology now known or hereafter developed.
The use of general descriptive names, registered names, trademarks, service marks, etc. in this publication does not imply, even in the absence of a specific statement, that such names are exempt from the relevant protective laws and regulations and therefore free for general use.
The publisher, the authors and the editors are safe to assume that the advice and information in this book are believed to be true and accurate at the date of publication. Neither the publisher nor the authors or the editors give a warranty, express or implied, with respect to the material contained herein or for any errors or omissions that may have been made.

Printed on acid-free paper

This Humana Press imprint is published by Springer Nature
The registered company is Springer Science+Business Media LLC New York

Preface

Lentiviral vectors (LVs) are very popular tools for stable cell engineering. The evolution of gene engineering of eukaryotic cells by LVs took great advantage from the establishment of innovative genetic and microbiologic technologies. In the present book, a consistent number of novel approaches based on the LV technology have been gathered, including new LV design and construction concepts, and improved strategies for cell targeting.

In many instances, a time-restricted expression of the desired product in target cells in the absence of potentially dangerous transfer of genetic material is desirable, as in the case of immune adjuvant strategies. Exosomes, whose biogenesis is highly reminiscent of that of lentiviruses, can fill this gap. Notably, methods and reagents for exosome production and detection largely overlap those currently in use for lentiviral vectors. The inclusion in the same book of protocols for LV and exosome production can offer a wide range of affordable experimental alternatives to scientists interested in gene and/or protein delivery.

The present collection of protocols begins with a chapter by Dankort and colleagues who, exploiting a commercially available recombination technology, describe a simple method to rapidly and efficiently construct LVs avoiding the traditional, time-consuming restriction enzyme and ligation-dependent methods. Schambach and colleagues introduce a regulatable, site-specific LV recombination technique based on the use of a single ("all-in-one") vector whereas, regarding the optimization of LV production, Fenard and colleagues describe how LV production can be increased through a slight decrease in the pH of the medium of the LV-producer cells. A method to target selected cell populations is described by Thirion and colleagues, who show how the fusion of single-chain antibodies with the LV envelope fusion protein can be instrumental for a selective LV delivery.

The second part of protocols dedicated to LVs includes techniques devoted to the optimization of the engineering of specific cell types, i.e., hematopoietic stem cells (Kustikova and colleagues), hepatocytes (Thomas and colleagues), T lymphocytes (Cribbs and colleagues), and spermatozoa (Chandrashekran and colleagues). In addition, Schmidt and colleagues describe a method to sequence LV integration sites rapidly and efficiently, and Geley and colleagues report the construction of drug-regulatable LVs for the production of RNAi through the expression of double-stranded short hairpin RNA. Finally, Schneider and colleagues provide technical details on the transduction of LVs for the production of monoclonal antibodies in cells to be implanted upon protection from the attacks of host immune system by encapsulation devices.

In the last section devoted to LV methods, protocols on the use of vectors mutated in the LV integrase function are reported. In particular, Nordin and colleagues offer an overview on the use of nonintegrating LVs (IDLVs) whose phenotype is dictated by a single amino acid substitution in the integrase catalytic core domain. Both functionality and flexibility of IDLVs have been proven by Yanez-Munoz and colleagues, who describe methods for their delivery into the striatum of a rat model of Parkinson's disease. Finally, Yla-Hertualla and colleagues give details regarding protocols aimed at the delivery of foreign proteins into target cells upon fusion with the LV integrase.

The last frontier in terms of macromolecule delivery by natural nanovesicles is represented by engineered exosomes. Biogenesis and structural features of exosomes are described in a great detail in the review of Baur and colleagues, whereas Sargiacomo and colleagues report original methods to produce, detect, and characterize fluorescently labeled exosomes. Knowlton and colleagues provide methods to purify and characterize exosomes isolated from cardiac myocytes. Finally, the last two chapters provide novel applications of exosome-based biotechnologies for the delivery of macromolecules. In particular, Manfredi and colleagues describe methods to incorporate full-length foreign proteins into both exosomes produced by eukaryotic cells and exosome-like nanovesicles released by insect cells, whereas Kuroda and colleagues give details on protocols devoted to the use of exosomes as carriers of miRNAs.

Overall, this book provides an exhaustive picture of current gene and protein delivery based on both lentivirus-generated and spontaneously released nanovesicles. The methods of macromolecule delivery based on engineered exosomes are basically novel, and the here described LV-based protocols of gene engineering represent, together with those published in the previous two editions of *Lentivirus gene engineering protocols* of the MiMB series, an almost complete guide for scientists approaching the universe of lentiviral vectors.

Rome, Italy   Maurizio Federico

Contents

Contributors

NATAŠA ANASTASOV • *Institute of Radiation Biology, Helmholtz Center Munich, German Research Center for Environmental Health, Neuherberg, Germany*

SIMONA ANTICOLI • *National AIDS Center, Istituto Superiore di Sanità, Rome, Italy*

CLAUDIA ARENACCIO • *National AIDS Center, Istituto Superiore di Sanità, Rome, Italy; Department of Science, University Roma Tre, Rome, Italy*

CYNTHIA C. BARTHOLOMAE • *Department of Translational Oncology, National Center for Tumor Diseases and German Cancer Research Center, Heidelberg, Germany*

ANDREAS BAUR • *Department of Dermatology, University Hospital Erlangen, Friedrich-Alexander University of Erlangen-Nürnberg, Erlangen, Germany*

MAURO BIFFONI • *Department of Hematology, Oncology and Molecular Medicine, Istituto Superiore di Sanità, Rome, Italy*

M.K. AZAHAM A. HAMID • *Cell Therapy Centre, University Kebangsaan Malaysia Medical Centre (UKMMC), Kuala Lumpur, Malaysia*

PAOLA DI BONITO • *Department of Infectious, Parasitic and Immunomediated Diseases, Istituto Superiore di Sanità, Rome, Italy*

ZAIRA BOUSSADIA • *Department of Hematology, Oncology and Molecular Medicine, Istituto Superiore di Sanità, Rome, Italy*

MARTIN BROADSTOCK • *School of Biological Sciences, Royal Holloway, University of London, Egham, UK; Wolfson Centre for Age-Related Diseases, King's College London, London, UK*

ANGELINE DE BRUYNS • *Department of Biology, McGill University, Montréal, QC, Canada*

COLIN CASIMIR • *Department of Natural Sciences, School of Science & Technology, Middlesex University, London, UK*

LUCAS CHAN • *Department of Haematological Medicine, School of Medicine, The Rayne Institute, King's College London, London, UK*

ANIL CHANDRASHEKRAN • *Division of Cancer, Department of Surgery and Cancer, Hammersmith Campus, Institute of Reproductive and Developmental Biology (IRDB), Imperial College London, London, UK*

CAROLINA COSCIA • *Department of Hematology, Oncology and Molecular Medicine, Istituto Superiore di Sanità, Rome, Italy*

ADAM P. CRIBBS • *Kennedy Institute of Rheumatology, University of Oxford, Oxford, UK; Botnar Research Centre, Nuffield Orthopaedic Centre, Oxford, UK; Department of Physiology, Anatomy and Genetics, MRC Functional Genomics Unit, Computational Genomics and Training Centre (CGAT), Oxford, UK*

DAVID DANKORT • *Department of Biology, McGill University, Montréal, QC, Canada*

ANNETTE DEICHMANN • *Department of Translational Oncology, National Center for Tumor Diseases and German Cancer Research Center, Heidelberg, Germany*

NICK DIBB • *Division of Cancer, Department of Surgery and Cancer, Hammersmith Campus, Institute of Reproductive and Developmental Biology (IRDB), Imperial College London, London, UK*

FLORIAN DREYER • *Department of Dermatology, University Hospital Erlangen, Friedrich-Alexander University of Erlangen-Nürnberg, Erlangen, Germany*

FARZIN FARZANEH • *Department of Haematological Medicine, School of Medicine, The Rayne Institute, King's College London, London, UK*

MAURIZIO FEDERICO • *National AIDS Center, Istituto Superiore di Sanità, Rome, Italy*

DAVID FENARD • *Généthon, Evry, France; INSERM, UMR_S951, Généthon, Evry, France; Université Evry Val d'Essonne, UMR_S951, Evry, France*

MARIA LUISA FIANI • *Department of Hematology, Oncology and Molecular Medicine, Istituto Superiore di Sanità, Rome, Italy*

RICHARD GABRIEL • *Department of Translational Oncology, National Center for Tumor Diseases and German Cancer Research Center, Heidelberg, Germany*

BEN GEILING • *Department of Biology, McGill University, Montréal, QC, Canada*

STEPHAN GELEY • *Division of Molecular Pathophysiology, Biocenter, Innsbruck Medical University, Innsbruck, Austria*

ZARIYANTEY ABDUL HAMID • *Biomedical Science Programme, School of Diagnostic & Applied Health Sciences, Faculty of Health Sciences, Universiti Kebangsaan Malaysia, Kuala Lumpur, Malaysia*

INES HÖFIG • *Institute of Radiation Biology, Helmholtz Center Munich, German Research Center for Environmental Health, Neuherberg, Germany*

NATHALIE HOLIC • *Généthon, Evry, France; INSERM, UMR_S951, Généthon, Evry, France; Université Evry Val d'Essonne, UMR_S951, Evry, France*

ALAN KENNEDY • *Division of Infection and Immunity, Institute of Immunity and Transplantation, University College London, London, UK*

ANNE A. KNOWLTON • *Molecular & Cellular Cardiology, Division of Cardiovascular Medicine, University of California, Davis, CA, USA; Pharmacology Department, University of California, Davis, CA, USA; The Department of Veteran's Affairs, Northern California VA, Sacramento, CA, USA*

ANGELA M. KRACKHARDT • *Medizinische Klinik III, Klinikum Rechts der Isar, Technical University Munich, Munich, Germany*

MASAHIKO KURODA • *Department of Molecular Pathology, Tokyo Medical University, Tokyo, Japan*

OLGA S. KUSTIKOVA • *Institute of Experimental Hematology, Hannover Medical School, Hannover, Germany*

AURÉLIEN LATHUILIÈRE • *Brain Mind Institute, Ecole Polytechnique Fédérale de Lausanne (EPFL), Lausanne, Switzerland*

TINGTING T. LIU • *Molecular & Cellular Cardiology, Division of Cardiovascular Medicine, University of California, Davis, CA, USA*

NGOC B. LU-NGUYEN • *School of Biological Sciences, Royal Holloway, University of London, Egham, UK*

TOBIAS MAETZIG • *Institute of Experimental Hematology, Hannover Medical School, Hannover, Germany*

ZULFIQAR A. MALIK • *Molecular & Cellular Cardiology, Division of Cardiovascular Medicine, University of California, Davis, CA, USA; Pharmacology Department, University of California, Davis, CA, USA*

SABINE MALL • *Medizinische Klinik III, Klinikum Rechts der Isar, Technical University Munich, Munich, Germany*

FRANCESCO MANFREDI • *National AIDS Center, Istituto Superiore di Sanità, Rome, Italy*

FAZLINA NORDIN • *Cell Therapy Centre, University Kebangsaan Malaysia Medical Centre (UKMMC), Kuala Lumpur, Malaysia*

SHIN-ICHIRO OHNO • *Department of Molecular Pathology, Tokyo Medical University, Tokyo, Japan*

ISABELLA PAROLINI • *Department of Hematology, Oncology and Molecular Medicine, Istituto Superiore di Sanità, Rome, Italy*

ELISABETH PFEIFFENBERGER • *Division of Molecular Pathophysiology, Biocenter, Innsbruck Medical University, Innsbruck, Austria*

CAROL READHEAD • *Translational Imaging Center, University of Southern California, Los Angeles, CA, USA*

JESSICA K. RIEGER • *Dr. Margarete Fischer-Bosch Institute of Clinical Pharmacology, Stuttgart, Germany; University of Tuebingen, Tuebingen, Germany*

MASSIMO SANCHEZ • *Department of Cell Biology and Neurosciences, Istituto Superiore di Sanità, Rome, Italy*

MASSIMO SARGIACOMO • *Department of Hematology, Oncology and Molecular Medicine, Istituto Superiore di Sanità, Rome, Italy*

AXEL SCHAMBACH • *Institute of Experimental Hematology, Hannover Medical School, Hannover, Germany; Division of Hematology/Oncology, Children's Hospital Boston, Harvard Medical School, Boston, MA, USA*

DIANA SCHENKWEIN • *Department of Biotechnology and Molecular Medicine, A.I. Virtanen Institute for Molecular Sciences, University of Eastern Finland, Kuopio, Finland*

MANFRED SCHMIDT • *Department of Translational Oncology, National Center for Tumor Diseases and German Cancer Research Center, Heidelberg, Germany*

BERNARD L. SCHNEIDER • *Brain Mind Institute, Ecole Polytechnique Fédérale de Lausanne (EPFL), Lausanne, Switzerland*

REINHARD SIGL • *Division of Molecular Pathophysiology, Biocenter, Innsbruck Medical University, Innsbruck, Austria*

MAIKE STAHLHUT • *Institute of Experimental Hematology, Hannover Medical School, Hannover, Germany*

CHRISTIAN THIRION • *SIRION Biotech GmbH, Martinsried, Germany*

MARIA THOMAS • *Dr. Margarete Fischer-Bosch Institute of Clinical Pharmacology, Stuttgart, Germany; University of Tuebingen, Tuebingen, Germany*

WEI WANG • *Department of Translational Oncology, National Center for Tumor Diseases and German Cancer Research Center, Heidelberg, Germany*

ROBERT WINSTON • *Department of Surgery and Cancer, Division of Cancer, Hammersmith Campus, Institute of Reproductive and Developmental Biology (IRDB), Imperial College London, London, UK*

RAFAEL J. YÁÑEZ-MUÑOZ • *School of Biological Sciences, Royal Holloway, University of London, Egham, UK*

SEPPO YLÄ-HERTTUALA • *Department of Biotechnology and Molecular Medicine, A.I. Virtanen Institute for Molecular Sciences, University of Eastern Finland, Kuopio, Finland*

CRISTIANA ZANETTI • *Department of Hematology, Oncology and Molecular Medicine, Istituto Superiore di Sanità, Rome, Italy*

Part I

Recent Improvements in LV Construction, Production, and Transduction

Chapter 1

Construction of Modular Lentiviral Vectors for Effective Gene Expression and Knockdown

Angeline de Bruyns, Ben Geiling, and David Dankort

Abstract

Elucidating gene function is heavily reliant on the ability to modulate gene expression in biological model systems. Although transient expression systems can provide useful information about the biological outcome resulting from short-term gene overexpression or silencing, methods providing stable integration of desired expression constructs (cDNA or RNA interference) are often preferred for functional studies. To this end, lentiviral vectors offer the ability to deliver long-term and regulated gene expression to mammalian cells, including the expression of gene targeting small hairpin RNAs (shRNAmirs). Unfortunately, constructing vectors containing the desired combination of cDNAs, markers, and shRNAmirs can be cumbersome and time-consuming if using traditional sequence based restriction enzyme and ligation-dependent methods. Here we describe the use of a recombination based Gateway cloning strategy to rapidly and efficiently produce recombinant lentiviral vectors for the expression of one or more cDNAs with or without simultaneous shRNAmir expression. Additionally, we describe a luciferase-based approach to rapidly triage shRNAs for knockdown efficacy and specificity without the need to create stable shRNAmir expressing cells.

Key words Gateway cloning, Lentiviral vectors, Short hairpin RNA (shRNA), Dual-luciferase reporter, shRNA triage, Design, Delivery, Lentivirus

1 Introduction

The last few decades have been revolutionary in the extensive amount of genomic data that has become available to researchers for the study of gene expression and function. This wealth of knowledge and other technological advances have made it possible to interrogate the biological role of genes in both diseased and normal tissues. Using gene sequence information, researchers have been able to introduce DNA into in vitro or in vivo study systems for the overexpression or suppression of genes of interest. For cell culture based studies, often delivery of these elements has relied on transient expression from plasmid-based technology, using transfection or electroporation. Unfortunately, this type of delivery method does not provide long-term gene expression or gene

Maurizio Federico (ed.), *Lentiviral Vectors and Exosomes as Gene and Protein Delivery Tools*, Methods in Molecular Biology, vol. 1448, DOI 10.1007/978-1-4939-3753-0_1, © Springer Science+Business Media New York 2016

knockdown. Furthermore, some cell types are not amenable to DNA uptake in this manner. Fortunately, retroviral and lentiviral vectors provide the means to yield stable integration of genetic components for the sustained expression or knockdown of genes of interest [1–3]. Lentiviruses additionally provide the ability to transduce dividing and non-dividing cells [4]. For their utility in producing stable vector integration into a host genome, retroviral and lentiviral constructs have been used extensively in the functional analysis of genes. As such, several vendors now provide retroviral and lentiviral constructs for cDNA overexpression or the expression of RNA interference (RNAi) for gene knockdown (reviewed in refs. [2, 5]).

Constructing lentiviral vectors for the expression of cDNA or RNAi using restriction and ligation strategies can be a constraining and time-consuming undertaking. Recently, the cloning process has been simplified by the use of ligation-independent methods for vector construction [6–12]. To avoid the use of traditional cumbersome methods of subcloning, one crucial step has been the implementation of recombination-based cloning systems such as Gateway technologies (Invitrogen). Gateway cloning technology is based on the site-specific recombination properties of bacteriophage λ [12, 13]. This phage inserts its DNA into the bacterial genome in between specific DNA attachment sites termed attPx (*p*hage *att*achment site) and attBx (*b*acterial *att*achment site), creating attLx (left end of prophage) and attRx (right end of prophage) sites. This phenomenon has been harnessed and commercialized as Gateway® cloning technology to allow for the efficient and precise transfer of desired DNA sequences from one plasmid to another by site-specific recombination. Using LR recombination (between attL and attR sites), recombinant expression plasmids can be created by transferring a desired attL flanked DNA fragment from an entry plasmid(s) into a destination plasmid containing an attR flanked bacterial lethal gene, *ccdB* [14]. The *ccdB* cassette ensures any non-recombinant destination plasmids or recombinant entry plasmids that carry it would be negatively selected against. Furthermore, entry plasmids are typically kanamycin resistant, whereas destination plasmids are ampicillin resistant, thus allowing for positive selection of the desired recombinant expression plasmid [15]. The specificity of Gateway cloning allows for the rapid construction of the plasmids containing cDNA and/or RNAi elements that are inserted unidirectionally by virtue of variants made to the attL and attR sequences. Increasing the number of attL/attR variants has expanded the utility of this system to permit directional, ordered cloning of multiple DNA inserts into an expression plasmid [16].

In recent years, RNAi has been used as a powerful investigative tool to elucidate the function of nearly any gene whose sequence is available. The simplest approach of delivering gene silencing RNAi is the transfection of short interfering RNA oligonucleotides (siRNA) [17, 18]. This can be an effective way to study the short-term effects of gene expression knockdown, although potential off-target effects due to initial high cytosolic siRNA concentrations occur (reviewed in ref. [19]). Additionally, knockdown is transient since siRNA concentration is diluted after several rounds of cell division. Alternatively, vector driven expression of short hairpin RNAs (shRNAs) may be used to create stable knockdown [19, 20]. shRNA expression can be driven from RNA Polymerase II or III promoters. While Pol III driven shRNA expression from promoters such as U6 and H1 were initially used [21, 22], the high levels of shRNA expression delivered can saturate the endogenous shRNA processing machinery [23–26]. Moreover, Pol III driven transcripts are less amenable to driving tissue-specific or inducible expression (reviewed in ref. [27], with exceptions noted). Newer Pol II driven shRNA vectors, mimic the structure of microRNAs (miRNAs), with shRNA sequences typically embedded in the human based miRNA-30 element (shRNAmir) [28–30]. Pol II driven shRNA expression has many advantages over the Pol III equivalent including the feasibility of inducible or tissue-specific expression and simultaneous expression of several shRNAmirs from a single polycistronic transcript [27, 29, 31]. While vectors for the stable shRNAmir expression are commercially available they are typically costly and are limited to a few selectable markers. In the construction of these vectors, shRNA target sites are selected using algorithms designed to predict target sequences that should produce effectual knockdown [32–34]. Moreover, because the precise sequence requirements for effective shRNA processing and targeting are still incompletely understood, commercially available targeting constructs are not guaranteed to successfully suppress gene expression [35].

Here we describe a novel method for the design and rapid triage of shRNA without the need to create stable shRNAmir expressing cell lines. Using a luciferase-based approach, shRNA efficacy and specificity can be assessed in a medium-throughput fashion to yield candidates for functional knockdown in vitro (Fig. 1). Furthermore, the shRNAmir expression vectors utilized in the triaging process are compatible with the Gateway cloning system. Using Multisite Gateway technology, we additionally describe techniques to rapidly construct and use lentiviral expression vectors that are capable of delivering one or more cDNAs along with simultaneous shRNAmir expression (Fig. 2). This system was constructed to facilitate efficient and flexible cloning of various elements (cDNA, markers, and shRNAmirs) into lentiviral vectors for desired combinations of gene expression and knockdown [36].

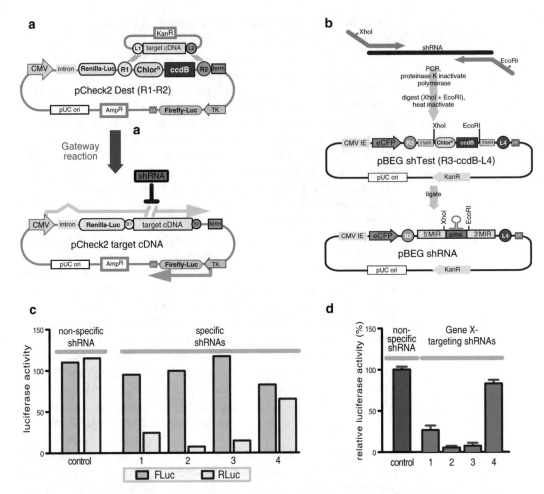

Fig. 1 Rapid triage of novel shRNAs. (**a**) Target cDNAs are cloned into pCheck2 Dest (R1–R2) through Gateway recombination between attR1–attR2 sites and attL1–attL2 compatible with all standard cDNA pEntry plasmids (attL1–attL2). The resulting plasmid produces two transcripts: a CMV-driven transcript (*yellow arrow*) encoding Renilla luciferase and a non-translated cDNA target and a TK-driven transcript (*green arrow*) encoding firefly luciferase to serve as an internal transfection control. (**b**) General method for the PCR amplification of novel shRNAs from a ~100 bp oligonucleotide core (e.g., shRNA2) with two universal primers (*red arrows*). After high fidelity PCR, the polymerase is inactivated by proteinase K treatment; the proteinase K is heat inactivated and then the PCR product is digested with XhoI/EcoRI. The restriction enzymes are subsequently heat inactivated and the fragment is cloned into the corresponding sites of pBEGshTest (R3-ccdB-L4) to create an attR3-attL4 based Entry vector pBEG shRNA. (**c**) Firefly and Renilla luciferase activities are measured sequentially for lysates derived from pCheck2 and pBEG shRNA coexpressing cells. Different shRNAs are compared by normalizing for transfection efficiency via Firefly Luciferase and then for specific knockdown by assessing Renilla luciferase levels. (**d**) This data is normalized to the luciferases observed for the nonspecific shRNA control

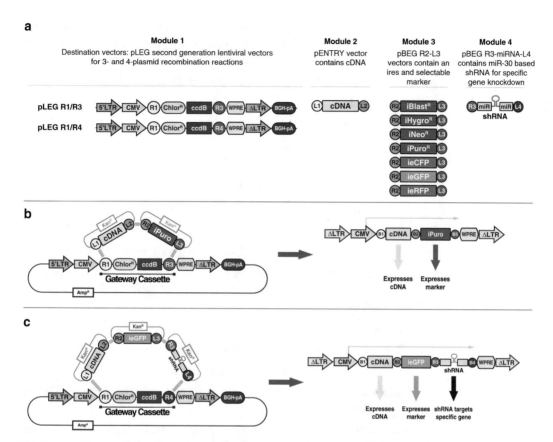

Fig. 2 A modular lentiviral vector system. (**a**) This modular system consists of a lentiviral vector backbone (Module 1), a cDNA contained in a standard ENTRY vector (Module 2), genetic markers or florescent proteins encoded downstream of internal ribosome entry sequences and are flanked by attR2 and attL3 sites contained in a pBEG vector (Module 3), and an optional miR30-embedded shRNA flanked by attR3 and attL4 sites (Module 4). (**b**) A three-way Gateway LR recombination reaction to insert a cDNA and marker of choice into the pLEG R1–R3 Destination vector. (**c**) A four-way Gateway LR Recombination reaction to insert a cDNA, marker, and shRNA of choice into the pLEG R1–R4 Destination vector

2   Materials

Prepare all solutions using ultrapure water and analytical grade reagents. Prepare and store all reagents at room temperature (unless indicated otherwise).

2.1 Design and Cloning of shRNA into pBEG Expression Vector

1. Primers for 3 primer PCR:

    (a) 10 µM shRNA template.

    (b) 10 µM universal primers:

    Fwd: 5′-CACCCTCGAGAAGGTATATTGCTGTTG ACAGTGAG-3′.

    Rev: 5′-CCCCTTGAATTCCGAGGCAGTAGGCA-3′.

2. Phusion® High-Fidelity DNA Polymerase, or other proofreading polymerase with comparable low error rate (New England BioLabs).

3. 5× HF Buffer (provided with Phusion polymerase).

4. DMSO.

5. 10 mM dNTP mix.

6. PCR plate or tubes.

7. Thermocycler.

8. 20 mg/mL Proteinase K.

9. XhoI and EcoRI restriction enzymes.

10. Agarose.

11. TAE buffer: 40 mM Tris–acetate and 1 mM EDTA.

12. pBEG shTest plasmid, or other shRNAmir expression plasmid with XhoI/EcoRI sites flanked by a miRNA-30 cassette (*see* **Note 1**).

13. Gel purification kit.

14. T4 DNA Ligase (New England BioLabs).

15. 10× T4 DNA Ligase Reaction Buffer.

16. Chemically competent, ccdB-sensitive bacteria (e.g., DH5α, DH10B).

17. SOC medium: 2% w/v tryptone, 0.5% w/v yeast extract, 10 mM NaCl, 2.5 mM KCl, 10 mM $MgCl_2$, and 20 mM glucose.

18. LB agar plates with 50 μg/mL kanamycin.

19. Miniprep plasmid DNA isolation kit.

2.2 Luciferase Assay Triaging of shRNAs

1. Target cDNA sequence flanked with L1–L2 Gateway recombination sites in an entry plasmid (*see* **Note 2**).

2. pCheck2 Dest (R1–R2) plasmid (Addgene #48955) (*see* **Note 2**).

3. LR Clonase II (Invitrogen).

4. 293T cells.

5. 24-well cell culture plates.

6. Dulbecco's modified Eagle's medium (DMEM) supplemented with 10% fetal bovine serum and 1% penicillin–streptomycin.

7. 1.5 mL microtubes.

8. Opti-MEM (Invitrogen).

9. 1 mg/mL polyethylenimine (PEI).

10. Dual-Luciferase® Reporter Assay System (Promega).

11. Phosphate buffered saline (PBS).

12. Luminometer (single-sample or a multi-sample/plate-reader).

13. Luminometer compatible tubes or multi-well plates.

2.3 Construction of Recombinant Lentiviral Vectors

1. Entry vectors as required by your application:

    (a) 2 component lentiviral vector: L1–L2 entry plasmid (e.g., cDNA of choice), R2–L3 entry plasmid (e.g., marker of choice).

    (b) 3 component lentiviral vector: L1–L2 entry plasmid (e.g., cDNA of choice), R2–L3 entry plasmid (e.g., marker of choice).

2. Destination vector: pLEG (R1–R3) or pLEG (R1–R4).

3. LR Clonase II Plus (Invitrogen).

4. Tris–EDTA (TE) pH 8.0: 10 mM Tris–Cl and 1 mM EDTA.

5. 20 mg/mL proteinase K.

6. Chemically competent, ccdB-sensitive bacteria.

7. SOC medium.

8. LB agar plates with 50 μg/mL carbenicillin.

9. Miniprep plasmid isolation kit.

10. Glycerol.

11. Midiprep plasmid isolation kit.

2.4 Production of Lentivirus

1. 293T cells.

2. 10 cm cell culture plates.

3. Lentiviral vector, Gag-Pol plasmid (e.g., pAX2), and VSV-G plasmid (e.g., pMDG).

4. Opti-MEM (Invitrogen).

5. 1 mg/mL polyethylenimine (PEI).

6. 0.45 μM syringe filter.

2.5 Stable Transduction of Cells with Lentivirus

1. Viral supernatant from Subheading 2.4.

2. Cells to be transduced.

3. Growth medium for the cells.

4. 10 mg/mL stock polybrene (Hexadimethrine bromide, Sigma H9268).

5. Appropriate agent for drug selection if lentiviral vector contains a drug-resistance gene.

6. Materials for confirmation of lentiviral construct expression (e.g., Western blot or real-time PCR equipment).

3 Methods

3.1 Design and Cloning of shRNA into pBEG shRNA Expression Vector

1. Select potential target sites in your gene of interest by finding published siRNA or shRNA sequences that have been functionally validated. If no sequences are found in the published literature, consult online RNAi database(s) for deposited shRNA sequences or design the shRNA anew using online design tools (*see* **Note 3**). Select at least two different targeting sequences to control for the possible effects due to off-target knockdown.

2. Select a control shRNA. Design either a non-targeting scramble shRNA or an shRNA targeting another gene, preferably in a different species. BLAST the shRNA sequence to ensure there are no additional homologies to the chosen sequence.

3. Format the target sequences in an shRNA template as follows: tgctgttgacagtgagCG-**X**(**N18–22**—*TAGTGAAGCCACA-GATGTA*—**N′18-22**)**X′**-tgcctactgcctcgaat (*see* **Note 4**). Order this DNA oligonucleotide for use in the next step.

4. To add the flanking XhoI/EcoRI sites to the shRNA template, perform a three primer PCR reaction between the shRNA template and the two universal primers (*see* **Note 5**). Prepare a PCR master mix including the following components per shRNA template to be amplified:

   5.0 μL HF buffer.

   1.0 μL 10 μM Fwd universal primer.

   1.0 μL 10 μM Rev universal primer.

   0.5 μL of 10 mM dNTP stock.

   15.0 μL ddH$_2$O.

   1.25 μL DMSO.

   0.25 μL (0.5 U) Phusion polymerase (add last).

   Add 24 μL of the master mix to 1.0 μL of each shRNA template (dilute shRNA template DNA to 10 μM first). Perform PCR using the following thermal cycler program:

   Step 1. 98 °C × 2 min.

   Step 2. 98 °C × 10 s.

   Step 3. 60 °C × 30 s.

   Step 4. 72 °C × 1 min.

   Repeat **steps 2–4** for a total of 30 cycles.

   Step 5. 72 °C × 10 min.

   Step 6. Cool to 4 °C.

5. Inactivate Phusion polymerase by adding 1 μL of proteinase K to each PCR reaction and incubate in the thermal cycler with the following program:

   37 °C × 30 min.

   95 °C × 30 min (to inactivate the proteinase K).

6. Digest the 10 μL of the PCR product with XhoI/EcoRI in a 20 μL total reaction volume for 1 h at 37 °C. Incubate the digests at 85 °C for 20 min to heat inactivate the restriction enzymes.

7. Digest 1–5 μg of pBEG shTest plasmid with XhoI/EcoRI for 2–4 h. Run the digest on a 0.8 % agarose-TAE gel for 40 min at a constant voltage of 120 V. Gel purify the 4333 bp fragment in a final elution volume of 30 μL.

8. Ligate the digested shRNA templates to the gel purified pBEG shTest backbone in a 20 μL total reaction volume from 4 h to overnight at room temperature. If performing the ligation using T4 DNA Ligase, prepare the following reaction recipe per ligation reaction:

   3.0 μL digested shRNA template.

   3.0 μL gel purified shTest backbone.

   11.0 ddH$_2$O.

   2.0 μL 10× Ligation Buffer.

   1.0 μL Ligase.

9. Transform 2–4 μL of the ligation reaction into 50 μL of chemically competent ccdB-sensitive bacteria in a 1.5 mL microtube on ice for 30 min.

10. Add 700 μL of antibiotic-free SOC medium to the microtube and grow the bacteria in a 37 °C shaker before plating on kanamycin-containing LB agar plates.

11. Incubate plates overnight at 37 °C and inoculate colonies into LB-kanamycin for overnight growth in a 37 °C shaker.

12. Miniprep the pBEG shTest R3-shRNA-L4 DNA using a miniprep kit. Use a protocol for the isolation of a low-copy plasmid (*see* **Note 6**).

3.2 Luciferase Assay Triaging of shRNAs

1. Clone the intended target cDNA into the pCheck2 Dest (R1–R2) vector (*see* **Note 2**) and midiprep the DNA for use in the luciferase assays.

2. The day before transfection (Day 1), seed 293T cells into 24-well plates at 5 × 10^4 cells/well (*see* **Note 7**). Seed 3 wells as technical replicates for each shRNA to be tested. Allow the cells to adhere overnight.

3. Prepare the pBEG shTest and pCheck2 DNA for co-transfection of the 293T cells (Day 2). Standardize pBEG shTest and pCheck2 DNA to 100 ng/uL (*see* **Note 8**). For each well to be transfected, combine 0.46 µg of pBEG shTest and 0.20 µg of pCheck2 DNA in a microtube (*see* **Note 9**). In a sterile cell culture hood, add 100 µL of Opti-MEM and 2 µL of PEI to each tube (*see* **Note 10**). Mix by inverting. DO NOT vortex. Incubate the DNA–Opti-MEM–PEI mix for 30 min at room temperature.

4. Before transfecting, replace the medium on the 293T cells with 500 µL/well of fresh DMEM. Add the transfection mix to the cells dropwise. Incubate the cells at 37 °C overnight.

5. The morning following transfection (Day 3), remove the transfection medium and replace with 500 µL/well of fresh DMEM.

6. About 48 h post-transfection (Day 4), prepare the reagents for the luciferase assay (1× Passive Lysis Buffer, LAR II, and Stop & Glo®) as instructed by the Promega Dual-Luciferase Assay System protocol (*see* **Note 11**). Prepare enough of each reagent to use 100 µL per replicate/well. Make sure all the reagents have reached room temperature before use.

7. Rinse the 293T cells with 500 µL of 1× PBS (*see* **Note 12**). Remove PBS. Add 100 µL of 1× Passive Lysis Buffer to each well and shake/rock the plate gently at room temperature for 30 min.

8. Read luminescence using either a single-sample luminometer or a multi-sample/plate-reading luminometer (*see* **Note 13**). If using a manual luminometer or a luminometer fitted with one reagent injector use the following instructions:

   (a) Predispense 100 µL of the LAR II reagent into the appropriate number of luminometer compatible tubes required to assay all of the samples.

   (b) Pipette 5 µL of 293T lysate into the LAR II reagent and pipette up and down 10 times to mix (*see* **Note 14**). DO NOT vortex.

   (c) Count 2 s (or program luminometer to delay 2 s) to allow the sample to equalize before measuring Firefly luciferase luminescence with a read time of 10 s in the luminometer. If the luminometer is not connected to a computer or a printer, manually record the luminescence measurement.

   (d) Remove the sample from the instrument and pipette 100 µL of Stop & Glo® reagent (or use reagent injector to dispense this) into the tube. Vortex for 2 s then count 2 s before measuring the Renilla luciferase luminescence with a read time of 10 s in the luminometer. Record the luminescence measurement.

   (e) Repeat **steps b–d** for the remaining samples.

9. To assess shRNA knockdown efficiency, divide the Renilla luciferase activity measurement by the Firefly luciferase activity measurement for each sample and normalize these ratios to the Renilla–Firefly ratio for the non-targeting control shRNA.

3.3 Construction of Recombinant Lentiviral Vectors

1. For your application, decide upon the combination of components (cDNA and marker, with or without shRNAmir) you will need to express with the lentiviral construct (*see* **Note 15**):

    (a) For a 2 component lentiviral vector you require three plasmids for the LR reaction (three-way recombination): (1) An entry plasmid with an L1–L2 flanked cDNA sequence, (2) An entry plasmid with an R2–L3 flanked marker (drug selection or fluorophore), and (3) the lentiviral destination plasmid pLEG R1–R3.

    (b) If shRNAmir expression is desired, a 3 component lentiviral vector can be constructed for which you require four plasmids for the LR reaction (four-way recombination): (1) An entry plasmid with an L1–L2 flanked cDNA sequence, (2) An entry plasmid with an R2–L3 flanked marker (drug selection or fluorophore), (3) An entry plasmid with an R3–L4 flanked shRNAmir (e.g., pBEG shTest), and (4) the lentiviral destination plasmid pLEG R1–R4.

2. Prior to use in Gateway LR recombination reactions, dilute entry plasmid DNA to 10 fmol/μL and destination plasmid DNA to 20 fmol/μL in ddH$_2$O.

3. To set up the LR recombination reactions, in a microtube add 0.5 μL of each entry plasmid and 0.5 μL of the destination plasmid to 0.5 μL of LR Clonase II Plus, and make up the reaction volume to 5 μL with TE. Incubate at room temperature for 16–24 h.

4. Add 1 μL of Proteinase K to the reaction and incubate at 37 °C for 20–30 min to terminate the reaction.

5. Transform the entire reaction into 50–100 μL of chemically competent, ccdB-sensitive bacteria in a 1.5 mL microtube on ice for 30 min (*see* **Note 16**).

6. Add 700 μL of antibiotic-free SOC medium to the microtube and grow the bacteria in a 37 °C shaker for 1 h. Plate the bacteria on carbenicillin LB agar plates.

7. Miniprep at least six colonies, saving an aliquot of bacteria from each prep to freeze at −80 °C in 15 % glycerol. The frozen stock will be used to inoculate a midiprep culture once the miniprep DNA has been screened.

8. Midiprep the correct recombinant plasmid for the production of lentivirus.

3.4 Production of Lentivirus Vector Particles

1. On Day 1, plate 5×10^6 293T cells in a 10 cm plate in DMEM. Allow cells to adhere overnight.

2. On Day 2, replace the medium on the 293T cells with 9 mL of fresh DMEM.

3. Aliquot the lentiviral vector and the packaging vectors into a 1.5 mL microtube in the following amounts: 8 μg of lentiviral vector, 5.2 μg of Gag-Pol plasmid (e.g., pAX2), and 2.8 μg of a VSV-G plasmid (e.g., pMDG).

4. In a sterile cell culture hood, add 550 μL of Opti-MEM to the DNA followed by the dropwise addition of 43 μL PEI. Invert to mix. Incubate the DNA–Opti-MEM–PEI mixture for 30 min at room temperature.

5. Add the transfection mixture to the plate of 293T cells dropwise. Incubate the cells overnight at 37 °C.

6. On Day 3, remove the transfection medium and replace with 7 mL of fresh DMEM.

7. On Day 4, harvest the lentivirus vector particles by collecting the medium off the cells and filtering the harvested medium through a 0.45 μM filter. Use the harvested medium immediately for transduction of recipient cells or store at 4 °C for up to 2 weeks. For long-term storage, keep at −80 °C.

3.5 Stable Transduction of Cells with Lentivirus Vector Particles

1. On Day 1, seed 5×10^5 of the cells to be transduced in a 10 cm plate. Let the cells adhere overnight (*see* **Note 17**).

2. On Day 2, change the medium on the cells for 5 mL of culture medium containing polybrene at 10 mg/mL and 5 mL of viral supernatant. Transduce the cells overnight at the appropriate growth temperature.

3. On Day 3, replace the medium on the cells with the regular growth medium.

4. On Day 5, replace the medium on the cells with growth medium containing the appropriate selection drug. Culture cells as needed in selection drug.

5. Confirm expression (e.g., shRNA knockdown) of the lentiviral construct with Western blot or real-time PCR analysis (Fig. 3).

4 Notes

1. We recommend the use of the pBEG shTest plasmid for shRNA triaging purposes since its efficacy has been validated within this experimental design and it will make subsequent cloning into lentiviral vectors much simpler. (Available through Addgene.)

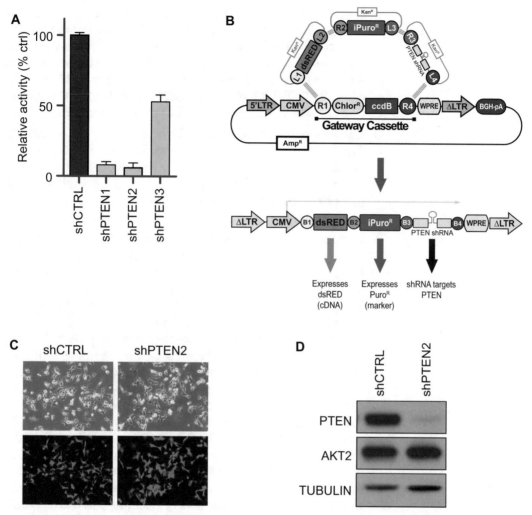

Fig. 3 *PTEN* shRNA triage, Gateway cloning, and in vitro validation. (**a**) Luciferase assay triage of PTEN specific shRNAs. (**b**) A Multisite Gateway LR recombination reaction to create a lentiviral vector expressing the dsRed fluorophore, a puromycin resistance gene, and a PTEN targeting shRNA (pLEG-dsRed-iPuro-shPTEN2). (**c**) dsRed expression in WM1617 melanoma cells infected with pLEG-dsRed-iPuro-shRNA lentivirus (post-puromycin selection). (**d**) Western blot analysis of PTEN specific knockdown in WM1617 pLEG-dsRed-iPuro-shRNA cells

2. If possible, obtain a plasmid that contains the target cDNA sequence flanked by attL1–attL2 Gateway recombination sites. The cDNA sequence can then be inserted downstream of Renilla luciferase in between the pCheck2 R1-R2 sites using a two-plasmid Gateway LR recombination reaction. For this Gateway recombination reaction use 10 fmol entry plasmid, 20 fmol pCheck2 R1–R2, and 1 μL LR Clonase II in a total of 5 μL and follow the rest of the instructions as laid out in Subheading 3.3. For commercially available cDNAs or ORFs

in attL1–attL2 entry plasmids, consult plasmid repositories at https://dnasu.org/DNASU/Home.do, http://www.add-gene.org, or http://www.genecopoeia.com. If such a plasmid does not exist, the target cDNA should first be cloned into the attL1–attL2 sites of the Gateway compatible pENTR1A or pENTR/D-TOPO plasmids (Life Technologies) via restriction enzyme site cloning or TOPO cloning, respectively.

3. Database of pre-constructed shRNA target sites are available at The RNAi Consortium http://www.broadinstitute.org/rnai/public/ or RNAi Codex http://cancan.cshl.edu/cgi-bin/Codex/Codex.cgi. To design shRNAs anew consult websites that offer algorithms for shRNA target site selection such as the one available here http://www.genelink.com/sirna/shrnai.asp.

4. Designing the shRNA template as follows: 5′-tgctgttg-acagtgag**CG**-$\underline{\textbf{X}}$(**N18-22**–*TAGTGAAGCCACAGATGTA*-**N′18-22**)$\underline{\textbf{X}}$′-tgcctactgcctcgaat (Fig. 4). Here, the portion in italics represents the constant 19 bp "loop sequence" flanked by 19–23 bp sense ($\underline{\textbf{X}}$-**N**) and antisense (**N′**-**X′**) target sequences (loop structure based on [37, 38]). Bolded nucleotides vary depending on the target sequence. The $\underline{\textbf{X}}′$ represents the last 3′ nucleotide of the antisense sequence and should compliment the intended target sequence because it is the antisense strand that binds to the target mRNA to elicit knockdown. The $\underline{\textbf{X}}$ represents the first 5′ nucleotide of the sense sequence that should be changed to be uncomplimentary to whatever nucleotide replaces the $\underline{\textbf{X}}′$ in the antisense sequence. If $\underline{\textbf{X}}′$ is an A or a T, change $\underline{\textbf{X}}$ to a C and if $\underline{\textbf{X}}′$ is a C or a G, change $\underline{\textbf{X}}$ to an A. This creates a bubble that is required for the proper endogenous processing of the shRNA by Dicer [38]. The small case sequences share homology with the universal primers to be used for PCR. For example to target human *PTEN* the following shRNA template was used: 5′-tgctgttgacagtgagCG-$\underline{\textbf{A}}$(**AGGAACAATATT-GATGATGTA***TAGTGAAGCCACAGATGTA***TACAT-CATCAATATTGTTCCT**)$\underline{\textbf{G}}$-tgcctactgcctcggaat. Note the $\underline{\textbf{A}}$(…)$\underline{\textbf{G}}$ mismatch outside the parenthesis The $\underline{\textbf{G}}$ represents the antisense sequence that will target a cytosine in the *PTEN* mRNA (CAGGAACAATATTGATGATGTA).

5. The universal primers, (Fwd) 5′-CACC**CTCGAG**AAG GTATAT<u>tgctgttgacagtgag</u>-3′ and (Rev) 5′-CCCCTT**GA att**<u>ccgaggcagtaggca</u>-3′, add flanking XhoI/EcoRI sites for subsequent cloning into pBEG shTest (primers based on those used by Chang et al. [37]). Bolded are the XhoI/EcoRI sites and small case are the portions of the primers homologous to the shRNA template. The expected PCR product has a CCAC at the 5′ end so it may be cloned into a TOPO vector if major problems are encountered when trying to clone the PCR product directly into the pBEG shTest vector.

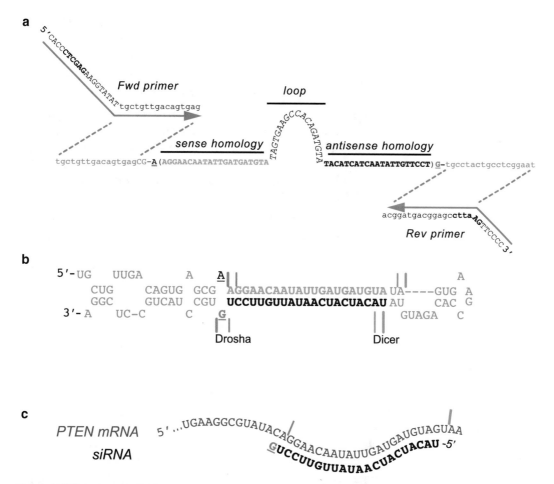

Fig. 4 shRNA design. (**a**) PTEN shRNA template DNA is depicted along with the forward and reverse primers for cloning. *Bolded* are gene specific sequences with *blue* and *black* being the sense and antisense sequences respectively. Sequences in *green* represent vector derived sequences not homologous to the target mRNA. *Lower case nucleotides* represent sequences the PCR primers bind to. *Underlined bases* are mismatched with the 3′ most underlined sequence being complementary to the target RNA (here a G). (**b**) Predicted structure of the shRNA and flanking sequence along with the predicted Drosha/Dicer cut sites. (**c**) Predicted binding of processed shRNA (now siRNA) and cleavage sites of endogenous mRNA (here PTEN)

6. The resultant colonies from the ligation transformation are generally (>99 %) correct, therefore, typically picking one colony to miniprep will suffice. It is however advised to pick at least two colonies in case the quality or concentration of one of the preps is not sufficient for use in the luciferase assays. The concentration of the pBEG shTest DNA is standardized before using it for transfections in the luciferase assays. Thus, clean DNA that is quantifiable is required. This is why use of a miniprep kit is recommended for the isolation of pBEG shTest DNA. Use a miniprep protocol for low-copy plasmids DNA isolation since the DNA yield for shRNA plasmids is usually low.

7. 293T cells are highly recommended although other efficiently transfectable mammalian cell lines can be used.

8. Standardizing the concentration of the DNA to be transfected is highly recommended to reduce variability that could be introduced by using variable transfection volumes.

9. The transfected ratio of pCheck2 to pBEG shTest plasmid DNA is 1:4. Amount of DNA to transfect is calculated according to plasmid size (i.e., bp). Take this into consideration if using another type of shRNA expression plasmid. Transfect the cells with up to 0.74 µg of DNA. Using more DNA can cause toxicity [39].

10. Prepare a master mix of Opti-MEM and PEI to dispense into the microtubes containing the pBEG shTest and pCheck2 DNA. Alternative transfection reagents can be used but we have found that PEI works very well and is the most cost-effective for this purpose.

11. The luciferase assay solutions (LAR II and Stop & Glo® Reagent) can be made in the lab instead of buying the Promega Dual-Luciferase Assay kit. These can be prepared as described previously [40, 41]. Cells should be lysed using the Promega lysis procedure with Promega Passive Lysis Buffer, which is available to purchase separately from the kit.

12. Before lysis, the 293T cells can be checked microscopically for expression of eCFP from the pBEG shTest plasmid to ensure the cells were transfected efficiently. The best results are obtained when ≥30 % of the cells are expressing eCFP.

13. The most efficient method to collect the luciferase assay measurements from a large number of samples is by using a luminometer configured to read multiple sample tubes or a 96-well plate in a plate-reader format. Furthermore, sample processing is much faster if the luminometer is equipped with two reagent injectors. If this is the case, the desired volume of sample lysate is first dispensed into the sample tubes or 96-well plate followed by sequential injection of LAR II and Stop & Glo® Reagent by the luminometer instrument. If using an automated program for the injection, shaking, and measurement steps, program the instrument to inject 100 µL of LAR II, shake for 2 s, acquire the Firefly luminescence reading over 10 s, inject 100 µL of Stop & Glo® Reagent, shake for 2 s, and acquire the Renilla luminescence reading over 10 s, in that order.

14. Up to 20 µL of lysate can be used for luminescence measurement. For high efficiency transfections (293T), do not use more than 10 µL of lysate since readings are beyond the linear range of detection for the luminometer. It is important to verify the luminometer is set to display a diagnostic error when

the luminescence exceeds the linear range of the detector. For low efficiency transfections (other cell lines), up to 20 μL of lysate can be used.

15. See pBEG entry plasmids and pLEG destination plasmids our lab has deposited at http://www.addgene.org/browse/article/7497/ (constructed as described in ref. [36]). Available pBEG R2-L3 plasmids contain a drug selection cassette (puromycin, neomycin, hygromycin, and blasticidin) or a fluorophore cassette (eGFP, eCFP, or dsRed) (Fig. 2).

16. Depending on the strain of bacteria used, white/clear screening of transformed bacterial colonies can help with selecting colonies containing the correct recombinant pLEG plasmid [42]. For example, if transforming DH10B bacteria with the recombination reaction, clear colonies will nearly always (>99%) contain the desired recombinant plasmid, whereas opaque colonies will never contain the correct construct. The colonies must be checked 13–16 h after plating otherwise they will all begin to appear white as they grow denser. This method of screening permits the medium/high-throughput production recombinant lentiviral vectors.

17. It is recommended to seed an extra plate of cells that will not be transduced but will be cultured in the selection drug during the selection period. This will serve as a control that can be monitored to determine when all the non-transduced cells have died from incubation in the selection drug.

Acknowledgements

This work was supported by the Canadian Institutes of Health Research [operating grant MOP-97925 to DD, Graduate scholarship to AdB]; the Canadian Cancer Society [CCSRI# 2011-700876] and the Canadian Cancer Society [CRS #19087]. The funders had no role in study design, data collection and analysis, decision to publish, or preparation of the manuscript.

References

1. Vannucci L, Lai M, Chiuppesi F et al (2013) Viral vectors: a look back and ahead on gene transfer technology. New Microbiol 36(1):1–22

2. Sakuma T, Barry MA, Ikeda Y (2012) Lentiviral vectors: basic to translational. Biochem J 443(3):603–618. doi:10.1042/BJ20120146, BJ20120146 [pii]

3. Palu G, Parolin C, Takeuchi Y et al (2000) Progress with retroviral gene vectors. Rev Med Virol 10(3):185–202, doi:10.1002/(SICI)1099-1654(200005/06)10:3<185::AID-RMV285>3.0.CO;2-8 [pii]

4. Naldini L, Blomer U, Gallay P et al (1996) In vivo gene delivery and stable transduction of nondividing cells by a lentiviral vector. Science 272(5259):263–267

5. Fewell GD, Schmitt K (2006) Vector-based RNAi approaches for stable, inducible and

genome-wide screens. Drug Discov Today 11(21–22):975–982. doi:10.1016/j. drudis.2006.09.008,S1359-6446(06)00369-2 [pii]

6. Aslanidis C, de Jong PJ (1990) Ligation-independent cloning of PCR products (LIC-PCR). Nucleic Acids Res 18(20):6069–6074

7. Berrow NS, Alderton D, Sainsbury S et al (2007) A versatile ligation-independent cloning method suitable for high-throughput expression screening applications. Nucleic Acids Res 35(6), e45. doi:10.1093/nar/gkm047, gkm047 [pii]

8. Li C, Evans RM (1997) Ligation independent cloning irrespective of restriction site compatibility. Nucleic Acids Res 25(20):4165–4166, doi:gka645 [pii]

9. Li MZ, Elledge SJ (2012) SLIC: a method for sequence- and ligation-independent cloning. Methods Mol Biol 852:51–59. doi:10.1007/978-1-61779-564-0_5

10. Shuman S (1994) Novel approach to molecular cloning and polynucleotide synthesis using vaccinia DNA topoisomerase. J Biol Chem 269(51):32678–32684

11. Yang J, Zhang Z, Zhang XA et al (2010) A ligation-independent cloning method using nicking DNA endonuclease. Biotechniques 49(5):817–821. doi:10.2144/000113520, 000113520 [pii]

12. Hartley JL, Temple GF, Brasch MA (2000) DNA cloning using in vitro site-specific recombination. Genome Res 10(11):1788–1795

13. Nash HA, Mizuuchi K, Enquist LW et al (1981) Strand exchange in lambda integrative recombination: genetics, biochemistry, and models. Cold Spring Harb Symp Quant Biol 45(Pt 1):417–428

14. Bernard P, Couturier M (1991) The 41 carboxy-terminal residues of the miniF plasmid CcdA protein are sufficient to antagonize the killer activity of the CcdB protein. Mol Gen Genet 226(1–2):297–304

15. Sasaki Y, Sone T, Yoshida S et al (2004) Evidence for high specificity and efficiency of multiple recombination signals in mixed DNA cloning by the Multisite Gateway system. J Biotechnol 107(3):233–243, doi:S0168165603002657 [pii]

16. Cheo DL, Titus SA, Byrd DR et al (2004) Concerted assembly and cloning of multiple DNA segments using in vitro site-specific recombination: functional analysis of multi-segment expression clones. Genome Res 14(10):2111–2120. doi:10.1101/gr.2512204, 14/10b/2111 [pii]

17. Xia H, Mao Q, Paulson HL et al (2002) siRNA-mediated gene silencing in vitro and in vivo. Nat Biotechnol 20(10):1006–1010. doi:10.1038/nbt739, nbt739 [pii]

18. Yu JY, DeRuiter SL, Turner DL (2002) RNA interference by expression of short-interfering RNAs and hairpin RNAs in mammalian cells. Proc Natl Acad Sci U S A 99(9):6047–6052. doi:10.1073/pnas.092143499, 092143499 [pii]

19. Rao DD, Vorhies JS, Senzer N et al (2009) siRNA vs. shRNA: similarities and differences. Adv Drug Deliv Rev 61(9):746–759. doi:10.1016/j.addr.2009.04.004, S0169-409X(09)00096-9 [pii]

20. Manjunath N, Wu H, Subramanya S et al (2009) Lentiviral delivery of short hairpin RNAs. Adv Drug Deliv Rev 61(9):732–745. doi:10.1016/j.addr.2009.03.004, S0169-409X(09)00060-X [pii]

21. Brummelkamp TR, Bernards R, Agami R (2002) A system for stable expression of short interfering RNAs in mammalian cells. Science 296(5567):550–553. doi:10.1126/science.1068999, 1068999 [pii]

22. Paddison PJ, Caudy AA, Bernstein E et al (2002) Short hairpin RNAs (shRNAs) induce sequence-specific silencing in mammalian cells. Genes Dev 16(8):948–958. doi:10.1101/gad.981002

23. Grimm D, Streetz KL, Jopling CL et al (2006) Fatality in mice due to oversaturation of cellular microRNA/short hairpin RNA pathways. Nature 441(7092):537–541. doi:10.1038/nature04791, nature04791 [pii]

24. Yi R, Doehle BP, Qin Y et al (2005) Overexpression of exportin 5 enhances RNA interference mediated by short hairpin RNAs and microRNAs. RNA 11(2):220–226. doi:10.1261/rna.7233305, rna.7233305 [pii]

25. Boudreau RL, Monteys AM, Davidson BL (2008) Minimizing variables among hairpin-based RNAi vectors reveals the potency of shRNAs. RNA 14(9):1834–1844. doi:10.1261/rna.1062908, rna.1062908 [pii]

26. An DS, Qin FX, Auyeung VC et al (2006) Optimization and functional effects of stable short hairpin RNA expression in primary human lymphocytes via lentiviral vectors. Mol Ther 14(4):494–504. doi:10.1016/j.ymthe.2006.05.015,S1525-0016(06)00213-9 [pii]

27. Wiznerowicz M, Szulc J, Trono D (2006) Tuning silence: conditional systems for RNA interference. Nat Methods 3(9):682–688. doi:10.1038/nmeth914, nmeth914 [pii]

28. Dickins RA, Hemann MT, Zilfou JT et al (2005) Probing tumor phenotypes using stable and regulated synthetic microRNA precursors. Nat Genet 37(11):1289–1295. doi:10.1038/Ng1651

29. Stegmeier F, Hu G, Rickles RJ et al (2005) A lentiviral microRNA-based system for single-copy polymerase II-regulated RNA interference in mammalian cells. Proc Natl Acad Sci U S A 102(37):13212–13217. doi:10.1073/pnas.0506306102, 0506306102 [pii]

30. Zeng Y, Cullen BR (2005) Efficient processing of primary microRNA hairpins by Drosha requires flanking nonstructured RNA sequences. J Biol Chem 280(30):27595–27603. doi:10.1074/jbc.M504714200, M504714200 [pii]

31. Xia XG, Zhou H, Xu Z (2006) Multiple shRNAs expressed by an inducible pol II promoter can knock down the expression of multiple target genes. Biotechniques 41(1):64–68, doi:000112198 [pii]

32. Taxman DJ, Livingstone LR, Zhang J et al (2006) Criteria for effective design, construction, and gene knockdown by shRNA vectors. BMC Biotechnol 6:7. doi:10.1186/1472-6750-6-7, 1472-6750-6-7 [pii]

33. Bassik MC, Lebbink RJ, Churchman LS et al (2009) Rapid creation and quantitative monitoring of high coverage shRNA libraries. Nat Methods 6(6):443–445. doi:10.1038/nmeth.1330, nmeth.1330 [pii]

34. Li L, Lin X, Khvorova A et al (2007) Defining the optimal parameters for hairpin-based knockdown constructs. RNA 13(10):1765–1774. doi:10.1261/rna.599107, rna.599107 [pii]

35. Fellmann C, Zuber J, McJunkin K et al (2011) Functional identification of optimized RNAi triggers using a massively parallel sensor assay. Mol Cell 41(6):733–746. doi:10.1016/j.molcel.2011.02.008, S1097-2765(11)00091-8 [pii]

36. Geiling B, Vandal G, Posner AR et al (2013) A modular lentiviral and retroviral construction system to rapidly generate vectors for gene expression and gene knockdown in vitro and in vivo. PLoS One 8(10), e76279. doi:10.1371/journal.pone.0076279, PONE-D-13-22537 [pii]

37. Chang K, Elledge SJ, Hannon GJ (2006) Lessons from Nature: microRNA-based shRNA libraries. Nat Methods 3(9):707–714. doi:10.1038/nmeth923, nmeth923 [pii]

38. Dow LE, Premsrirut PK, Zuber J et al (2012) A pipeline for the generation of shRNA transgenic mice. Nat Protoc 7(2):374–393. doi:10.1038/nprot.2011.446, nprot.2011.446 [pii]

39. Li LH, Sen A, Murphy SP et al (1999) Apoptosis induced by DNA uptake limits transfection efficiency. Exp Cell Res 253(2):541–550. doi:10.1006/excr.1999.4666, S0014-4827(99)94666-9 [pii]

40. Hampf M, Gossen M (2006) A protocol for combined Photinus and Renilla luciferase quantification compatible with protein assays. Anal Biochem 356(1):94–99. doi:10.1016/j.ab.2006.04.046, S0003-2697(06)00307-1 [pii]

41. Dyer BW, Ferrer FA, Klinedinst DK et al (2000) A noncommercial dual luciferase enzyme assay system for reporter gene analysis. Anal Biochem 282(1):158–161. doi:10.1006/abio.2000.4605, S0003-2697(00)94605-0 [pii]

42. Kwan KM, Fujimoto E, Grabher C et al (2007) The Tol2kit: a multisite gateway-based construction kit for Tol2 transposon transgenesis constructs. Dev Dyn 236(11):3088–3099. doi:10.1002/dvdy.21343

Chapter 2

Development of Inducible Molecular Switches Based on All-in-One Lentiviral Vectors Equipped with Drug Controlled FLP Recombinase

Tobias Maetzig and Axel Schambach

Abstract

Drug-inducible recombination based on flippase (FLP) is frequently used in animal models and in transgenic cell lines to initiate or to abrogate gene expression. Although the system is highly efficient, functional gene analyses depend on the availability of suitable animal models. In contrast, lentiviral vectors are readily available and versatile tools for the transfer of genetic information into a wide variety of target cells, and can be produced at high titer in a timely manner. To combine the advantages of both approaches, we generated a tight, drug-controlled FLP recombinase consisting of a 5′ FKBP12 derived conditional destruction domain and a 3′ estrogen receptor ligand binding (ERT2) domain. We successfully constructed lentiviral vectors expressing drug-controlled FLP in combination with a fluorescent reporter for recombination of FLP recognition target (FRT) sites located *in trans* as well as with target alleles located *in cis* (all-in-one configuration). In this chapter, we describe the design of the drug controlled FLP recombinase, the construction of molecular switches consisting of FLP expressing lentiviral vectors for inducible recombination of target sites located *in cis* and *in trans*, as well as the details for the characterization of lentiviral FLP vectors in cell lines.

Key words FLP recombinase, FRT, FKBP12, ERT2, Lentiviral vector, Gene transfer, Codon optimization

1 Introduction

Lentiviral gene transfer allows for stable and conditional transgene expression in a wide variety of target cells, including non-dividing hematopoietic stem and neuronal cells [1–4]. While stable expression is driven from constitutively active promoters of cellular, viral, or artificial origin, conditional expression depends on drug-inducible promoters (e.g., doxycycline regulated) or elements controlling gene function on the posttranslational level. For example, fusion proteins containing the G400V/M543A/L544A triple mutant of the human estrogen receptor ligand binding domain (ERT2) are retained in the cytoplasm until nuclear translocation is

Maurizio Federico (ed.), *Lentiviral Vectors and Exosomes as Gene and Protein Delivery Tools*, Methods in Molecular Biology, vol. 1448, DOI 10.1007/978-1-4939-3753-0_2, © Springer Science+Business Media New York 2016

triggered by binding to the β-estradiol receptor antagonist 4-hydroxy-tamoxifen (4-OHT) [5]. An alternative system exploits conditional destruction domains like the FKBP12 F36V/L106P double mutant that causes proteasomal degradation of fusion proteins in the absence of the cell permeable, stabilizing ligand Shield-1 [6, 7]. While the former posttranslational regulation mechanism is mainly suitable for control of nuclear acting proteins like transcription factors and recombinases, the latter seems universally applicable.

One of the prime examples for site-specific recombinases is the flippase (FLP) derived from the 2 μm plasmid of *S. cerevisiae*, which commonly mediates recombination between FLP recognition target (FRT) sites. Although a minimal 34 bp FRT site is sufficient for excision, an extended 48 bp FRT site consisting of two 13 bp repeat elements separated by a single interspersed nucleotide, an 8 bp spacer granting directionality, and a third 13 bp arm allows both excision and integration of appropriate target/donor molecules [8].

The FLP/FRT system is widely utilized for gene function analysis in transgenic animals and in recombinant cell lines [9, 10]. For *spatiotemporal* control of recombination, FLP can be expressed as a fusion protein with ERT2, thus allowing for 4-OHT induced recombination of target alleles harboring FRT sites [5, 11]. The outcome of the recombination event depends on the orientation of the FRT sites: (a) excision, if two FRT sites share the same orientation or (b) inversion, if two FRT sites are arranged in opposing orientations [8]. Theoretically, the excision reaction is reversible, however, practically it is mainly unidirectional since integration into a single FRT site requires an excess of donor molecules. In contrast, repeated cycles of inversion can occur for as long as FLP gains access to the nuclear chromatin.

The FLP-ERT2 transgene cassette can be inserted into the silencing resistant ROSA26 locus under control of the endogenous or an heterologous promoter to achieve uniform expression levels in various organs, tissues, and developmental stages of transgenic mice [12, 13]. This allows optimal induction of recombination in the presence of 4-OHT and minimal leakiness under steady-state conditions.

Despite a large panel of mouse models for FLP mediated targeted deletion/activation of genes, forward genetic screens could greatly benefit from the availability of lentiviral vectors equipped with a tight, drug-controlled FLP recombinase and a respective target allele expressed from the same viral backbone. The system would thus function as a unidirectional switch between the "off" and the "on" (or vice versa) state of gene expression, thereby preventing leaky expression of the target locus prior to recombination. The construction of such lentiviral vectors was so far elusive, due to the inability of ERT2 to fully prevent premature FLP-mediated recombination. The reasons for this are associated with the requirement for high expression levels of lentiviral genomic RNA and the inevitable translation of the transgene cassette in producer cells as well as the unpredictable influence of the integration site on vector performance in target cells.

By flanking FLP-ERT2 with an additional 5′ FKBP12 derived conditional destruction domain, we succeeded in generating a FLP expression cassette with limited leakiness in the absence of inducing drugs [14]. Here, we describe the development of this tight, drug-controlled FLP recombinase expression cassette and its application for the construction of lentiviral vectors for inducible recombination of FRT flanked target loci *in cis* (all-in-one configuration) and *in trans* as needed for the generation of drug controlled molecular switches for biomedical and biotechnological applications.

2 Materials

2.1 Plasmid Preparation

1. Third generation lentiviral packaging system:

    (a) pRRL.PPT.SF.mCherry.i2.EBFP2.pre, pRRL.PPT. SF.HA.NLS.FLPs.i2.F-EBFP2-F3.pre*, and pRRL.PPT. SF.FlpR.pre third generation lentiviral transfer vectors. These plasmids encode for lentiviral vectors with a self-inactivating deletion in their 3′ U3 (enhancer/promoter) region. Therefore, expression of various transgenes in target cells depends on an internal *Spleen Focus Forming Virus* (SFFV) promoter. An original (pre) or modified (pre*) *Woodchuck Hepatitis Virus* post-transcriptional regulatory element stabilizes the lentiviral RNA, and thus increases titer and expression [15]. Details on vector elements are provided in the suitable subsections.

    (b) pMD.G. This plasmid encodes for the envelope glycoprotein (g) from *Vesicular Stomatitis Virus* (VSV). VSVg-pseudotyped vector preparations have a broad tropism and high stability.

    (c) pRSV-Rev. This plasmid encodes for the *Human Immunodeficiency Virus* (HIV-1) Rev protein expressed from a *Rous Sarcoma Virus* (RSV) promoter. In packaging cells, Rev improves the nuclear export of full length lentiviral vector RNA by binding to the Rev responsive element (RRE) and exploiting the cellular CRM-1 nuclear export pathway.

    (d) pcDNA3.gag/pol.4xCTE. This plasmid encodes for the lentiviral structural (gag) and enzymatic (pol) proteins required for viral particle formation in packaging cells. Nuclear export of this gag/pol mRNA is independent from the Rev/RRE system normally employed for export of HIV RNA from the nucleus. Instead, multiple copies of the constitutive transport element (CTE) of *Mason Pfizer Monkey Virus* (MPMV) facilitate gag/pol mRNA export via interaction with the cellular protein TAP1 [16].

2. Self-produced chemically competent *E. coli* XL1-blue bacteria cells.

3. Ampicillin.

4. LB and LB agar medium.

5. Restriction enzymes, and T4 DNA ligase.

6. Gel extraction, mini and maxi prep kits.

7. Sequencing primer *pUC57rv*: 5'-GGA AAC AGC TAT GAC CAT G-3'.

2.2 Cell Culture

1. 293T cell line.

2. SC-1 and SC-1 FLP reporter cell lines.

3. High glucose Dulbecco's modified Eagle's medium (DMEM) supplemented with 10% fetal bovine serum, 0.1 mg/ml sodium pyruvate, and 100 U/ml penicillin–streptomycin.

4. Phosphate buffered saline (PBS).

5. 0.05% trypsin–EDTA.

6. Chloroquine: 25 mM (1000×) stock.

7. 1 M Hepes.

8. Protamine sulfate: 4 mg/ml (1000×) stock.

9. 4-hydroxy-tamoxifen (4-OHT): 1 mM (1000×) stock in EtOH.

10. Shield-1: 1 mM (1000×) stock in EtOH.

11. EtOH.

2.3 Calcium Phosphate-Mediated Transfection

1. 2× HEPES buffered saline (HeBS), pH 7.05.

2. 2.5 M $CaCl_2$ (calcium chloride).

3. Sterile double-distilled H_2O.

3   Methods

In the following sections, we describe (1) the design of a transgene cassette encoding for a drug controlled human codon-optimized FLP (FLPs) recombinase, (2) the generation of the FLP cassette in the pUC57 plasmid backbone, the cloning of of lentiviral vectors expressing drug-inducible FLPs for recombination of target alleles (3) *in trans* and (4) *in cis* (all-in-one configuration), and (5) the characterization of the vectors in cell lines.

3.1 Design of a Human Codon-Optimized and Drug-Controlled FLPs Recombinase cDNA

In order to generate a tight, drug-controlled FLP mutant with strong expression in mammalian cells, a cDNA with a 5′ Kozak consensus sequence for optimal translational initiation was designed to encode for a fusion protein consisting of the FKBP12 F36V/L106P mutant (FKBP12) [6], a hemagglutinin tag (HA), nuclear localization signal (NLS), a murine codon-optimized FLPo [17] and ERT2 [5] with each module flanked by restriction sites. In the next step, the coding sequence was adapted to human codon usage (*see* **Note 1**) intended to maximize protein expression as well as to remove inhibitory RNA motifs potentially interfering with retroviral production and expression (e.g., cryptic splice and polyadenylation signals). Notably, intermodule restriction sites were protected from modification during the optimization procedure, and their status as unique sites in the optimized transgene cassette was verified. The codon optimized cDNA termed "FKBP12.HA.NLS.FLPs-ERT2" was purchased embedded into the pUC57 plasmid backbone from a commercial vendor (Fig. 1).

3.2 Cloning of Tight, Drug-Controlled FLPs in the pUC57 Plasmid Backbone

The presence of intermodule restriction sites in the pUC57-FKBP12.HA.NLS.FLPs-ERT2 plasmid allowed construction of various FLPs permutations (Table 1), prior to transfer into lentiviral expression vectors. For the sake of simplicity, we focus on the generation of the tightest, drug-controlled FLPs permutation (FKBP12.HA.FLPs-ERT2) in the pUC57 plasmid.

1. Prepare a 20 μl restriction reaction (Table 2) with the parental pUC57-FKBP12.HA.**NLS**.FLPs-ERT2 plasmid using the blunt-end restriction endonucleases *Eco47*III/*Sna*BI for removal of the nuclear localization signal 5′ of FLPs (Table 1 and Fig. 1; *see* **Note 2**).

2. Incubate the reaction for 1 h at 37 °C in a water bath.

3. Perform agarose gel electrophoresis, and excise the digested plasmid backbone with a size of 5381 bp on a UV table using a scalpel.

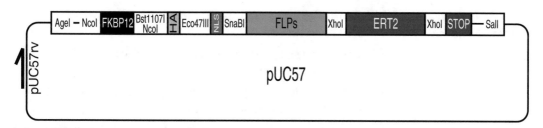

Fig. 1 pUC57-FKBP12.HA.NLS.FLPs-ERT2 plasmid design. The human codon-optimized transgene cassette consists of FKBP12, hemagglutinin (HA) tag, nuclear localization signal (NLS), FLP recombinase (FLPs), and mutant estrogen receptor ligand binding domain (ERT2). Restriction sites flanking individual modules and the whole transgene cassette are indicated. *pUC57rv*, sequencing primer for the 5′ region of the transgene cassette

Table 1
Cloning details for pUC57-FKBP12.HA.NLS.FLPs-ERT2 derived FLPs permutations

Parental pUC57 plasmid	RE	Backbone (bp)	Insert (bp)	Daughter pUC57 plasmid	Insert (bp)
FKBP12.HA.**NLS.** FLPs-ERT2	*Eco47*III/ *Sna*BI	5381	33	FKBP12. HA.FLPs-ERT2	2649
FKBP12.HA.FLPs-ERT2	*Nco*I	5024	357	HA.FLPs-ERT2	2292
FKBP12.HA.NLS. FLPs-**ERT2**	*Xho*I	4463	951	FKBP12.HA.NLS. FLPs	1731
FKBP12.HA.NLS.FLPs	*Nco*I	4106	357	HA.NLS.FLPs	1374

Modules excised by restriction digest are indicated in **bold**. Sizes for the backbone and the insert of the parental plasmids after digestion with the indicated restriction enzyme(s) are indicated in base pairs (bp). The insert sizes of the resulting "daughter pUC57 plasmids" generated by self-ligation of the parental plasmid backbone are indicated for the *Age*I/*Sal*I excised transgene cassette. *RE* restriction enzyme, *bp* base pairs

Table 2
Restriction digest reaction setup

Volume/concentration	Reagent
1 μg	Plasmid DNA
1 μl (10 U)	RE 1
1 μl (10 U)	RE 2 (optional)
2 μl	10× Restriction enzyme buffer
To 20 μl	H_2O

RE restriction endonuclease, *U* units

    4. Transfer the agarose fragment into a 1.7 ml collection tube, and extract DNA using a gel extraction kit according to the manufacturer's instructions, and elute DNA in 30 μl elution buffer.

3.3 DNA Ligation and Transformation

    1. Prepare ligation reaction (Table 3), and incubate for 1 h at room temperature.

    2. Thaw self-generated chemically competent *E. coli* XL1-blue bacteria cells on ice.

    3. On ice, gently mix 6 μl of the ligation reaction with 60 μl bacteria in a 1.7 ml reaction tube.

    4. Incubate for 5 min on ice before heat shocking the cells for 50 s at 42 °C.

    5. Put bacteria back on ice and immediately add 250 μl ice-cold LB-medium (without antibiotics).

Table 3
DNA ligation reaction protocol for one (backbone self-ligation) and three fragments

Reagent	Backbone self-ligation	3-Fragment ligation
Backbone	4 μl	3 μl
"Large insert"		5 μl
"Small insert"		8 μl
T4-DNA ligase buffer (10×)	2 μl	2 μl
T4-DNA ligase	2 μl	2 μl
H₂O	12 μl	

6. Shake bacteria for 60 min at 220 rpm and 37 °C prior to plating on prewarmed LB-agar plates supplemented with 100 μg/ml ampicillin (LB-Amp plates).

7. After overnight incubation at 37 °C, store LB-Amp plates in fridge until further use.

3.4 Screening for Bacteria Colonies with Correctly Assembled Plasmids

1. Transfer up to four bacteria colonies from LB-Amp plates into separate tubes with 3 ml LB medium supplemented with 100 μg/ml ampicillin (LB-Amp medium) using a sterile pipette tip/tooth pick.

2. Let liquid cultures shake overnight at 220 rpm and 37 °C.

3. Pour 1.5 ml liquid culture into a 1.7 ml collection tube, spin down at $16{,}100 \times g$ in a tabletop centrifuge for 30 s, discard the supernatant and proceed with extraction of plasmid DNA using a plasmid mini prep kit according to the manufacturer's instructions.

4. Perform control digest of mini-prep plasmid DNA, e.g., with *Age*I/*Sal*I, and analyze restriction pattern by agarose gel electrophoresis (Tables 1 and 2). For the pUC57-FKBP12.HA.FLPs-ERT2 construct, verify the removal of the NLS element by sequencing with the *pUC57rv* primer (Fig. 1).

5. Store mini-prep DNA of correct plasmids for subsequent subcloning at 4 °C.

3.5 Construction of Lentiviral Vectors for Coexpression of FKBP12.HA.FLPs-ERT2 and EBFP2

Since the pUC57 plasmid backbone lacks elements that facilitate transgene expression in mammalian cells, the FKBP12.HA.FLPs-ERT2 transgene cassette should be cloned into a third generation lentiviral vector equipped with a strong *Spleen Focus Forming Virus* (SF) promoter and an internal ribosome entry site (IRES, i2)-enhanced blue fluorescent protein 2 (EBFP2) marker cassette for functional characterization (Fig. 2) [1, 18]. The resulting vector "pRRL.PPT.SF.FKBP12.HA.FLPs-ERT2.i2.EBFP2.pre*" allows

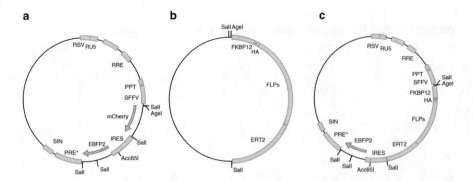

Fig. 2 Plasmid maps for the construction of a lentiviral vector coexpressing drug-inducible FLPs and EBFP2. Schematic plasmid maps of the parental vectors (**a**) pRRL.PPT.SF.mCherry.i2.EBFP2.pre* and (**b**) pUC57-FKBP12.HA.FLPs-ERT2 required for cloning of (**c**) pRRL.PPT.SF.FKBP12.HA.FLPs-ERT.i2.EBFP2.pre*. RSV, *Rous Sarcoma Virus* promoter; R-U5, "repeat" and "unique" region from the 5′ long terminal repeat; RRE, Rev responsive element; PPT, polypurine tract; SFFV, *Spleen Focus Forming Virus* promoter (SF); IRES, internal ribosome entry site (i2); EBFP2, enhanced blue fluorescent protein 2; pre*, post transcriptional regulatory element; SIN, 3′ long terminal repeat with self-inactivating deletion in U3; FKBP12, FKBP12 F36V/L06P mutant; HA, hemagglutinin tag; FLPs, human codon-optimized FLP; ERT2, G400V/M543A/L544A triple mutant of the human estrogen receptor ligand binding domain. Selected restriction sites are indicated

for fate tracking of transduced cells via the EBFP2 fluorescent marker and for drug-induced recombination of target alleles located *in trans*.

1. Prepare 20 μl restriction digest reactions (Table 2) with plasmids listed in Table 4.

2. Incubate the reactions for 1 h at 37 °C prior to agarose gel electrophoresis, excision of DNA fragments, and gel extraction.

3. Prepare 3-fragment ligation reactions (Table 3), incubate for 1 h at room temperature and transform competent *E. coli* XL1 blue bacteria cells as described in Subheading 3.3.

4. Identify bacteria clones containing correctly assembled plasmids by restriction digest of mini-prep DNA (e.g., *Age*I / *Sal*I restriction digest yields fragments of 12 bp, 345 bp, 984 bp, **2649 bp**, and 6574 bp with the **bold and underlined** fragment resembling the inserted FKBP12.HA.FLPs-ERT2 cassette as indicated in Table 1, *see* **Note 3**).

5. Amplify correct plasmids in 250 ml LB-Amp bacteria liquid cultures for purification of maxi prep DNA for virus production.

Table 4
Restriction scheme for cloning of pRRL.PPT.SF.FKBP12.HA.FLPs-ERT2.i2.EBFP2.pre*

Parental plasmids	RE	Fragment size (bp)
pRRL.PPT.SF.mCherry.i2.EBFP2.pre*	AgeI / Acc65I	7463
pRRL.PPT.SF.mCherry.i2.EBFP2.pre*	Acc65I / SalI	454
pUC57-FKBP12.HA.FLPs-ERT2	AgeI / SalI	2649

Parental plasmids, restriction endonucleases (RE), and the size of the bands required for ligation are indicated

3.6 Construction of All-in-One Lentiviral Vectors as Conditional Molecular Switches

To construct a lentiviral vector that functions as a conditional molecular switch, the drug-inducible FKBP12-HA.FLPs-ERT2 transgene cassette and a target locus must be located on the same backbone (all-in-one configuration). Therefore, the IRES-EBFP2 cassette from pRRL.PPT.SF.FKBP12.HA.FLPs-ERT.i2.EBFP2. pre* has to be replaced by a FLP reporter allele (FlpR) (Fig. 3) resulting in pRRL.PPT.SF.FKBP12.HA.FLPs-ERT.i2.FlpR.pre [19]. This vector reports drug-induced FLPs mediated recombination with a change from eGFP to dTomato expression (*see* **Note 4**). For cloning of pRRL.PPT.SF.FKBP12.HA.FLPs-ERT.i2.FlpR.pre perform the following steps:

1. Prepare 20 μl restriction digest reactions (Table 2) for plasmids listed in Table 5.

2. Perform a stepwise digest of (a) pRRL.PPT.SF.FKBP12. HA.FLPs-ERT.i2.EBFP2.pre* with Acc65I (37 °C) and SfiI (50 °C), and a regular digest of (b) pRRL.PPT.SF.HA.NLS. FLPs.i2.F-EBFP2-F3.pre* with Acc65I / XbaI.

3. Perform a partial digest of (c) pRRL.PPT.SF.FlpR.pre by first digesting for 1 h at 50 °C with SfiI, before digesting for 1 min and 5 min at 37 °C with XbaI (*see* **Note 5**).

4. Perform agarose gel electrophoresis and extract DNA from bands with lengths of (a) 8441 bp, (b) 182 bp, and (c) 2713 bp.

5. Prepare a 3-fragment ligation (Table 3) reaction, and transform bacteria as described in Subheading 3.3.

6. Screen for correctly assembled plasmids by control digest (Table 2; e.g., AgeI / SalI digestion results in fragments with sizes of 12 bp, 2136 bp, **2649 bp**, and 6539 bp), and perform maxi-preps for subsequent virus production.

3.7 Production of Lentiviral Particles by Calcium Phosphate Mediated Transfection of 293T Cells

High quality plasmid DNA as well as 293T cells of superior quality are of utmost importance for production of high titer viral particles. 293T cells are maintained in DMEM (high glucose) supplemented with 10% fetal bovine serum, 100 U/ml penicillin–streptomycin and 0.1 mg/ml sodium pyruvate (DMEM^{+++}), and are kept in a

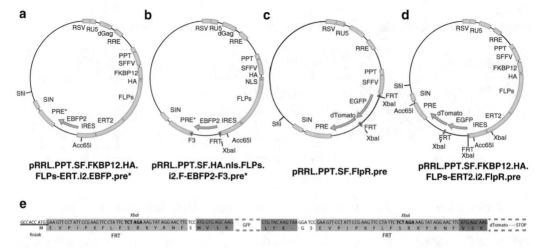

Fig. 3 Plasmid maps for the construction of the all-in-one lentiviral FLP reporter construct. (**a**) Schematic plasmid maps of the parental lentiviral vectors (**a**) pRRL.PPT.SF.FKBP12.HA.FLPs-ERT.i2.EBFP.pre*, (**b**) pRRL. PPT.SF.HA.NLS.FLPs.i2.F-EBFP2-F3.pre*, and (**c**) pRRL.PPT.SF.FlpR.pre for cloning of the all-in-one lentiviral FLP reporter (**d**) pRRL.PPT.SF.FKBP12.HA.FLPs-ERT2.FlpR.pre. (**e**) Schematic representation of the FLP reporter cassette (FlpR). The 5′ located GFP is expressed prior to recombination. After FLP-mediated excision of the FRT flanked GFP, dTomato will be translated. The 5′ Kozak consensus sequence is underlined. FRT sites are boxed in grey, and eGFP and dTomato are boxed in *green* and *red*, respectively. The nucleotide sequence and corresponding amino acids of the individual elements are indicated. RSV, *Rous Sarcoma Virus* promoter; R-U5, "repeat" and "unique" region from the 5′ long terminal repeat; RRE, Rev responsive element; PPT, polypurine tract; SFFV, *Spleen Focus Forming Virus* promoter (SF); IRES, internal ribosome entry site (i2); EBFP2, enhanced blue fluorescent protein 2; pre and pre*, *wild-type* and mutated post transcriptional regulatory element; SIN, 3′ long terminal repeat with self-inactivating deletion in U3; FKBP12, FKBP12 F36V/L06P mutant; HA, hemagglutinin tag; NLS, nuclear localization signal; FLPs, human codon-optimized FLP; ERT2, G400V/M543A/L544A triple mutant of the human estrogen receptor ligand binding domain. FRT, *wild type* FLP recognition target site; F3, mutant FRT site. Selected restriction sites are indicated

Table 5
Restriction digest for cloning all-in-one lentiviral FLP vectors

Plasmid	μg	Digest 1	*t* (min)	Digest 2	*t* (min)
(a) pRRL.PPT.SF.FKBP12.HA.FLPs-ERT.i2. EBFP2.pre*	1	*Acc65*I	60	*Sfi*I	60
(b) pRRL.PPT.SF.HA.NLS.FLPs.i2.F-EBFP2-F3.pre*	1	*Acc65*I/*Xba*I	60		
(c1) pRRL.PPT.SF.FlpR.pre	5	*Sfi*I	60	*Xba*I	1
(c2) pRRL.PPT.SF.FlpR.pre	5	*Sfi*I	60	*Xba*I	5

Plasmids to be digested, the amount of plasmids, restriction enzymes, and the time for digestion are indicated. Stepwise digestion of DNA is required due to different temperature optimums for *Acc65*I/*Xba*I (37 °C) and *Sfi*I (50 °C), and for partial digests

humidified incubator at 37 °C and atmosphere of 5% CO_2. Use prewarmed medium and buffers for 293T culture.

1. On day 1, dissociate 293T cells by removal of medium, washing with 10 ml PBS, and addition of 2 ml (T75 flask)—5 ml (T175 flask) 0.05% trypsin–EDTA. Put cells back into incubator until cells detach (typically after ~5 min). If needed, gently tap the flask to support detachment of cells.

2. Add medium to a total volume of 10 ml, and create a homogenous cell suspension by pipetting the medium up and down using a 10 ml pipette and a pipette boy.

3. Seed 5×10^6–6×10^6 cells in 10 ml DMEM^{+++} in a 10 cm tissue culture dish (*see* **Note 6**).

4. On day 2, exchange the 293T culture medium for 7 ml fresh DMEM^{+++} supplemented with 1:100 1 M HEPES and 25 μM chloroquine per 10 cm plate.

5. For transfection, mix plasmids encoding for the lentiviral transfer vector, gag/pol, Rev, and the VSVg envelope according to Table 6. Fill up with double-distilled water to a total volume of 450 μl. In this split packaging system, the presence of Rev is required for nuclear export of unspliced vector RNA, but is dispensable for nuclear export of gag/pol mRNA linked to a 4×CTE, which depends on cellular TAP1 (*see* Subheading 2.1). If more than one plate is to be transfected with the same construct, increase the volumes of all transfection reagents, respectively.

6. Add 50 μl 2.5 M $CaCl_2$ to plasmid mixture; mix by pipetting up and down until solution is "clear".

Table 6
Plasmid mixture for lentiviral vector production by calcium phosphate mediated transfection per 10 cm plate

Plasmid	Amount (μg)
LV transfer vector	5–10
pcDNA3.g/p.4xCTE	12
pRSV-Rev	6
pMD.G (VSVg)	1.5

Packaging of lentiviral transfer vector RNA depends on its Rev mediated nuclear export, while the export of lentiviral gag/pol is due to the presence of the 4xCTE Rev independent. Vector RNA, gag/pol, and the VSVg envelope components assemble at the plasma membrane prior to budding into the culture medium

7. Pipette 500 μl 2× HEPES buffered saline solution (2×HeBS) into a 15 ml tube, and add the DNA-CaCl₂ solution drop-wise while blowing air (30 s) into the 2×HeBS buffer ("air bubbling") using a pipette boy and a 2 ml pipette (*see* **Note 7**).

8. Let sit for 15–20 min before adding the solution drop-wise to the 293T cells while gently swirling the plate to facilitate optimal mixture of the DNA-calcium phosphate complexes within the medium.

9. 12–16 h later (day 3), exchange medium for 8 ml DMEM⁺⁺⁺ supplemented with 1:100 1 M HEPES.

10. Collect viral supernatants 24 and 36 h (day 4) later by aspiration of medium with a 10 ml syringe; add 8 ml fresh DMEM⁺⁺⁺ supplemented with 1:100 1 M HEPES to the cells after the first harvest. Filter supernatants through a 0.45 μm filter (low protein binding) into a 50 ml tube. Freeze supernatants at −80 °C for long term storage. Alternatively, store supernatants from the first harvest at 4 °C, pool with supernatants from the second harvest and proceed with ultracentrifugation in a SW 32 Ti rotor (Beckman Coulter) at 76,800×*g* rpm for 2 h at 4 °C (*see* **Note 8**).

11. After ultracentrifugation, completely remove the medium from the centrifugation tube without disturbing the vector pellet, and resuspend viral vector particles in 300 μl fresh DMEM⁺⁺⁺ (*see* **Note 9**).

12. Make 30–50 μl aliquots and store at −80 °C for later use.

3.8 Characterization of Lentiviral FLPs Vectors in SC-1 FLP Reporter and Wild-Type SC-1 Cells

Two different cell lines are required to characterize lentivirally expressed drug-inducible FKBP12.HA.FLPs-ERT2: (1) SC-1 FLP reporter (FlpR) cells that undergo green to red conversion upon recombination of at least one of its three reporter alleles [19], and (2) *wild-type* SC-1 cells. While the former are required to characterize FKBP12.HA.FLPs-ERT2 coexpressed with EBFP2, the latter serve for the analysis of lentiviral all-in-one constructs harboring FKBP12.HA.FLPs-ERT2 and a *cis*-acting reporter (*see* **Note 10**).

1. On day 1, trypsinize SC-1 and SC-1 FlpR cells grown in T75 tissue culture treated cell culture flasks by removal of medium, washing with PBS and addition 0.05 % trypsin–EDTA.

2. Resuspend cells in 10 ml DMEM⁺⁺⁺, and seed 7×10^4 wild type SC-1 or SC-1 FlpR cells per well of a tissue culture treated 12-well plate in 1 ml DMEM⁺⁺⁺. Culture cells in an incubator at fully humidified atmosphere at 37 °C and 5 % CO₂.

3. On day 2, exchange the medium for 500 μl fresh DMEM⁺⁺⁺ supplemented with 4 μg/ml protamine sulfate, and add concentrated lentiviral particles in triplicates in increasing concen-

trations to the appropriate wells. Start by adding 3×1 µl, 3×3 µl, and 3×10 µl supernatant to reach gene transfer rates of ~5 % (*see* **Note 11**). Mix by gently pipetting the medium up and down.

4. On day 3, after overnight transduction, replace the protamine sulfate containing medium with 1 ml fresh DMEM^{+++}.

5. On day 5, dissociate cells by trypsin–EDTA treatment. Split cells 1:10 into four wells of a tissue culture treated 12 well plate in a total volume of 1 ml DMEM^{+++} each. Treat one well each with 1 µM 4-OHT, 1 µM Shield-1, 1 µM 4-OHT + 1 µM Shield-1, and 1:500 EtOH for the next 7 days (*see* **Note 12**). Use the remaining cells for flow cytometric analysis of gene transfer and recombination rates (day 2 after transduction) (*see* **Note 13**). Flow cytometric analysis of all-in-one vector transduced SC-1 cells requires plotting of eGFP (non-recombined) vs dTomato (recombined) expressing cells; flow cytometric analysis of pRRL.PPT.SF.FKBP12.HA.FLPs-ERT2.i2.EBFP2. pre* vector transduced SC-1 FlpR cells requires plotting of EBFP vs dTomato with EBFP$^+$/dTomato$^+$ cells reporting specific recombination events (*see* **Note 14**).

6. Split cells every 2–3 days 1:10 for a total of up to 30 days and perform flow cytometric analyses on days 9, 16, 23, and 30 after transduction. This schedule allows monitoring drug-induced recombination and leaky activation of the FKBP12. HA.FLPs-ERT2 cassette over time (Fig. 4).

4   Notes

1. Codon optimization and gene synthesis of custom made DNA is available through various commercial vendors of recombinant DNA.

2. Constructs containing the ERT2 conditional nuclear translocation domain need to be freed from the endogenous NLS to render nuclear import of fusion proteins solely dependent on the presence of 4-OHT.

3. The cloning strategy for the construction of pRRL.PPT. SF.FKBP12.HA.FLPs-ERT2.i2.EBFP2.pre* can also be utilized for the construction of lentiviral vectors coexpressing any other FLPs permutation listed in Table 1 in combination with EBFP2. Control digest of mini prep DNA with *Age*I/*Sal*I results in fragment sizes of 12, 345, 984, and 6574 bp along with the respective FLPs insert size indicated in Table 1.

4. IRES mediated expression of the FlpR cassette downstream of FKBP12.HA.FLPs-ERT2 commonly results in weak fluorescent signals for eGFP prior to recombination and for dTomato

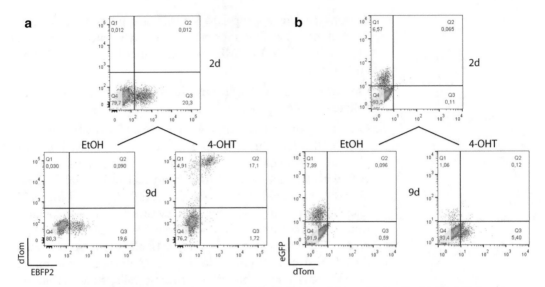

Fig. 4 Drug-inducible FLPs vector performance in SC1 FlpR and *wild-type* SC-1 cells. (**a**) SC-1 FlpR cells were transduced with pRRL.PPT.SF.FKBP12.HA.FLPs-ERT2.i2.EBFP2.pre*. Two days after transduction, cells were split into two wells and subsequently treated with EtOH or 1 μM 4-OHT for 7 days. Flow cytometric analysis for gene transfer (EBFP2⁺) and recombination (dTomato⁺) occurred 2 (*upper panel*) and 9 (*lower panel*) days after transduction. (**b**) *Wild-type* SC-1 cells were transduced with pRRL.PPT.SF.FKBP12.HA.FLPs-ERT2.i2.FlpR.pre vectors and subsequently treated as cells from (**a**). Transduced cells are eGFP⁺ and switch to dTomato⁺ after recombination. dTom, dTomato

after recombination. If higher expression levels, for example of a gene of interest, are needed, a transgene cassette consisting of FRT—FKBP12.HA.FLPs-ERT2-IRES-GFP—FRT can be constructed upstream of a second untranslated transgene cassette [14]. FLPs-mediated recombination will excise the upstream cassette and place the second transgene cassette under direct control of the SFFV promoter, providing a strong increase in gene expression. This configuration is especially useful when transplanting gene modified cells (e.g., hematopoietic stem and progenitor cells) for in vivo analysis of gene function in recipient mice.

5. Partial digest of 5 μg plasmid DNA normally results in a faint band of the required size in agarose gel electrophoresis. If no such band is detected due to suboptimal cleavage of DNA, digestion time should be increased; if no such band is detected due to complete cleavage of DNA, digestion in a suboptimal buffer, at room temperature or in a suboptimal buffer at room temperature might result in generation of the correct fragment.

6. Expect to seed 6–10 cell culture treated 10 cm plates from a single T175 cell culture flask. If the total cell count is markedly higher than ~6 × 10⁷, cells became too confluent and virus pro-

duction might be hampered. If virus production with the same batch of cells produces lower than expected titers twice in a row, repeat virus production with a new batch of cells. If supernatants should be subjected to ultraconcentration, transfect at least two plates per construct, and pool supernatants from the 36 and 48 h harvests in a single tube prior to centrifugation.

7. Air bubbling can be efficiently performed for up to four transfection reactions in the same tube.

8. To prevent tubes from collapsing, ultraconcentration tubes should be loaded with 32–35 ml of medium.

9. We commonly use DMEM^{+++} for resuspension of viral particles, but any other cell culture medium will also work for this purpose, especially if the pH for freezing is buffered.

10. The lentiviral vectors described here will presumably also function in any other cell type susceptible to lentiviral transduction and supportive of strong FKBP12.HA.FLPs-ERT2 expression from the SFFV promoter.

11. Although FKBP12.HA.FLPs-ERT2 lacks activity in the absence of 4-OHT and Shield-1 over a wider range of viral integrations per cell, for analysis of vector performance at the single copy level, low gene transfer rates between 3–30 % are recommended. This seems especially important when using the all-in-one vector configuration to exclude recombination between lentiviral integration sites of the same cell. If pure populations of vector expressing cells are required, enrichment of the desired cell population by FACS sorting is recommended.

12. Drug-inducible activation of FKBP12.HA.FLPs-ERT2 is cell type dependent. While treatment of SC-1 fibroblasts with 1 μM 4-OHT provides maximal recombination efficiency, hematopoietic 32D and K562 cell lines required treatment with 1 μM 4-OHT + 1 μM Shield-1 for the same effect. Treatment with 1 μM Shield-1 alone commonly only results in suboptimal recombination rates. Most recombination events occur during the first 7 days of treatment. Extension of this period will have little effect on the overall recombination rate.

13. Since in flow cytometry, EBFP2 is excited by the 405 nm violet laser line, FITC by the 488 nm blue laser line, and dTomato by the 561 nm violet laser line, there is limited spectral overlap between the different channels. However, single positive compensation controls for all fluorescent markers should be used to set up the photomultipliers and compensations prior to acquisition of flow cytometry data. Since EBFP2 and the viability marker DAPI share similar fluorescent characteristics, propidium iodide (PI) can be used for exclusion of dead cells from analyses.

14. Transduction of pRRL.PPT.SF.FKBP12.HA.FLPs-ERT2. i2.EBFP2.pre* into SC-1 FlpR cells frequently results in a population of cells that undergoes recombination as reported by dTomato expression, but lacks EBFP2 expression. An accurate representation of FLPs activity can be obtained when restricting the analysis of recombination events to EBFP2 expressing cells.

Acknowledgements

This work was supported by the German Research Foundation (DFG, Cluster of Excellence REBIRTH Exc 62/1 and the SFB738), the European Union (PERSIST FP7-HEALTH-2007-B-222878, CellPID FP7-HEALTH-2010-261387), the DAAD and the BMBF (Modern Applications in Biotechnology, German–Chinese JRG). We thank Michael Morgan for critically reading the final version of the manuscript.

References

1. Dull T, Zufferey R, Kelly M et al (1998) A third-generation lentivirus vector with a conditional packaging system. J Virol 72(11):8463–8471

2. Naldini L, Blomer U, Gage FH et al (1996) Efficient transfer, integration, and sustained long-term expression of the transgene in adult rat brains injected with a lentiviral vector. Proc Natl Acad Sci U S A 93(21):11382–11388

3. Zufferey R, Dull T, Mandel RJ et al (1998) Self-inactivating lentivirus vector for safe and efficient in vivo gene delivery. J Virol 72(12):9873–9880

4. Maetzig T, Brugman MH, Bartels S et al (2011) Polyclonal fluctuation of lentiviral vector-transduced and expanded murine hematopoietic stem cells. Blood 117(11):3053–3064. doi:10.1182/blood-2010-08-303222

5. Feil R, Wagner J, Metzger D et al (1997) Regulation of Cre recombinase activity by mutated estrogen receptor ligand-binding domains. Biochem Biophys Res Commun 237(3):752–757. doi:10.1006/bbrc. 1997.7124

6. Banaszynski LA, Chen LC, Maynard-Smith LA et al (2006) A rapid, reversible, and tunable method to regulate protein function in living cells using synthetic small molecules. Cell 126(5):995–1004. doi:10.1016/j. cell.2006.07.025

7. Banaszynski LA, Sellmyer MA, Contag CH et al (2008) Chemical control of protein stability and function in living mice. Nat Med 14(10):1123–1127. doi:10.1038/nm.1754

8. Turan S, Bode J (2011) Site-specific recombinases: from tag-and-target- to tag-and-exchange-based genomic modifications. FASEB J 25(12):4088–4107. doi:10.1096/fj.11-186940

9. Skarnes WC, Rosen B, West AP et al (2011) A conditional knockout resource for the genome-wide study of mouse gene function. Nature 474(7351):337–342. doi:10.1038/nature 10163

10. Schnutgen F, De-Zolt S, Van Sloun P et al (2005) Genomewide production of multipurpose alleles for the functional analysis of the mouse genome. Proc Natl Acad Sci U S A 102(20):7221–7226. doi:10.1073/pnas. 0502273102

11. Hunter NL, Awatramani RB, Farley FW et al (2005) Ligand-activated Flpe for temporally regulated gene modifications. Genesis 41(3):99–109. doi:10.1002/gene.20101

12. Lao Z, Raju GP, Bai CB et al (2012) MASTR: a technique for mosaic mutant analysis with spatial and temporal control of recombination using conditional floxed alleles in mice. Cell Rep 2(2):386–396. doi:10.1016/j.celrep. 2012.07.004

13. Zambrowicz BP, Imamoto A, Fiering S et al (1997) Disruption of overlapping transcripts in the ROSA beta geo 26 gene trap strain leads to widespread expression of beta-galactosidase in mouse embryos and hematopoietic cells. Proc Natl Acad Sci U S A 94(8):3789–3794

14. Maetzig T, Kuehle J, Schwarzer A et al (2014) All-in-One inducible lentiviral vector systems based on drug controlled FLP recombinase. Biomaterials 35(14):4345–4356. doi:10.1016/j.biomaterials.2014.01.057

15. Schambach A, Bohne J, Baum C et al (2006) Woodchuck hepatitis virus post-transcriptional regulatory element deleted from X protein and promoter sequences enhances retroviral vector titer and expression. Gene Ther 13(7):641–645. doi:10.1038/sj.gt.3302698

16. Wodrich H, Schambach A, Krausslich HG (2000) Multiple copies of the Mason-Pfizer monkey virus constitutive RNA transport element lead to enhanced HIV-1 Gag expression in a context-dependent manner. Nucleic Acids Res 28(4):901–910

17. Raymond CS, Soriano P (2007) High-efficiency FLP and PhiC31 site-specific recombination in mammalian cells. PLoS One 2(1):e162. doi:10.1371/journal.pone.0000162

18. Ai HW, Shaner NC, Cheng Z et al (2007) Exploration of new chromophore structures leads to the identification of improved blue fluorescent proteins. Biochemistry 46(20):5904–5910. doi:10.1021/bi700199g

19. Voelkel C, Galla M, Maetzig T et al (2010) Protein transduction from retroviral Gag precursors. Proc Natl Acad Sci U S A 107(17):7805–7810. doi:10.1073/pnas.0914517107

Chapter 3

Production of Retrovirus-Based Vectors in Mildly Acidic pH Conditions

Nathalie Holic and David Fenard

Abstract

Gene transfer vectors based on *retroviridae* are increasingly becoming a tool of choice for biomedical research and for the development of biotherapies in rare diseases or cancers. To meet the challenges of preclinical and clinical production, different steps of the production process of self-inactivating γ-retroviral (RVs) and lentiviral vectors (LVs) have been improved (e.g., transfection, media optimization, cell culture conditions). However, the increasing need for mass production of such vectors is still a challenge and could hamper their availability for therapeutic use. Recently, we observed that the use of a neutral pH during vector production is not optimal. The use of mildly acidic pH conditions (pH 6) can increase by two- to threefold the production of RVs and LVs pseudotyped with the vesicular stomatitis virus G (VSV-G) or gibbon ape leukemia virus (GALV) glycoproteins. Here, we describe the production protocol in mildly acidic pH conditions of GALVTR- and VSV-G-pseudotyped LVs using the transient transfection of HEK293T cells and the production protocol of GALV-pseudotyped RVs produced from a murine producer cell line. These protocols should help to achieve higher titers of vectors, thereby facilitating experimental research and therapeutic applications.

Key words Lentiviral vector, γ-Retroviral vector, Vector production, Mildly acidic pH, Gibbon ape leukemia virus glycoprotein, Vesicular stomatitis virus G glycoprotein

1 Introduction

Gene transfer vectors based on the use of *retroviridae* are commonly used in biomedical research, especially γ-retroviral (RVs) and human immunodeficiency virus type 1 (HIV-1)-derived lentiviral vectors (LVs) which are highly efficient tools for gene transfer in a broad variety of experimental models and in human cells [1]. Numerous preclinical studies and clinical trials are currently under way in ex vivo and in vivo gene and cell therapies for the treatment of various diseases, such as cancers, blood disorders, neurological disorders, and inherited or acquired immunodeficiencies [2–8].

One key feature of retrovirus-based vectors is the possibility to pseudotype viral particles with a panel of glycoproteins (GPs)

Maurizio Federico (ed.), *Lentiviral Vectors and Exosomes as Gene and Protein Delivery Tools*, Methods in Molecular Biology, vol. 1448, DOI 10.1007/978-1-4939-3753-0_3, © Springer Science+Business Media New York 2016

derived from heterologous viruses [9]. This molecular flexibility allows the specific retargeting of viral particles. To date, the most widely used GP for RVs and LVs is the vesicular stomatitis virus G GP (VSV-G), because of its stability during production/purification processes and its broad tropism [10, 11]. Vectors can also be efficiently pseudotyped with other GPs, harboring a more specific hematopoietic tropism, such as the gibbon ape leukemia virus GP (GALV) for RVs or the modified GALV GP (GALVTR) for LVs [12–15]. However, mass production of clinical grade retroviral vectors is still a challenge in terms of quantity and also quality [10, 16].

Over the last years, some improvements in RV and LV production protocols have already been possible by acting on multiple steps of the production process like transfection, cell culture, or media optimization [10, 16, 17]. Although the pH is a critical physicochemical parameter with variable values in the human body and subcellular compartments, this parameter has never been modified in viral vector culture protocols since it is commonly considered that mammalian cell cultures must be performed at neutral pH to prevent cellular toxicity. However, we recently published that neutral pH is not the optimal condition to produce high quantities of LVs or RVs pseudotyped with GALVTR or VSV-G GPs [18]. Our data showed that the culture of HEK293T cells in pH 6-buffered medium augments the production of RVs or LVs by two- to threefold. Viral particles produced at pH 6 were as stable as the one produced in neutral pH medium, either in culture at 37 °C or after multiple freeze/thaw cycles. pH 6-produced LVs are also highly efficient for the transduction of target cells like hCD34+ hematopoietic stem/progenitor cells [18].

Here we describe a detailed production protocol of GALVTR- and VSV-G-pseudotyped LVs by transient transfection of HEK293T cells, and the production protocol of GALV-pseudotyped RVs from a producer cell line (PG13-MFG-GFP) [19] in mildly acidic pH conditions.

2   Materials

2.1   Components for LV Production

1. Human embryonic kidney HEK293T cells [20].

2. Complete DMEM: Dulbecco's modified Eagle's medium, high glucose, GlutaMax™ Supplement, pyruvate (GIBCO® DMEM) supplemented with 10 % of heat-inactivated fetal calf serum and 1 % penicillin-streptomycin (5000 U/ml-5000 μg/ml). The pH value of the solution is around 7.2. Filter through a 0.22 μm syringe filter and keep at 4 °C (*see* **Note 1**).

3. pH 6-buffered DMEM: Using a pH meter, adjust complete DMEM to pH 6 by adding few drops of hydrochloric acid 37 % and sterilize using 0.22 μm size syringe filter. This solution has to be prepared extemporaneously (*see* **Note 1**).

4. Dulbecco's phosphate-buffered saline.

5. TrypLE™ Express Enzyme (1×) with Phenol Red (Life Technologies).

6. 2.5 M CaCl$_2$: Filter through a 0.22 μm filter and keep at −20 °C.

7. 0.1× TE: 1 mM Tris–HCl pH 8, 0.1 mM EDTA pH 8.

8. 2× HEPES-buffered saline (HBS) solution: 280 mM NaCl, 100 mM HEPES, 1.5 mM Na$_2$HPO$_4$. Adjust pH value to 7.12. Filter through a 0.22 μm filter and store at −20 °C (*see* **Note 2**).

9. Distilled H$_2$O.

10. Plasmids: pCCLsin.cPPT.hPGK.eGFP.WPRE, pMDG, pBA. GALV/Ampho-Kana, pKrev, pKLgagpol [20, 21] (*see* **Note 3**).

11. NucleoBond® Xtra Maxi Plus EF kit (Macherey Nagel).

12. T175 cell culture flask.

13. 0.2 μm CA Minisart® NML syringe filter (Sartorius).

14. 0.45 μm CA syringe filter.

15. Screw-capped cryotubes.

16. 37 °C Incubator with 5 % CO$_2$ humidified atmosphere.

17. Type II laminar flow hood.

18. Nikon Eclipse TE200 inverted fluorescent microscope.

2.2 Components for RV Production

1. Moloney-derived retrovirus producer cell line PG13-MFG-GFP [19].

3 Methods

Biosafety considerations are important while working with retroviral vectors. Production, handling, and storage of retroviral vectors may be subjected to authorization and regulations varying in different countries.

To reduce the risks, general guidelines include (1) the use of protective equipment to reduce the mucosal exposure to the vector (lab coat/gowns, gloves, masks, and safety glasses); (2) confinement of the genetically modified organisms and cells in a type II laminar flow hood and in laboratory areas with appropriate signage and restricted access; (3) work practice that minimizes aerosols and avoids the use of sharp objects; (4) appropriate waste handling including waste decontamination before disposal (bleach for liquid waste, autoclave for solid waste); and (5) surface decontamination after work using appropriate chemical disinfectants.

The first method details the optimization of the classical protocol of production of GALVTR-LVs and VSV-G-LVs by transient transfection of HEK293T cells [17, 20]. Transfection is classically carried out; about 16–20 h post-transfection, cells are washed and incubated in culture medium buffered at pH 6. Viral particles accumulate in this culture medium and are collected after 24 h. A second part explains the production protocol of GALV-pseudotyped RVs from the PG13-MFG-GFP producer cell line in mildly acidic pH conditions.

3.1 GALVTR- and VSV-G-Pseudotyped LV Production

1. Forty-eight hours prior transfection, plate one T175 flask with 10×10^6 HEK293T cells in 22.5 ml of fresh complete DMEM. Incubate in a 37 °C incubator with 5 % CO_2 (*see* **Notes 4** and **5**).

2. At the time of transfection (day 0), the cell density should be around 25×10^6 cells/flask (Fig. 1a) (*see* **Note 6**).

3. Three hours prior to transfection, discard medium and add 22.5 ml of fresh complete DMEM (*see* **Note 7**).

4. To prepare the transfection mix, add in a 1.5 ml tube plasmids pKLgagpol (14.6 µg), pKrev (5.6 µg), pCCLsin.cPPT.hPGK.eGFP.WPRE (22.5 µg), pBA.GALV/Ampho-Kana (24 µg), and complete with nuclease-free water to a final volume of 347 µl. Vortex the solution and combine with 660 µl of $0.1\times$ TE and 113 µl of 2.5 M $CaCl_2$ (*see* **Notes 8** and **9**).

5. In a 15 ml tube, prepare 1120 µl of $2\times$ HBS.

6. While vortexing, add drop by drop the 1120 µl of transfection mix to HBS tube. Leave the tube for 5 min at room temperature with no agitation to allow precipitate formation.

7. Add 2.24 ml of the HBS/transfection mix drop by drop to the plated cells and gently swirl the plate to ensure homogeneous dispersal of the calcium phosphate precipitate (*see* **Note 10**).

8. Incubate cells overnight in a 37 °C/5 % CO_2 incubator.

9. About 16–20 h post-transfection (day 1), prepare 14 ml of pH 6-buffered complete DMEM. This solution has to be extemporaneously prepared. Compared to the classical pH 7.2 complete DMEM, the color of the medium is yellow (Fig. 1b).

10. Remove the medium with precipitate and gently replace with 14 ml of pH 6-buffered complete DMEM obtained in **step 9** (*see* **Note 11**).

11. Incubate cells in a 37 °C/5 % CO_2 incubator.

12. The following day (day 2), observe the cells under a fluorescent microscope. The cells should be confluent and more than 90 % of these latter should express GFP (Fig. 1c) (*see* **Note 12**).

13. Harvest the GALVTR-LV supernatant. The viral suspension obtained from producer cells cultured in pH 6-buffered complete DMEM appears more orange than the one obtained in the pH 7.2 classical medium (Fig. 1d).

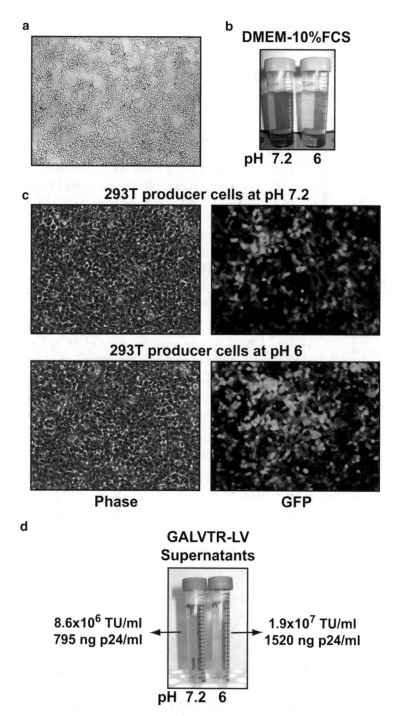

Fig. 1 GALVTR-LV production in the neutral versus mildly acidic complete DMEM medium. (**a**) Low-magnification (4×) photomicrograph of the typical HEK293T cell density in a T175 flask at the time of plasmid transfection (day 0). (**b**) Representative image of the classical pH 7.2 complete DMEM medium (*red*) and the pH 6 complete DMEM medium (*yellow*) after acidification with hydrochloric acid. (**c**) Photomicrographs (10× magnification) of HEK293T cells, transfected with GFP-expressing GALVTR-LV, at the time of viral harvest (day 2) in pH 7.2 or pH 6 conditions. Bright-field images are showing confluent HEK293T cells. GFP+ cells are typically >90 %. (**d**) Representative image of harvested GALVTR-LV supernatants (day 2) after low-speed centrifugation and filtration (0.45 μ). Infectious (TU/ml) and physical titers (ng of p24/ml) of pH 7.2- and pH 6-produced GALVTR-LV supernatants produced concomitantly from HEK293T cells represented in (**a**) and (**c**) using the medium in (**b**) are depicted

14. To remove cellular debris, centrifuge the viral suspension at $250 \times g$ for 5 min and filter it through a 0.45 μm membrane.

15. Aliquot the raw lentiviral suspension in screw-capped cryo-tubes and store at –80 °C (*see* **Note 13**).

16. Quantify infectious and/or physical particles by classical methods of titration at neutral pH [17] (*see* **Note 14**). GALVTR-LVs produced in pH 6 medium and harvested from HEK293T cells photographed in Fig. 1 correspond to an infectious titer of 1.9×10^7 TU/ml and to a physical titer of 1520 ng p24/ml (Fig. 1d). This titer is approximately twofold higher than the one obtained concomitantly in pH 7.2 conditions.

3.2 GALV-Pseudotyped RV Production

1. Dissociate PG13-MFG-GFP producer cell line and seed 1.5×10^7 cells into a T175 flask in a 20 ml final volume of complete DMEM (*see* **Note 4**).

2. Incubate cells overnight in a 37 °C/5 % CO_2 incubator.

3. The following day (day 0), prepare 14 ml of pH 6-buffered complete medium as described above (see **step 9** for GALVTR-LVs and VSV-G-LVs production procedure).

4. Inspect the cells under a microscope. They should be around 80 % confluent.

5. Aspirate medium from cells and add 14 ml of pH 6-buffered complete medium prepared in **step 3**.

6. Twenty-four hours later (day 1), harvest the viral supernatant (*see* **Note 15**).

7. Next, proceed as in **steps 14**, **15**, and **16**, Subheading 3.1.

---

4   Notes

1. Before use, prewarm complete DMEM or pH 6-buffered DMEM at 37 °C.

2. The pH value of the 2× HBS solution is critical; it has to be exactly adjusted at 7.12. Store the solution at –20 °C.

3. Endotoxin-free plasmids are purified using NucleoBond® Xtra Maxi Plus EF kit. Ratio A260/A280 should be between 1.8 and 2 and ratio A260/A230 between 1.8 and 2.2. The absence of contaminating RNA has to be checked by agarose electrophoresis.

4. HEK293T and PG13-MFG-GFP cells are routinely maintained at 37 °C in complete DMEM in a humidified atmosphere with 5 % CO_2. When cells are reaching 70–80 % confluence, they have to be passaged by dissociation with trypsin. Be sure that cells are correctly dispersed. Cells are then split at a 1:10 to 1:15 ratio twice a week. Avoid the use of cells that have been over-confluent and passaged more than 20 times.

5. This protocol can be adapted to different flasks or dishes by seeding a density of 5.5×10^4 cells/cm^2 in a final volume of complete DMEM recommended by the manufacturer.

6. At the time of transfection, the cell density is critical and should be approximately 1.5×10^5 cells/cm^2 (around 80% confluence). Check that cells are well attached and homogeneously distributed.

7. HEK293T are semi-adherent cells. Do not disturb the cell monolayer when discarding or changing medium.

8. 0.1× TE, 2.5 mM CaCl$_2$ and 2× HBS must be equilibrated at room temperature before use.

9. To produce VSV-G-pseudotyped LVs, replace 24 μg pBA. GALV/Ampho-Kana with 8 μg of pMDG.

10. It is important to slowly mix the transfection mix to 2× HBS solution. This step is critical to form a fine precipitate in order to obtain an optimal transfection efficiency. The volume of DNA/CaCl$_2$/HBS precipitate equals 1/10th of the volume of medium in which cells are incubated.

11. Before removing the transfection mix, inspect the cells under a microscope. A fine precipitate is observable in areas where there are no cells.

12. The transfection efficiency could also be precisely determined by monitoring GFP expression by FACS analysis. More than 90% of the cells should be GFP positive.

13. For the following step of target cell transduction with these vectors, do not use aliquots that have been subjected to more than one or two freeze-thaw cycles.

14. Infectious titers can be determined by two different methods. Target cells (e.g., HCT116, HT1080) are transduced with serially diluted viral supernatants. Few days later, the transduction efficiency is determined either by following the expression of a fluorescent protein like GFP using flow cytometry (titers are expressed as the number of transduction unit per milliliter (TU/ml)) or by monitoring the number of integrated proviral DNA into the genomic DNA of target cells using a quantitative polymerase chain reaction (titers are expressed as the number of infectious genome per milliliter (ig/ml)). Physical titers can be measured by quantifying HIV-1 p24 capsid content using a commercial ELISA kit [17, 20].

15. If a second harvest is desired, PG13-MFG-GFP cells have to be seeded at a lower density (10^7 cells/T175 flask). After the first harvest, carefully add 14 ml of fresh pH 6-buffered complete DMEM to the flask and incubate cells in a 37 °C/5% CO$_2$ incubator. The next day, collect the second supernatant and pool supernatants from both harvests.

Acknowledgment

This work was supported by the Association Française contre les Myopathies (AFM). We thank Anne Galy for the critical reading of the manuscript.

References

1. Sakuma T, Barry MA, Ikeda Y (2012) Lentiviral vectors: basic to translational. Biochem J 443(3):603–618. doi:10.1042/BJ20120146

2. Biffi A, Aubourg P, Cartier N (2011) Gene therapy for leukodystrophies. Hum Mol Genet 20(R1):R42–R53. doi:10.1093/hmg/ddr142

3. Di Nunzio F, Felix T, Arhel NJ et al (2012) HIV-derived vectors for therapy and vaccination against HIV. Vaccine 30(15):2499–2509. doi:10.1016/j.vaccine.2012.01.089

4. Balaggan KS, Ali RR (2012) Ocular gene delivery using lentiviral vectors. Gene Ther 19(2):145–153

5. Emeagi PU, Goyvaerts C, Maenhout S et al (2013) Lentiviral vectors: a versatile tool to fight cancer. Curr Mol Med 13(4):602–625

6. Wagemaker G (2014) Lentiviral hematopoietic stem cell gene therapy in inherited metabolic disorders. Hum Gene Ther 25(10):862–865. doi:10.1089/hum.2014.102

7. Fischer A, Hacein-Bey Abina S, Touzot F et al (2015) Gene therapy for primary immunodeficiencies. Clin Genet 88:507–515. doi:10.1111/cge.12576

8. Gill S, June CH (2015) Going viral: chimeric antigen receptor T-cell therapy for hematological malignancies. Immunol Rev 263(1):68–89. doi:10.1111/imr.12243

9. Frecha C, Szecsi J, Cosset FL et al (2008) Strategies for targeting lentiviral vectors. Curr Gene Ther 8(6):449–460

10. Ansorge S, Henry O, Kamen A (2010) Recent progress in lentiviral vector mass production. Biochem Eng J 48(3):362–377

11. Cronin J, Zhang XY, Reiser J (2005) Altering the tropism of lentiviral vectors through pseudotyping. Curr Gene Ther 5(4):387–398

12. Christodoulopoulos I, Cannon PM (2001) Sequences in the cytoplasmic tail of the gibbon ape leukemia virus envelope protein that prevent its incorporation into lentivirus vectors. J Virol 75(9):4129–4138

13. Horn PA, Topp MS, Morris JC et al (2002) Highly efficient gene transfer into baboon marrow repopulating cells using GALV-pseudotype oncoretroviral vectors produced by human packaging cells. Blood 100(12):3960–3967. doi:10.1182/blood-2002-05-1359

14. Sandrin V, Boson B, Salmon P et al (2002) Lentiviral vectors pseudotyped with a modified RD114 envelope glycoprotein show increased stability in sera and augmented transduction of primary lymphocytes and CD34+ cells derived from human and nonhuman primates. Blood 100(3):823–832

15. Hennig K, Raasch L, Kolbe C et al (2014) HEK293-based production platform for gamma-retroviral (self-inactivating) vectors: application for safe and efficient transfer of COL7A1 cDNA. Hum Gene Ther Clin Dev 25(4):218–228. doi:10.1089/humc.2014.083

16. Segura MM, Mangion M, Gaillet B et al (2013) New developments in lentiviral vector design, production and purification. Expert Opin Biol Ther 13(7):987–1011. doi:10.1517/14712598.2013.779249

17. Kutner RH, Zhang XY, Reiser J (2009) Production, concentration and titration of pseudotyped HIV-1-based lentiviral vectors. Nat Protoc 4(4):495–505

18. Holic N, Seye AK, Majdoul S et al (2014) Influence of mildly acidic pH conditions on the production of lentiviral and retroviral vectors. Hum Gene Ther Clin Dev 25(3):178–185. doi:10.1089/humc.2014.027

19. Merten OW (2004) State-of-the-art of the production of retroviral vectors. J Gene Med 6(Suppl 1):S105–S124

20. Merten OW, Charrier S, Laroudie N et al (2011) Large-scale manufacture and characterization of a lentiviral vector produced for clinical ex vivo gene therapy application. Hum Gene Ther 22(3):343–356

21. Fenard D, Ingrao D, Seye A et al (2013) Vectofusin-1, a new viral entry enhancer, strongly promotes lentiviral transduction of human hematopoietic stem cells. Mol Ther Nucleic Acids 2:e90. doi:10.1038/mtna.2013.17

Chapter 4

Optimized Lentiviral Transduction Protocols by Use of a Poloxamer Enhancer, Spinoculation, and scFv-Antibody Fusions to VSV-G

Nataša Anastasov, Ines Höfig, Sabine Mall, Angela M. Krackhardt, and Christian Thirion

Abstract

Lentiviral vectors (LV) are widely used to successfully transduce cells for research and clinical applications. This optimized LV infection protocol includes a nontoxic poloxamer-based adjuvant combined with antibody-retargeted lentiviral particles. The novel poloxamer P338 demonstrates superior characteristics for enhancing lentiviral transduction over the best-in-class polybrene-assisted transduction. Poloxamer P338 exhibited dual benefits of low toxicity and high efficiency of lentiviral gene delivery into a range of different primary cell cultures. One of the major advantages of P338 is its availability in pharma grade and applicability as cell culture medium additive in clinical protocols. Lentiviral vectors pseudotyped with the vesicular stomatitis virus glycoprotein (VSV-G) can be produced to high titers and mediate high transduction efficiencies in vitro. For clinical applications the need for optimized transduction protocols, especially for transduction of primary T and stem cells, is high. The successful use of retronectin, the second lentivirus enhancer available as GMP material, requires the application of specific coating protocols not applicable in all processes, and results in the need of a relatively high multiplicity of infection (MOI) to achieve effective transduction efficiencies for hematopoietic cells (e.g., CD34+ hematopoietic stem cells). Cell specificity of lentiviral vectors was successfully increased by displaying different ratios of scFv-fused VSV-G glycoproteins on the viral envelope. The system has been validated with human CD30+ lymphoma cells, resulting in preferential gene delivery to CD30+ cells, which was increased fourfold in mixed cell cultures, by presenting scFv antibody fragments binding to respective surface markers. A combination of spinoculation and poloxamer-based chemical adjuvant increases the transduction of primary T-cells by greater than twofold. The combination of poloxamer-based and scFv-retargeted LVs increased transduction of CD30+ lymphoma cells more than tenfold, and has the potential to improve clinical protocols.

Key words Lentiviral vector, Antibody fragments fused to VSV-G, scFv-CD30-VSV-G, scFv-EGFR-VSV-G, Envelope glycoprotein, Poloxamers, T-cells, B-cells, Hematopoietic cells

---

* These authors are contributed equally.

Maurizio Federico (ed.), *Lentiviral Vectors and Exosomes as Gene and Protein Delivery Tools*, Methods in Molecular Biology, vol. 1448, DOI 10.1007/978-1-4939-3753-0_4, © Springer Science+Business Media New York 2016

1   Introduction

The use of retroviral vectors is the method of choice for genetic modifications of primary cells. Lentiviral expression vectors deliver stable gene expression and have become important tools for research and recently gene therapeutic applications. Lentiviral vectors (LV) pseudotyped with glycoproteins of the vesicular stomatitis virus (VSV-G) are widely used for transduction of human and other mammalian cells, and integrate stably into the chromosomes of both proliferating and non-proliferating cells [1]. Currently, there is great interest in providing optimal transduction conditions for efficient LV gene delivery into therapeutic cells, mostly for stem and primary hematopoietic target cells [2]. Successful transduction of a specific cell type depends on a number of factors, including cell density, passage number, purity of lentiviral preparation, the multiplicity of infection (MOI), and the presence of adjuvants that facilitate transduction [3, 4]. Gene transfer into primary lymphocytes, hematopoietic tumor cells, and cell lines of the lymphoid lineage is known to be difficult [5, 6]. Gene transfer in these cell types often requires the use of a highly concentrated and high-purity-grade lentivirus preparation. Consequently, large-scale transduction of patient cells in clinical trials requires substantial upscaling of lentivirus production and complex downstream processing to obtain high titer and concentrated vector stocks, rendering the production expensive [7]. Improvements in lentiviral transduction rates thus would lead to a reduction in virus production volumes, and reduce the costs of good for clinical trials. Moreover, reducing the MOI may decrease the risk of insertional mutagenesis upon insertion of multiple LV genome copies per cell. Higher efficiency of gene transfer can be achieved by different strategies. These include the use of concentrated virus preparations obtained through ultracentrifugation [8] or by ultrafiltration [5]. Another alternative strategy is to enhance lentiviral gene transfer rates through the addition of transduction-promoting adjuvants, such as polycations or cationic liposomes. However, most of these adjuvant treatments have toxic effects, limiting their use especially in sensitive target cells of primary origin [7, 9].

Presently, clinical retrovirus transduction protocols include the use of the fibronectin fragment retronectin known as retroviral transduction enhancer, with limitations for Retrovirus vectors [10]. Polybrene (a linear polycationic polymer) is the best-in-class adjuvant in use for retrovirus, improving gene transduction rates for a broad range of target cells [11, 12]. Unfortunately, polybrene can only be used over short application times and at low concentrations between 5 and 10 µg/ml (dependent on the target cell type) due to its cellular toxicity acting through disruption of the transmembrane potential [13]. This severely limits its applicability in clinical trials, especially when involving sensitive primary cells, such as those of the hematopoietic lineage.

Recently, we identified the poloxamer P338 that possesses superior activity than polybrene [14], with the added benefits of being nontoxic and available in pharma grade. Poloxamers are large nonionic amphiphilic molecules, with two hydrophilic ethylene oxide branches and a hydrophobic propylene oxide core region. They are known to interact with cellular membranes promoting the sealing of lesions [15, 16] and the delivery of macromolecules such as drugs or nucleic acids [16, 17]. Genetic modification of the surface of viral vectors is an alternative way to enhance viral vector gene delivery. By adding an antibody fragment (single-chain antibody scFv) to the lentivirus surface we generated transduction-enhanced lentivirus particles with gain in specificity. Combining the use of P338 with scFv-modified lentivirus particles and spinoculation allowed us to develop optimized protocols for transduction of hematopoietic cells in vitro [18].

VSV-G-pseudotyped LVs possess superior mechanical stability, allowing for spinoculation in transduction protocols [8]. The VSV-G protein is directed to the endoplasmatic reticulum by a signal sequence (SS). There it is glycosylated and forms trimers which are integrated into the cell membrane. Alterations in the protein structure of VSV-G commonly lead to inappropriate processing and unstable lentiviruses [19]. Low transduction rates and the use of high MOIs have been reported for hematopoietic cells including primary T-cells and lymphoma cells, and some epithelial cell lines [20, 21]. Genetic modification of the lentiviral VSV-G envelope for specific antigen binding has been reported as a means to increase contact time and lentiviral uptake rates [22–25].

In this chapter we describe how to produce VSV-G fusion proteins containing N-terminal single-chain antibody fragments (scFv) directed against surface antigens, exemplified for EGFR or CD30. Further on we describe an optimized protocol for transduction of clinically relevant cells in vitro, combining scFv-modified lentiviral particles with spinoculation and chemical adjuvant (P338) supplementation.

2   Materials

2.1   Plasmids

1. Transfer vector pGreenPuro (BioCat, Heidelberg, Germany).

2. Packaging plasmid pMDLg/pRRE (Addgene, Cambridge, MA, see Note 1).

3. Packaging plasmid pRSV/Rev (Addgene).

4. Envelope plasmid pMD2.G (Addgene).

5. Antibody-fused envelope plasmid scFv-αCD30-VSV-G-pMD2.G [18].

6. PureYield™ Plasmid Midiprep System (Promega, MA, USA), endotoxin free.

2.2 Cell Culture and Transfection

1. Human embryonic kidney HEK293T cell line.

2. DMEM complete medium supplemented with 10% fetal calf serum, containing 1 mM sodium pyruvate and 2 mM glutamine.

3. Solution of trypsin (0.25%) and EDTA.

4. Transient transfection reagent: Lipofectamine 2000 (Life Technologies, Carlsbad, CA, USA).

5. The anaplastic large-cell lymphoma cell lines KARPAS-299, SUDHL-1, and SUP-M2 (DSMZ, Braunschweig, Germany).

6. Lymphoma cell medium: RPMI 1640 medium supplemented with 10% FCS and 2 mM glutamine.

7. Transient transfection medium: Opti-MEM without FCS.

8. Blood of healthy donors as T-cell source after informed consent following requirements of the local ethical board and principles of the Helsinki declaration.

9. Ficoll/Hypaque.

10. T-cell medium: RPMI medium supplemented with 5% human serum, 5% FCS, sodium pyruvate (1 mM), L-glutamine (2 mM), nonessential amino acids (10 mM), HEPES (10 mM) penicillin/streptomycin (100 IU/ml), and gentamycin (16 μg/ml); 5 ng/ml interleukin (IL)-7 and 5 ng/ml IL-15 freshly added to the medium for expansion of lymphocytes in vitro.

11. T-cell activation medium: T-cell medium supplemented with Dynabeads human T-activator CD3/CD28 (Invitrogen, Carlsbad, USA) in a bead-to-cell ratio of 1:1 and 30 IU/ml IL-2 (PeproTech, London, UK) for activation of T-cells.

2.3 Virus Concentration

1. Filter system for cell debris: Radio-sterilized Stericup filter units (0.45 μm, Millipore, Billerica, MA, USA).

2. Lentiviral concentration: Vivaspin tubes (Sartorius, Göttingen, Germany).

3. PEG-it™ (5×) virus precipitation solution (BioCat, Heidelberg, Germany).

4. 25 mM HEPES buffer.

5. Phosphate-buffered saline (PBS).

2.4 Viral Titer Evaluation and Target Cell Transduction

1. Sterile adhesive six-well plates for cell culture.

2. Lentivirus transduction enhancer adjuvant P338 (available in pharma-grade LentiBoost™, *see* **Note 2**).

3. Lentivirus transduction enhancer adjuvant polybrene.

3   Methods

3.1   Engineering the scFv-CD30-VSV-G-pMD2.G Plasmid

As a backbone we used pMD2.G encoding wild-type VSV-G as pseudotyping glycoprotein in the LV membrane. To obtain an antibody fusion of VSV-G, a DNA sequence encoding a His-Tag and a single-chain fragment (scFv) against CD30 (or EGFR) was inserted N-terminally between the signal sequence and the wild-type VSV-G sequence using the flanking restriction sites *MfeI* and *XhoI* (Fig. 1).

3.2   Transfection of HEK293T Cell Line for Lentivirus (LV) Production

Preparation of plasmids used for lentivirus production should be done using endotoxin-free buffers and plasmid DNA Midiprep (Promega, MA, USA). Transfection should be done using optimal ratio of transfer:packaging:envelope plasmids as 10 μg:24 μg:4 μg, respectively. This ensures optimal recombinant viral particle production. Transfection must be performed following standard cell culture methods as indicated in any protocol for lentiviral vector production. Below is a brief outline of the method using the 293T cell line. Cells are usually plated on Monday so that all steps can be easily completed during the week.

Day 1: Plating

1. Plate 5×10^6 HEK293T cells per 10 cm petri dish in 7 ml complete DMEM medium. Use 5–10 petri dishes per lentiviral construct. Incubate overnight at 37 °C and 5 % CO_2 (around 70–80 % confluency next day before transfection is preferred).

Day 2: Transfection

2. Change the medium 1 h prior to transfection with 5 ml fresh complete DMEM medium containing 1 mM sodium pyruvate.

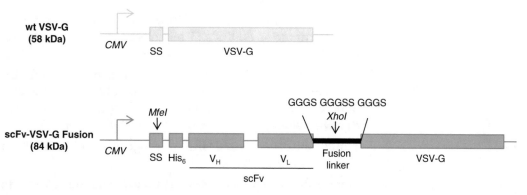

Fig. 1 Design of antibody-fused VSV-G. An scFv antibody fragment against CD30 consisting of a variable heavy (V_H) and light chain (V_L) was cloned between the signal sequence (SS) and the protein sequence of VSV-G using the flanking restriction sites *MfeI* and *XhoI*. For detection purposes, a His-tag (His$_6$) was fused to the N-terminus. Adapted from [18]

3. Pre-warm Lipofectamine 2000 and Opti-MEM medium at room temperature.

4. Prepare the first component of the transfection mix: Add 15 μl Lipofectamine 2000 to 485 μl Opti-MEM medium without FCS (Σ 500 μl) and incubate for 5 min.

5. In between prepare the second component of the transfection mix: Dilute 8 μg pRSV.Rev, 16 μg pMDLg/pRRE, 1.8 μg pMD2.G, 2.2 μg scFv-αCD30-VSV-G-pMD2.G (*see* **Note 3**), and 10 μg transfer vector (pGreenPuro) in Opti-MEM medium without FCS to a final volume of 500 μl.

6. Mix both components (prepared in **steps 4** and **5**), vortex DNA-lipid complex for 10 s, and incubate for 20 min at room temperature.

7. Add DNA-lipid complex to the HEK293T cells in 10 cm petri dish: Distribute 1 ml DNA-lipid complex dropwise in circles over the whole medium surface of the petri dish. Wave the petri dish gently three times. Incubate for 48–72 h at 37 °C and 5 % CO_2.

Day 4: Collection of supernatant containing lentiviral particles

1. Collect the viral supernatant containing medium in 50 ml Falcon tube.

2. Spin at $300 \times g$/5 min/room temperature.

3. Filter through Steri-Cup filters (0.45 μm pore size filters). It is recommended not to use the 0.22 μm pore size filters; otherwise viral titers will considerably decrease.

At this point virus can be used for transduction, aliquoted, and frozen at –80° or concentrated.

3.3 Lentiviral Vector Concentration

It is recommended to concentrate the virus and aliquot for longer storage at –80 °C (up to 1 year).

1. Load 5 ml of sterile water to Vivaspin viral concentration tubes and centrifuge at $3000 \times g$/5 min/room temperature to pre-treat the filter.

2. Discard water from bottom tube and put max. 18 ml viral supernatant in Vivaspin concentration tubes. Centrifuge at $3000 \times g$/for 15 min to 30 min/room temperature to concentrate viral supernatant from 18 ml to 500 μl (~30-fold).

3. Aliquot the concentrated virus in cryogenic vials (30–50 μl per vial) and store at –80 °C.

4. Optionally to **step 1** (*see* **Note 4**) transfer viral supernatant to sterile 50 ml Falcon tube. Example: Add 5 ml of PEG-it virus precipitation solution to 20 ml of viral supernatant.

5. Incubate overnight at 4 °C (at least 12 h). Lentiviral particle-containing supernatants mixed with PEG-it precipitation solution are stable for up to 4–5 days at 4 °C.

6. Centrifuge supernatant/PEG-it mixture at $1500 \times g$/30 min/room temperature. After centrifugation, the lentiviral particles appear as beige or white pellet at the bottom of the vessel.

7. Discard the supernatant and centrifuge residual PEG-it solution by centrifugation at $1500 \times g$/5 min/room temperature. Remove all traces of fluid by filter tips, taking care not to disturb the precipitated lentiviral particles in pellet.

8. Resuspend lentiviral pellets in ~500 μl of DMEM (containing 25 mM HEPES buffer) or using sterile cold PBS.

9. Aliquot the concentrated virus in cryogenic vials (30–50 μl per vial) and store at −80 °C.

3.4 Lentiviral Vector Titer Evaluation

Lentiviral vector preparations are always tested on 293T cells to evaluate the efficiency of recombinant virus recovery and to estimate the lentivital vector titer. This provides an indication of the quality of the preparation that is subsequently to be used in other systems (other cell line cultures, primary cells of interest or eventual in vivo applications, *see* **Note 5**).

1. Plate in six-well plates: 2×10^5 293T cells in 2 ml complete DMEM medium/well at the day before transduction.

2. Transduce 293T cells using serial dilutions of the lentiviral vector: undiluted; 10^{-1}; 10^{-2}; 10^{-3}; 10^{-4} and corresponding control (without lentiviral vector) and incubate overnight at 37 °C and 5 % CO_2.

3. After 24 h remove the media containing lentiviral vector dilutions, wash the cells two times, add 2 ml of fresh complete DMEM medium, and incubate at 37 °C and 5 % CO_2.

4. After 48–72 h check the efficiency of cell transduction using a fluorescent microscope or harvest the cells and analyze efficiency of transduction by flow cytometry (FACS).

5. Standard lentiviral vector titers range between 2×10^8 and 2×10^9 transduction units (TU) per ml.

3.5 Isolation of Peripheral Blood Mononuclear Cells from Blood of Healthy Donors

1. Isolate peripheral blood mononuclear cell (PBMC) from a healthy donor's blood sample by density gradient centrifugation. Dilute blood 1:1 in PBS and layer on 15 ml Ficoll/Hypaque in a 50 ml tube. Centrifuge at $880 \times g$/20 min/room temperature with brakes turned off.

2. After centrifugation, harvest the PBMC interface and wash twice with RPMI.

3. Count the cells and seed them in a concentration of 1×10^6 cells per ml using T-cell activation medium (*see* **Note 6**) in a 24-well plate.

4. Incubate the cells for 2–3 days at 37 °C and 5 % CO_2 followed by lentiviral transduction.

3.6 Transduction of Primary PBMC with P338

The transduction efficiency is extremely variable and donor dependent.

1. Prepare 1 ml T-cell medium and add polybrene to a final concentration of 10 μg/ml and P338 to a final concentration of 1000 μg/ml (*see* **Notes 7 and 8**).

2. Add the corresponding amount of concentrated lentiviral particles to obtain the desired MOI in the adjuvant-added medium of **step 1**. Mix gently.

3. Pellet 1×10^6 PBMC in an Eppendorf tube.

4. Resuspend PBMCs in the mix prepared in **step 2**, add 100 U/ml IL-2, and plate in a 24-well plate.

5. Centrifuge plate at $800 \times g$ for 90 min (*see* **Note 9**).

6. Incubate for 24 h at 37 °C and 5 % CO_2.

7. Transfer well content in an Eppendorf tube, and centrifuge at $500 \times g$ for 5 min. Wash with 1 ml RPMI (*see* **Note 10**).

8. Add fresh T-cell medium supplemented with IL-7 and IL-15 (each 5 ng/ml), and incubate for 24–72 h in a 24-well plate before subsequent analysis of GFP expression. Basic transduction rates can vary between donor samples (Fig. 2).

3.7 Transduction of CD30+ Lymphoma Cells with Adjuvants Polybrene and P338, Spinoculation, and a scFv-αCD30-VSV-G-Fused LV

1. Prepare 500 μl lymphoma cell medium and add polybrene to a final concentration of 10 μg/ml and P338 to a final concentration of 1000 μg/ml (*see* **Notes 7 and 8**).

2. Add corresponding amount of concentrated scFv-CD30-fused lentiviral particles (33 % scFv-αCD30-VSV-G) to obtain the desired MOI in the adjuvant-added medium of **step 1**. Mix gently.

3. Pellet 10^6 CD30+ lymphoma cells in an Eppendorf tube.

4. Resuspend lymphoma cells in the mix prepared in **step 2** and plate in a 24-well plate.

5. Centrifuge plate at $800 \times g$ for 90 min (*see* **Note 9**).

6. Incubate for 24 h at 37 °C and 5 % CO_2 (*see* **Note 11**).

7. Transfer well content in an Eppendorf tube, and centrifuge at $500 \times g$ for 5 min. Wash with 500 μl lymphoma cell medium.

8. Add fresh lymphoma cell medium, and incubate for 24 h in a 24-well plate before subsequent analysis of GFP expression (Fig. 3).

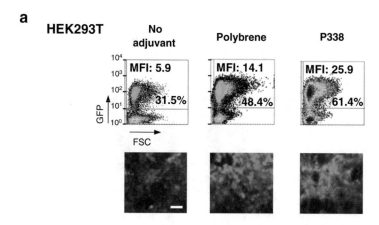

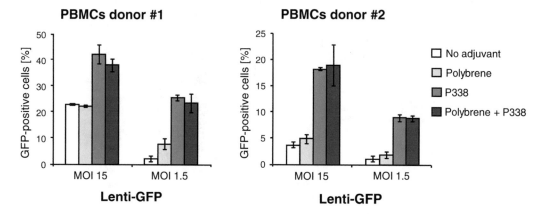

Fig. 2 Adjuvant-assisted lentiviral infection of HEK293T and PMBCs. GFP-coding lentiviral particles (Lenti-GFP) were added to HEK293T cells (**a**) at a MOI of 0.25 without and with polybrene (10 μg/ml) or P338 (1000 μg/ ml) and to IL2/OKT3-stimulated PBMCs (**b**) from healthy donors (#1 and #2) incubated at a MOI of 15 or 1.5 with polybrene (10 μg/ml), P338 (1000 μg/ml), and a combination of both (two different experiments, mean ± SD; adapted from [14])

4 Notes

1. The www.addgene.org website contains a number of commercially available different lentiviral packaging and envelope-expressing plasmids in addition to several transfer vector plasmids for RNAi purpose or transgene overexpression.

2. The non-proprietary name "Poloxamer" is used for a number of block copolymers that are listed in the US Pharmacopoeia [26]. Among them, BASF offers P338 in pharma-grade with an average number of ethylene oxide units of 265.45 and pro-

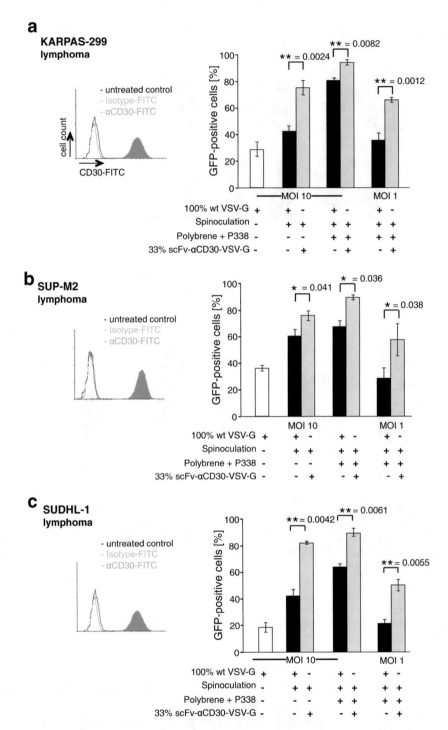

Fig. 3 Transduction of CD30+ lymphoma cells with chemical adjuvants, spinoculation, and scFv-αCD30-added LV. Quantification of transduction of CD30+ lymphoma cells KARPAS-299 (**a**), SUP-M2 (**b**), and SUDHL-1 (**c**) with MOI 10 and 1 of GFP-coding lentiviral particles (100 % wt-VSV-G and 33 % scFv-αCD30-VSV-G) with or without spinoculation and a mix of polybrene and P338 (three different experiments, mean ± SD, *$p < 0.05$, **$p < 0.01$ by t-test; adapted from [18])

pylene oxide units of 50.34 resulting in an average molecular weight of 14,600. This product shows identical molecular properties in mass spectrometry with the block copolymer Synperonic F108 (trade name of, e.g., Sigma-Aldrich) and they are therefore considered as chemical equivalents. SIRION Biotech offers a commercially available kit for optimized retrovirus transduction (LentiBoost™). The use of P338 (Synperonic F108) in pharmacologic compositions for increasing gene transfer using retroviruses is patented and published as WO2013127964. Royalty-free licenses are available for academic customers for research use. Licenses for commercial and therapeutic applications are available from SIRION Biotech GmbH.

3. Due to mass differences in wt VSV-G and antibody-fused scFv-αCD30-VSV-G (Fig. 1) plasmid amounts for LV production must be calculated stoichiometrically to produce lentiviral particles with 33% scFv-αCD30-VSV-G on their envelope membranes.

4. Dependent on the experimental strategy of choice and also of further usage of lentiviral particles the method of virus concentration should be used. For standard cell culture transduction experiments viral concentration using Vivaspin tubes is a method of choice. For cells that are not growing properly in the presence of residual FCS after viral concentration, PEG-it is a method of choice. PEG-it has an advantage to allow for resuspension of the viral pellets in a buffer or medium of choice, compatible with transduction of specific primary cells or for use in vivo.

5. Particular care should be taken to the fitness of cells at the time point of transfection and transduction efficiency. Different cell types have different characteristics and growth efficiencies. The golden rule is that the cells should be placed in media freshly and not more than 2 weeks in culture if they are used for transfection or transduction experiments. In particular the 293T cells detach from the solid support very easily and many floating cells can readily survive. Different from parental 293 cells, they reach confluency without covering all the available space of the solid support, rather growing in faintly attached clumps. In any case, do not maintain the cell lines for more than 20–30 passages in culture.

6. Alternatively to the CD3/CD28 Dynabeads, the monoclonal anti-CD3-antibody (LGC Standards, Wesel, Germany) OKT3 (30 ng/ml) combined with 50 U/ml IL-2 can be used to activate PBMC.

7. For a number of cells with epithelial origin, a final concentration of P338 of 100 µg/ml results in higher LV transduction efficiency.

8. For a number of cell types, including the ones used in this chapter, the use of polycationic enhancers such as polybrene can be synergistic with the poloxamer P338 [18].

9. Spinoculation in 24-well plates is less stressful to cells than centrifugation in Eppendorf tubes which is why this method is preferred. For some sensitive cell types (e.g., Jurkat) spinoculation in Eppendorf cups results even in cell death.

10. For some cell types centrifugation in Eppendorf tubes is stressful. Instead of Eppendorf tubes, Falcon tubes (15 ml) can be used for gentle cell centrifugation and resuspension instead.

11. Among the anaplastic large-cell lymphoma cell lines used, SUDHL1 cells show lower growth efficiency and viability after overnight incubation with lentiviral particles. Therefore, LV-containing medium was replaced directly after centrifugation of SUDHL-1 cells.

Acknowledgments

This work was supported by the German Federal Ministry of Technology and Economics (ZIM-KOOP—KF2341801SB9). The authors would like to thank M. Salomon and S. Schrödel (Sirion Biotech GmbH, Martinsried, Germany) for technical support and J. Lintelmann (Cooperation Group Comprehensive Molecular Analytics, Helmholtz Center Munich, Germany) for performing mass spectrometric analyses. Published data was reprinted with kind permission from John Wiley & Sons Ltd. (Figs. 1 and 3) and Elsevier (Fig. 2).

Disclosures

C. Thirion is a founder and shareholder of Sirion Biotech GmbH. Other authors declare no conflict of interest.

References

1. Bukrinsky MI, Haggerty S, Dempsey MP et al (1993) A nuclear localization signal within HIV-1 matrix protein that governs infection of non-dividing cells. Nature 365:666–669

2. Millington M, Arndt A, Boyd M et al (2009) Towards a clinically relevant lentiviral transduction protocol for primary human CD34 hematopoietic stem/progenitor cells. PLoS One 4:e6461

3. Birmingham A, Anderson E, Sullivan K et al (2007) A protocol for designing siRNAs with high functionality and specificity. Nat Protoc 2:2068–2078

4. Takahashi K, Tanabe K, Ohnuki M et al (2007) Induction of pluripotent stem cells from adult human fibroblasts by defined factors. Cell 131:861–872

5. Anastasov N, Klier M, Koch I et al (2009) Efficient shRNA delivery into B and T lymphoma cells using lentiviral vector-mediated transfer. J Hematop 2:9–19

6. Anastasov N, Bonzheim I, Rudelius M et al (2010) C/EBPbeta expression in ALK-positive anaplastic large cell lymphomas is required for cell proliferation and is induced by the STAT3 signaling pathway. Haematologica 95:760–767

7. Wurm M, Schambach A, Lindemann D et al (2010) The influence of semen-derived enhancer of virus infection on the efficiency of retroviral gene transfer. J Gene Med 12:137–146

8. Burns JC, Friedmann T, Driever W et al (1993) Vesicular stomatitis virus G glycoprotein pseudotyped retroviral vectors: concentration to very high titer and efficient gene transfer into mammalian and nonmammalian cells. Proc Natl Acad Sci U S A 90:8033–8037

9. Lin P, Correa D, Lin Y et al (2011) Polybrene inhibits human mesenchymal stem cell proliferation during lentiviral transduction. PLoS One 6:e23891

10. Ingrao D, Majdoul S, Seye AK et al (2014) Concurrent measures of fusion and transduction efficiency of primary CD34+ cells with human immunodeficiency virus 1-based lentiviral vectors reveal different effects of transduction enhancers. Hum Gene Ther Methods 25:48–56

11. Hesse J, Ebbesen P, Kristensen G (1978) Correlation between polyion effect on cell susceptibility to in vitro infection with murine C-type viruses and polyion effect on some membrane-related functions. Intervirology 9:173–183

12. Castro BA, Weiss CD, Wiviott LD et al (1988) Optimal conditions for recovery of the human immunodeficiency virus from peripheral blood mononuclear cells. J Clin Microbiol 26:2371–2376

13. Aubin RJ, Weinfeld M, Paterson MC (1988) Factors influencing efficiency and reproducibility of polybrene-assisted gene transfer. Somat Cell Mol Genet 14:155–167

14. Höfig I, Atkinson MJ, Mall S et al (2012) Poloxamer synperonic F108 improves cellular transduction with lentiviral vectors. J Gene Med 14:549–560

15. Lee RC, River LP, Pan FS et al (1992) Surfactant-induced sealing of electropermeabilized skeletal muscle membranes in vivo. Proc Natl Acad Sci U S A 89:4524–4528

16. Hannig J, Zhang D, Canaday DJ et al (2000) Surfactant sealing of membranes permeabilized by ionizing radiation. Radiat Res 154:171–177

17. Lu GW, Jun HW, Dzimianski MT et al (1995) Pharmacokinetic studies of methotrexate in plasma and synovial fluid following i.v. bolus and topical routes of administration in dogs. Pharm Res 12:1474–1477

18. Höfig I, Barth S, Salomon M et al (2014) Systematic improvement of lentivirus transduction protocols by antibody fragments fused to VSV-G as envelope glycoprotein. Biomaterials 35:4204–4212

19. Li Y, Drone C, Sat E et al (1993) Mutational analysis of the vesicular stomatitis virus glycoprotein G for membrane fusion domains. J Virol 67:4070–4077

20. Lamb LS Jr, Bowersock J, Dasgupta A et al (2013) Engineered drug resistant gammadelta T cells kill glioblastoma cell lines during a chemotherapy challenge: a strategy for combining chemo- and immunotherapy. PLoS One 8:e51805

21. Strappe PM, Hampton DW, Cachon-Gonzalez B et al (2005) Delivery of a lentiviral vector in a Pluronic F127 gel to cells of the central nervous system. Eur J Pharm Biopharm 61:126–133

22. Waehler R, Russell SJ, Curiel DT (2007) Engineering targeted viral vectors for gene therapy. Nat Rev Genet 8:573–587

23. Guibinga GH, Hall FL, Gordon EM et al (2004) Ligand-modified vesicular stomatitis virus glycoprotein displays a temperature-sensitive intracellular trafficking and virus assembly phenotype. Mol Ther 9:76–84

24. Kameyama Y, Kawabe Y, Ito A et al (2008) Antibody-dependent gene transduction using gammaretroviral and lentiviral vectors pseudotyped with chimeric vesicular stomatitis virus glycoprotein. J Virol Methods 153:49–54

25. Padmashali RM, Andreadis ST (2011) Engineering fibrinogen-binding VSV-G envelope for spatially- and cell-controlled lentivirus delivery through fibrin hydrogels. Biomaterials 32:3330–3339

26. Kabanov A, Zhu J, Alakhov V (2005) Pluronic block copolymers for gene delivery. Adv Genet 53:231–261

Part II

New LV Targets and Applications

Chapter 5

Transduction of Murine Hematopoietic Stem Cells with Tetracycline-regulated Lentiviral Vectors

Maike Stahlhut, Axel Schambach, and Olga S. Kustikova

Abstract

Tetracycline-regulated integrating vectors allow pharmacologically controlled genetic modification of murine and human hematopoietic stem cells (HSCs). This approach combines the stable transgene insertion into a host genome with the opportunity for time- and dose-controlled reversible transgene expression in HSCs. Here, we describe the step-by-step protocol for transduction of murine stem-cell enriched populations of bone marrow cells, such as lineage negative cells (Lin⁻), with a lentiviral vector expressing the enhanced green fluorescent protein (EGFP) under the control of the tetracycline-regulated promoter. This chapter explains how to establish in vitro and in vivo systems to study transgene dose-dependent mechanisms affecting cell fate decisions of genetically modified hematopoietic cells.

Key words Tetracycline-regulated lentiviral vectors, Murine hematopoietic stem cells, Transduction, Gene transfer, Dose-dependent transgene expression

1 Introduction

Tetracycline-regulated retroviral vectors allow genetic modification of hematopoietic stem cells (HSCs) via drug-controlled transgene overexpression and are widely used to study determinants of normal and malignant hematopoiesis such as self-renewal, proliferation/survival, and impaired differentiation [1–3]. Furthermore, recently developed tetracycline-regulated RNAi technologies enable the study of loss-of-function phenotypes and thus characterization of genes encoding putative drug targets in hematopoietic disorders [3]. Tetracycline-regulated vectors based on lentiviral (LV) backbone integrate into the genome of target cells independently of cell division [4, 5] and thus allow further optimization of existing transduction protocols [6, 7]. Accumulating studies show that

Maurizio Federico (ed.), *Lentiviral Vectors and Exosomes as Gene and Protein Delivery Tools*, Methods in Molecular Biology, vol. 1448, DOI 10.1007/978-1-4939-3753-0_5, © Springer Science+Business Media New York 2016

tetracycline-regulated lentiviral vectors provide efficient dose- and time-controlled reversible transgene expression to investigate immediate [8, 9] and long-term effects of transgene upregulation and downregulation in murine HSCs [5, 10, 11] using in vitro and in vivo experimental systems. Importantly, long-term murine bone marrow (BM) transplantation (BMT) experiments demonstrated stable and reversible transgene expression in serial recipients with development of benign clonal selection, both in the presence and absence of doxycycline (DOX) induction [11]. Here, when lentiviral self-inactivating vectors were used to express enhanced green fluorescent protein (EGFP) under the control of the tetracycline-regulated promoter, the majority of tetracycline-regulated vector integration sites were identified in introns and exons of transcription units and in non-coding/repeat regions of the genome, as previously described for constitutively expressing lentiviral vectors [11–13]. However, there is no guarantee that insertional mutagenesis will be avoided in the case of increased vector copy numbers (VCN), prolonged animal observation time and particularly when fluorescent markers are co-expressed with potent proto-oncogenes or genes involved in signaling cascades [6, 11, 14, 15]. Nevertheless, the opportunities to control vector and doxycycline dose, to monitor background activity of tetracycline-regulated promoters (TRPs) and to characterize the vector insertional profile [11, 16] allow establishment of promising in vitro and in vivo systems to study the dose-dependent role of transgene overexpression in mechanisms triggering fate decisions of genetically modified HSCs.

In this chapter, we provide the detailed transduction protocol of lineage negative (Lin⁻) bone marrow cells from Rosa26rtTA-nls-Neo2 (Rosa26rtTA) mice expressing the reverse tetracycline-inducible transactivator (rtTA-M2) under the control of the ubiquitously active Rosa26 locus [8, 11, 17]. For transduction, we used a lentiviral self-inactivating vector expressing EGFP [11] under the control of the T11 tetracycline-regulated promoter [2], which is an improved version of the TRP originally described by Gossen and Bujard [18]. We present a detailed description of all steps, including pre-stimulation of the HSC-enriched fraction (Lin⁻) of Rosa26rtTA BM, transduction of (Lin⁻) Rosa26rtTA cells by tetracycline-regulated lentiviral vectors with different multiplicities of infection (MOIs), doxycycline dose-dependent induction of transgene overexpression and determination of gene transfer/expression levels. Emphasis is given to the important characteristics of tetracycline-regulated system, such as inducibility and background activity of TRPs in the absence of doxycycline. We describe the specific details of culturing transduced cells for in vitro expansion or transplantation into lethally irradiated mouse recipients for long-term in vivo murine transplantation studies (Fig. 1).

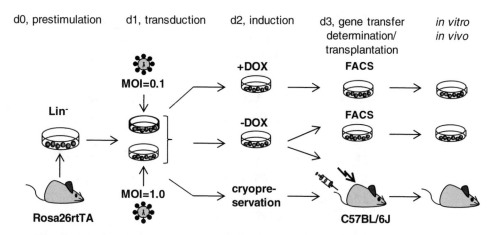

Fig. 1 Flow sheet of experimental procedures. *DOX* doxycycline, *MOI* multiplicity of infection, *d0–3* day 0–3

2 Materials

Prepare all solutions using ultrapure water (Biochrom, Berlin, Germany) under sterile conditions. Follow the appropriate S2 biosafety regulations when working with Vesicular Stomatitis Virus glycoprotein (VSVg)-pseudotyped LV vector particles.

2.1 Pre-stimulation of Purified Lineage Negative Rosa26rtTA Bone Marrow Cells

1. StemSpan medium (STEMCELL Technologies SARL, Cologne, Germany). For long-term storage, keep aliquots at –20 °C. Before use, thaw and store at 4 °C.

2. Cytokines (Peprotech, Hamburg, Germany): recombinant murine stem cell factor (mSCF), recombinant murine interleukin 3 (mIL-3), recombinant human FMS-like tyrosine kinase 3 ligand (hFlt-3), recombinant human interleukin 11 (hIL-11). Store aliquots at –20 °C.

3. 200 mM L-glutamin. For long-term storage, keep aliquots at –20 °C.

4. 10,000 U/mL penicillin/10 mg/mL streptomycin. Aliquots should be kept at –20 °C for long-term storage.

5. 20 μg/μL meropenem HEXAL (HEXAL AG, Holzkirchen, Germany). Keep aliquots at –20 °C.

6. Culturing medium: serum-free StemSpan medium with 2 % penicillin/streptomycin, 1 % L-glutamine, 20 μg/mL meropenem HEXAL, 50 ng/mL mSCF, 20 ng/mL mIL-3, 50 ng/mL hFlt-3, 50 ng/mL hIL-11 (*see* **Note 1**).

7. Türk's solution (Merck KGaA, Darmstadt, Germany).

8. APC-conjugated streptavidin antibody (eBioscience, San Diego, CA, USA).

9. Phosphate-buffered saline (PBS) (DPBS Dulbecco's Phosphate Buffered Salt Solution).

10. Fetal bovine serum (FBS) Standard Quality, heat inactivated for 30 min at 56 °C. For long-term storage, keep aliquots at –20 °C. Before use, thaw and store at 4 °C.

11. Staining buffer: 4% FBS in PBS.

12. FACS-buffer: 4% FBS, 2 mM EDTA in PBS.

13. Cell culture plastic ware: 48-well tissue plates for suspension cell culture, 50 mL tubes.

14. Cell culture incubator set at 37 °C, 5% CO_2, 100% humidity.

15. Neubauer counting chamber and cover glasses.

16. Automatic counter CASY-TT instrument (Roche Diagnostics, Mannheim, Germany).

17. Suitable Eppendorf centrifuge, e.g., Heraeus Fresco 17 Centrifuge (Thermo Fisher Scientific, Waltham, MA, USA).

18. FACSCalibur flow cytometer (Becton Dickinson, Heidelberg, Germany).

19. 100 μg/mL propidium iodide (PI) (100×).

20. Freezing medium: 10% DMSO in FBS.

2.2 Transduction of Lineage Negative Rosa26rtTA Bone Marrow Cells with Tetracycline-regulated Lentiviral Vectors

1. 48 μg/mL retronectin (RN) (TaKaRa, Saint-Germain-en-Laye, France), store at –20 °C.

2. 10× Hank's balanced salt solution (HBSS). To prepare 1× HBSS: add 5 mL 10× HBSS to 45 mL of water.

3. Bovine serum albumin (BSA).

4. 1 M Hepes buffer.

5. RN-blocking solution: 2% BSA in PBS. Weigh 1 g of BSA and transfer to 50 mL tube. Dissolve with 50 mL PBS. Sterilize by filtration with 0.22 μm MILLEX®-GP (Merck KGaA). Store at 4 °C.

6. RN-washing solution: 2.5% (volume/volume) 1 M Hepes in 1× HBSS. Dilute 1.25 mL of 1 M Hepes with 48.75 mL of 1× HBSS. Store at 4 °C.

7. Cooling centrifuge Heraeus Multifuge 3 S-R (Thermo Fisher Scientific) with tissue culture plate holders.

8. Cell-free tetracycline-regulated lentiviral vector supernatant (SNT) with known titer. Store aliquots at –80 °C. Ecotropic- or VSVg-pseudotyped LV vector particles are recommended. For example, concentrated ecotropic-pseudotyped (see **Note 2**) LV vector pRRL.PPT.T11.EGFP.pre [11] SNT with titer of 3.7×10^7 tu/mL (transducing units per milliliter) (see **Note 3**).

2.3 Doxycycline Induction of Transgene Expression

Doxycycline hyclate (Sigma-Aldrich, St. Louis, MO, USA), 1.0 mg/mL stock solution: dissolve 0.1 g of Doxycycline hyclate in 100 mL of water. Sterilize by filtration with 0.22 μm

MILLEX®-GP (Merck KGaA). For long-term storage, keep 1 mL aliquots at −20 °C. The working aliquot can be stored at 4 °C (*see* **Note 4**).

2.4 Determination of Gene Transfer/Expression Levels

1. 100 μg/mL propidium iodide (100×).
2. FACSCalibur flow cytometer.
3. FlowJo software (Tree Star, Ashland, OR, USA) or similar flow cytometry analysis program.

3 Methods

Here, we describe the step-by-step routine transduction protocol of lineage negative Rosa26rtTA bone marrow cells. Modification of this HSC-enriched fraction of murine bone marrow cells with tetracycline-regulated lentiviral vectors can be accomplished in four main steps: (Subheading 3.1) pre-stimulation of purified lineage negative Rosa26rtTA bone marrow cells; (Subheading 3.2) transduction of lineage negative Rosa26rtTA bone marrow cells with tetracycline-regulated lentiviral vectors; (Subheading 3.3) doxycycline induction of transgene expression; (Subheading 3.4) determination of gene transfer/expression levels.

3.1 Pre-stimulation of Purified Lineage Negative Rosa26rtTA Bone Marrow Cells

Work under sterile conditions (day 0) (Fig. 1).

1. Resuspend purified (Lin⁻) Rosa26rtTA BM cells (*see* **Note 5**) in 1 mL of culturing medium. Keep on ice.
2. Determine the number of vital purified (Lin⁻) Rosa26rtTA BM cells by diluting 1:100 in Türk's solution and counting in a Neubauer counting chamber. Alternatively, an automatic counter can be used.
3. Determine the purity of (Lin⁻) Rosa26rtTA bone marrow cells. To accomplish this, stain 10^5 lineage negative and lineage positive cells with 0.1 μg of APC-conjugated streptavidin antibody for 30 min at 4 °C in 0.1 mL of staining buffer. After staining add 1 mL of PBS, centrifuge for 2 min at $400 \times g$ in a Heraeus Fresco 17 Centrifuge and carefully discard the supernatant. Repeat the washing procedure and resuspend the pellet in 0.3 mL of FACS buffer. Add 3 μL of 100× PI solution to stain dead cells, mix by vortex. Acquire the amount of APC-positive cells on a FACSCalibur flow cytometer: a purity ≥85 % of APC negative cells in (Lin⁻) fraction is recommended.
4. Dilute the (Lin⁻) Rosa26rtTA cells at a density of $0.5 \times 10^6/0.5$ mL in culturing medium and plate in independent wells of a 48- or 24-well suspension culture plate (*see* **Note 6**). One well corresponds to one biological replicate.
5. Cultivate for 12–24 h in a cell culture incubator (Fig. 1).

3.2 Transduction of Lineage Negative Rosa26rtTA Bone Marrow Cells with Tetracycline-regulated Lentiviral Vectors

1. Define the size and number of wells for RN pre-coating. Considerations for this step include the cell number to be transduced, multiplicity of infection and number of replicates (*see* **Notes 7** and **8**). For example, to transduce 1×10^5 (Lin⁻) Rosa26rtTA cells with one vector but two different multiplicities of infection (MOI 0.1 and 1) in three biological replicates, pre-coat a total of six wells of a 48-well (1.1 cm²) suspension culture plate (*see* **Note 9**).

2. For RN pre-coating of 48-well plate, add 228 μL of 48 μg/mL RN solution per well (final concentration 10 μg/cm²) (*see* **Note 10**). Incubate for 2 h at room temperature (RT) to allow the RN to adhere to the plate (*see* **Note 11**). Before transduction, remove the RN solution and block with 500 μL of RN-blocking solution for at least 30 min at RT. Discard the blocking solution and add 700 μL of RN-washing solution.

3. Thaw LV vector SNT (*see* **Notes 2** and **12**), and store it on ice. In an Eppendorf tube, supplement the calculated amount of SNT to achieve the selected MOI with ice-cold pure StemSpan medium. For example, to obtain an MOI 1.0 in order to transduce 1×10^5 of (Lin⁻) Rosa26rtTA cells with the ecotropic vector pRRL.PPT. T11.EGFP.pre [11], supplement 100 μL of SNT (titer 2×10^6 tu/mL) with pure StemSpan medium to a final volume of 400 μL (for 48-well plate) (*see* **Note 13**). We recommend preparing a master mix for several biological replicates. Mix carefully.

4. Remove the washing solution from RN pre-coated wells.

5. Add prepared supernatant to RN pre-coated well. For instance, add SNT with a final volume of 400 μL to RN pre-coated well of 48-well tissue culture plate.

6. Centrifuge the plate at 2000 rpm ($800 \times g$) and 32 °C for 60 min in a Heraeus Multifuge to facilitate the binding of LV vector particles with RN (*see* **Notes 14** and **15**).

7. During the centrifugation step, carefully resuspend and count the pre-stimulated (Lin⁻) Rosa26rtTa cells. Calculate if any additional culture medium is needed to achieve the required density and amount of (Lin⁻) Rosa26rtTA cells for transduction. Have culture medium and cell suspension prepared in the sterile hood.

8. After the centrifugation step to bind the LV vector particles to the RN, carefully remove the supernatants from wells (LV vector particles are expected to be bound to RN on the bottom of the well). It is important to work fast and not allow the wells to dry. Add prepared cells to LV vector-coated wells. For instance, add 1×10^5 of (Lin⁻) Rosa26rtTA cells in 400 μL of culture medium to one LV vector-coated well of a 48-well tissue culture plate.

9. Incubate the cells in a cell culture incubator (day 1) (Fig. 1).

3.3 Doxycycline Induction of Transgene Expression

1. On day 2 (Fig. 1), carefully resuspend the transduced cells in each well (*see* **Notes 16** and **17**). Divide the volume of each well (400 μL for 48-well plate) into two aliquots (200 μL) and transfer into two wells of a new 48-well suspension culture plate.

2. Supplement the one culture aliquot with an additional equal volume of fresh culturing medium containing no DOX and the second culture aliquot with medium containing double the final DOX concentration. For example for 48-well plate, the first aliquot (200 μL) could be supplemented with 200 μL of 0 μg/mL DOX culturing medium ("no DOX" control), and the second aliquot with 200 μL of 2.0 μg/mL DOX culturing medium (final DOX concentration 1.0 μg/mL).

3. It is recommended to include intermediate DOX concentrations corresponding to final 0.01 and 0.1 μg/mL of DOX (*see* **Note 18**).

4. Identical DOX concentrations including the "no DOX" control are recommended to be applied when different MOIs of lentiviral tetracycline-regulated vector are used to transduce (Lin⁻) Rosa26rtTA cells (*see* **Note 18**).

5. Incubate the cells in a cell culture incubator (day 2) (Fig. 1).

3.4 Determination of Gene Transfer/Expression Levels

1. On day 3 (Fig. 1), carefully resuspend cells in each well.

2. Take an aliquot to count the number of living cells.

3. Take an aliquot for FACS analysis: 3×10^4 cells are sufficient (usually ~40 μL). Add 300 μL of FACS buffer and 3 μL of 100× PI solution, mix by vortex. Keep on ice.

4. Acquire EGFP-positive cells on a FACSCalibur flow cytometer and analyze with FlowJo or equivalent software (Fig. 2).

5. Determine the background activity of the tetracycline-regulated promoter in the absence of DOX (Figs. 2 and 3) (*see* **Note 19**).

6. Determine gene transfer (percent of EGFP⁺ cells) and expression (MFI of EGFP) levels after 24 h of DOX induction (Fig. 3).

7. Further in vitro expansion to determine gene transfer/expression levels in transduced (Lin⁻) Rosa26rtTA cells on days 5 and 10 after DOX induction is recommended (*see* **Note 20**). On days 8–10, material for DNA preparation and vector copy number identification could be taken (*see* **Note 19**).

8. Transplantation of transduced (Lin⁻) Rosa26rtTA donor cells, which were not treated with DOX, into lethally irradiated recipient mice (C57BL/6J) is recommended on day 3 (Fig. 1). Alternatively, the material cryopreserved on day 2 could be transplanted (Fig. 1, *see* **Notes 16** and **17**).

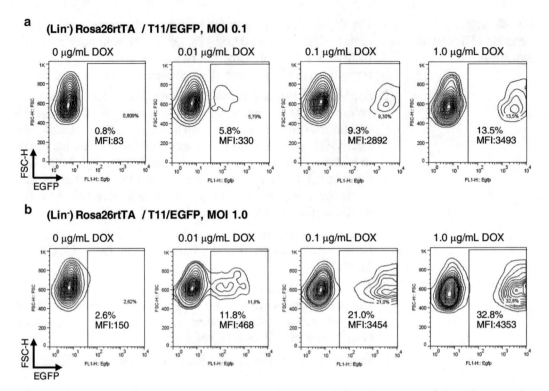

Fig. 2 Estimation of gene transfer/expression levels and background activity of the lentiviral T11/EGFP vector in transduced (Lin⁻) Rosa26rtTA cells. (**a**, **b**) T11 background activity (at 0 μg/mL of DOX) and transduction rate (percentage of EGFP⁺ cells; MFI of EGFP), when different concentrations of DOX (0.01, 0.1, 1.0 μg/mL) were applied for 24 h to induce EGFP expression in (Lin⁻) Rosa26rtTA cells transduced with the T11/EGFP vector using MOI = 0.1 (**a**) and MOI = 1.0 (**b**). Selected contour plots from three biological replicates are presented. *MFI* mean fluorescence intensity of EGFP, *DOX* doxycycline, *MOI* multiplicity of infection

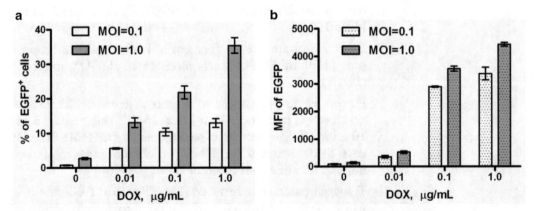

Fig. 3 T11 promoter inducibility in (Lin⁻) Rosa26rtTA cells transduced with lentiviral T11/EGFP vector. Gene transfer (percentage of EGFP⁺ cells) (**a**) and gene expression (MFI of EGFP) (**b**) levels, when different concentrations of DOX (0, 0.01, 0.1, 1.0 μg/mL) were applied for 24 h to induce EGFP expression in (Lin⁻) Rosa26rtTA cells transduced with the T11/EGFP vector using MOI = 0.1 and MOI = 1.0. Data are summarized from experiments performed in biological replicates and presented as mean ± SD, $n = 3$. *MFI* mean fluorescence intensity of EGFP, *DOX* doxycycline, *MOI* multiplicity of infection

4   Notes

1. In addition to the presently described cytokine composition of the culturing medium, others can also be used [8, 11, 19–21].

2. We recommend concentration of ecotropic- or VSVg-pseudotyped LV vector particles [22, 23] via ultracentrifugation at 10,000 rpm ($13,238 \times g$) 16–24 h or at 25,000 rpm ($82,740 \times g$) for 2 h at 4 °C, correspondingly (Ultracentrifuge Optima LE-80K, Beckman Coulter, Brea, CA, USA). Dissolve the concentrated LV vector particles in pure serum-free StemSpan medium to avoid exposure of HSCs to serum components resulting in unwanted differentiation. Store LV vector aliquots at –80 °C.

3. To estimate the titer of tetracycline-regulated lentiviral vectors, we use modified murine fibroblasts (SC1), which express rtTA2 (SC1/rtTA2) [8, 11, 24].

4. Doxycycline is light sensitive. For short-term usage, keep 1 mg/mL stock solution aliquots at 4 °C in Eppendorf tubes made from dark plastic or use aluminum foil to cover the Eppendorf tube and protect the DOX from light. For long-term storage, keep 1 mg/mL stock solution at –20 °C.

5. On average, we harvest ~4×10^7 BM cells from one mouse (age ≥8 weeks) when total BM is flushed out from femurs, tibiae and pelvis. For preparation of (Lin⁻) Rosa26rtTA BM cells, we use the Lineage Cell Depletion kit (Miltenyi Biotec, Bergisch Gladbach, Germany) and magnetic cell separation (MACS) technology. The expected amount of (Lin⁻) cells is ~1 % of the total BM cells [6], but may vary depending on the purity of isolated (Lin⁻) cells. Purity of (Lin⁻) cells ≥85 % is recommended depending on experimental purpose.

6. (Lin⁻) cell aliquots can be cryopreserved immediately after MACS purification in freezing medium at –80 °C and later transferred to liquid nitrogen. After thawing, it is important to count viable cell numbers: in our experience, the number of viable cells is usually about half of that estimated before freezing.

7. Tissue culture plate format and corresponding amounts of reagents depend on the amount of cells to be transduced [6]. When ≤2×10^4 cells are transduced (for example LSK: Lin⁻ Sca1⁺ cKit⁺) with tetracycline-regulated lentiviral vectors, the use of a 96-well plate is recommended.

8. For further in vitro experiments (Fig. 1), we recommend plating freshly prepared or thawed (Lin⁻) cells in triplicates (three biological replicates) [11].

9. We recommend using empty wells to separate experimental wells for mock untransduced cells and/or cells transduced with different vectors. When possible, different tissue culture plates could be used.

10. Amounts of RN depend on tissue culture plate format [6]. For instance, to achieve a final RN concentration of 10 $\mu g/cm^2$ to pre-coat one well in a 24-well plate (2.0 cm^2), add 420 μL of 48 $\mu g/mL$ RN stock to the well [6].

11. RN pre-coating could be started at day 0 (Fig. 1). If transduction is performed on the next day (day 1) RN pre-coated plates could be prepared by incubation for 2 h at RT at day 0, and then kept overnight at 4 °C.

12. If the titer is high but experimental MOI and amount of cells are low, dilute the calculated amount of SNT with ice-cold pure StemSpan medium in an Eppendorf tube to achieve the lower titer. For example, to transduce 1×10^5 of (Lin⁻) Rosa26rtTA cells with an ecotropic vector pRRL.PPT.T11.EGFP.pre [11] with a titer 3.7×10^7 tu/mL and an MOI = 1.0, we recommend diluting the SNT stock to a titer of 2×10^6 tu/mL.

13. We suppose that only half of the LV vector particles will bind to the RN pre-coated plate.

14. LV vector particles preloading (via spinoculation) can be performed at 4 °C, but the efficiency of (Lin⁻) transduction was observed to be increased at 32 °C.

15. LV vector particles preloading procedure can be repeated when the titer of the supernatant is low, but high MOIs are needed.

16. If further in vivo murine BMT experiments will be performed, we recommend culturing the majority of the transduced cells without DOX induction until day 3, when the transduced cells will be transplanted (Fig. 1). Alternatively, transduced material could be cryopreserved already at day 2 (Fig. 1). In both cases, we recommend using an aliquot of transduced cells for DOX treatment and transduction rate evaluation and/or for further in vitro expansion.

17. Cell differentiation during the culture period should be taken into consideration when calculating the amount of cells needed for BMT experiments [6].

18. For biological replicates within independent experiments [11], we recommend use of ecotropic- or VSVg-pseudotyped LV vector supernatants from the same preparation batch in order to minimize the "batch to batch" variability.

19. It was shown that transduction of (Lin⁻) Rosa26rtTA cells with increasing MOIs of tetracycline-regulated lentiviral vectors resulted in increased vector copy number and a linear increase

of background activity of tetP TRP in the absence of DOX [11, 18]. The level of "leakiness" could be decreased by using improved TRPs, for instance such as T11 [2, 11] (Figs. 2 and 3).

20. For further in vitro expansion, we give the cells fresh culturing medium (no DOX or final DOX concentration) 2–3 times per week. It could be necessary to split the cells into larger tissue culture plates to maintain the recommended cell density. For both feeding and splitting we include half fresh and half conditioned medium [6].

Acknowledgements

This work was supported by the German Research Foundation (DFG, Research priority program SPP 1230 Ba1837/7-2, cluster of excellence REBIRTH Exc 62/1, SFB7308) and the European Union (grants PERSIST FP7-HEALTH-2007-B-222878 and CellPID FP7-HEALTH-2010-261387). We thank Christopher Baum for his support. We thank Niels Heinz and Bernhard Schiedlmeier for useful advice on Tet-regulated vectors. We thank Michael Morgan for carefully reading the final draft.

References

1. Kenny PA, Enver T, Ashworth A (2002) Retroviral vectors for establishing tetracycline-regulated gene expression in an otherwise recalcitrant cell line. BMC Mol Biol 3:13

2. Heinz N, Schambach A, Galla M et al (2011) Retroviral and transposon-based tet-regulated all-in-one vectors with reduced background expression and improved dynamic range. Hum Gene Ther 22:166–176

3. Zuber J, McJunkin K, Fellmann C et al (2011) Toolkit for evaluating genes required for proliferation and survival using tetracycline-regulated RNAi. Nat Biotechnol 29:79–83

4. Vigna E, Naldini L (2000) Lentiviral vectors: excellent tools for experimental gene transfer and promising candidates for gene therapy. J Gene Med 2:308–316

5. Vigna E, Cavalieri S, Ailles L et al (2002) Robust and efficient regulation of transgene expression in vivo by improved tetracycline-dependent lentiviral vectors. Mol Ther 5:252–261

6. Modlich U, Schambach A, Li Z, Schiedlmeier B (2009) Murine hematopoietic stem cell transduction using retroviral vectors. In: Baum C (ed) Genetic modification of hematopoietic stem cells. Humana Press, New York, pp 23–31

7. Loew R (2009) The use of retroviral vectors for tet-regulated gene expression in cell populations. In: Baum C (ed) Genetic modification of hematopoietic stem cells. Humana Press, New York, pp 221–242

8. Kustikova OS, Schwarzer A, Stahlhut M et al (2013) Activation of Evi1 inhibits cell cycle progression and differentiation of hematopoietic progenitor cells. Leukemia 27:1127–1138

9. Konrad TA, Karger A, Hackl H et al (2009) Inducible expression of EVI1 in human myeloid cells causes phenotypes consistent with its role in myelodysplastic syndromes. J Leukoc Biol 86:813–822

10. Laurenti E, Barde I, Verp S et al (2010) Inducible gene and shRNA expression in resident hematopoietic stem cells in vivo. Stem Cells 28:1390–1398

11. Kustikova OS, Stahlhut M, Ha T-C et al (2014) Dose response and clonal variability of lentiviral tetracycline-regulated vectors in murine hematopoietic cells. Exp Hematol 42:505–515.e7

12. Beard BC, Dickerson D, Beebe K et al (2007) Comparison of HIV-derived lentiviral and MLV-based gammaretroviral vector integration sites in primate repopulating cells. Mol Ther 15:1356–1365

13. Kustikova OS, Schiedlmeier B, Brugman MH et al (2009) Cell-intrinsic and vector-related properties cooperate to determine the incidence and consequences of insertional mutagenesis. Mol Ther 17:1537–1547

14. Heckl D, Schwarzer A, Haemmerle R et al (2012) Lentiviral vector induced insertional haploinsufficiency of Ebf1 causes murine leukemia. Mol Ther 20:1187–1195

15. Montini E, Cesana D, Schmidt M et al (2009) The genotoxic potential of retroviral vectors is strongly modulated by vector design and integration site selection in a mouse model of HSC gene therapy. J Clin Invest 119:964–975

16. Kustikova OS, Modlich U, Fehse B (2009) Genetic modification of hematopoietic stem cells. In: Baum C (ed) Genetic modification of hematopoietic stem cells. Humana Press, New York, pp 373–390

17. Magnusson M, Brun ACM, Miyake N et al (2007) HOXA10 is a critical regulator for hematopoietic stem cells and erythroid/megakaryocyte development. Blood 109:3687–3696

18. Gossen M, Bujard H (1992) Tight control of gene expression in mammalian cells by tetracycline-responsive promoters. Proc Natl Acad Sci U S A 89:5547–5551

19. Schnabel CA, Jacobs Y, Cleary ML (2000) HoxA9-mediated immortalization of myeloid progenitors requires functional interactions with TALE cofactors Pbx and Meis. Oncogene 19:608–616

20. Zhang CC, Lodish HF (2005) Murine hematopoietic stem cells change their surface phenotype during ex vivo expansion. Blood 105:4314–4320

21. Li Z, Schwieger M, Lange C et al (2003) Predictable and efficient retroviral gene transfer into murine bone marrow repopulating cells using a defined vector dose. Exp Hematol 31:1206–1214

22. Schambach A, Bohne J, Baum C et al (2006) Woodchuck hepatitis virus post-transcriptional regulatory element deleted from X protein and promoter sequences enhances retroviral vector titer and expression. Gene Ther 13:641–645

23. Schambach A, Swaney WP, van der Loo JC (2009) Design and production of retro- and lentiviral vectors for gene expression in hematopoietic cells. In: Baum C (ed) Genetic modification of hematopoietic stem cells. Humana Press, New York, pp 191–205

24. Urlinger S, Baron U, Thellmann M et al (2000) Exploring the sequence space for tetracycline-dependent transcriptional activators: novel mutations yield expanded range and sensitivity. Proc Natl Acad Sci U S A 97:7963–7968

Chapter 6

Introduction of shRNAs, miRNAs, or AntagomiRs into Primary Human Liver Cells Through Lentiviral Vectors

Jessica K. Rieger and Maria Thomas

Abstract

RNA interference (RNAi) is a specific and efficient method to silence gene expression in mammalian cells. However, genetic manipulation of primary cells including human hepatocytes by RNAi remained challenging. Therefore an efficient gene transfer protocol to modify gene expression in primary cells by using VSV-G-pseudotyped, EGFP-expressing lentiviral vectors was established. The protocol comprises the production of lentiviral vectors as well as the steps for efficient delivery of short-hairpin RNAs (shRNAs), microRNAs, or antagomiRs to human hepatocytes. With this method the amount of preparative work is reduced, by achieving high transduction efficiencies with low multiplicity of infection (MOI). Depending on the laboratory equipment, we provide two alternative workflows. The procedure of lentiviral vector production with subsequent titer determination takes approx. 6–10 working days.

Key words RNAi, Lentiviral vector transduction, Primary human hepatocytes, miRNAs, AntagomiRs

1 Introduction

RNA interference (RNAi) is a recently established and powerful tool to reduce expression of endogenous mRNA or protein expression [1–3]. Moreover RNAi is being used to silence mRNAs encoding pathogenic proteins for therapy in vivo [4]. Despite several different protocols available, the efficiency of siRNA delivery by transfection techniques via lipophilic agents is still not satisfactory for many applications or cells such as primary cells.

A method, which achieves higher transfection rates, is the use of recombinant viruses, in particular adenoviral and lentiviral derivatives. Adenoviral methods to transduce cells exist, but the adenoviral vectors are non-replicating and remain episomal which results in only transient gene expression [5–8]. Human immunodeficiency virus (HIV)-based vectors are currently the most popular lentiviral-based expression systems and effectively transduce both dividing and nondividing cells by stable integration into the genome of the

Maurizio Federico (ed.), *Lentiviral Vectors and Exosomes as Gene and Protein Delivery Tools*, Methods in Molecular Biology, vol. 1448, DOI 10.1007/978-1-4939-3753-0_6, © Springer Science+Business Media New York 2016

host cells. Long-term transgene expression is facilitated by lentiviral transduction and the virus particles do not lead to any inflammatory response.

Our aim was to develop robust, comprehensive, and reliable protocols for the design, generation, and purification of lentiviral particles and their use for transduction of primary cells such as primary human hepatocytes. For the protocol validation, we generated a panel of vectors coding for active shRNAs targeting major nuclear receptors as well as known liver-specific microRNAs and antagomiRs. We successfully applied this protocol in our explorative studies on the function of nuclear receptors, PPARα and CAR [2, 3].

2 Materials

2.1 Reagents/Kits

1. HEK293FT cell line (Invitrogen R700-07).
2. BLOCK-iT™ Lentiviral RNAi Expression Kit (Invitrogen).
3. ViraPower™ Lentiviral Gateway Expression Kit (Invitrogen).
4. miRZip™ Lentivector-based AntagomiRs (System Biosciences#MZIPxxxPA/AA-1).
5. pMIRNA1 Lentivector-based microRNAs (System Biosciences#PMIRHxxxPA/AA-1).
6. G418 (Calbiochem).
7. TurboFect (Thermo Scientific).
8. 0.05 % Trypsin with EDTA (Life Technologies).
9. PEG-it™ Virus Concentration Solution (System Biosciences).
10. Corning® BioCoat™ Cellware, Collagen Type I, 12-well plates.

2.2 Equipment

1. Sterile filter 0.45 μm PVDF.
2. Single-use syringes, 50 ml.
3. Ultracentrifuge tubes.
4. Ultracentrifuge Beckmann Optima L-100XP.
5. Ultracentrifuge rotor SW28 (swing out) with buckets.
6. FACS Calibur.

2.3 Reagent Setup

2.3.1 Medium for Culturing HEK293FT and HT1080 Cells

1. D-MEM (high glucose) with 10 % FCS.
2. 1 % Penicillin/streptomycin (f.c. 10,000 U/10,000 μg).
3. 1 % Sodium pyruvate (f.c. 100 mM).
4. 1 % Glutamine (f.c. 200 mM).
5. 1 % MEM NEAA (nonessential amino acids, 100×, without L-glutamine).

6. BSA/PBS: 1% Solution of BSA in PBS, sterile filtered, aliquoted, and stored at –20 °C.

7. 6 mg/ml Polybrene for higher transduction efficiency: Dissolve 6 mg of polybrene in 1 ml of sterile water.

2.3.2 Medium for Culturing Primary Human Liver Cells

1. William's E Medium with 10% FBS Gold.

2. 1% Penicillin/streptomycin (f.c. 10,000 U/10,000 μg).

3. 1% L-Glutamine (f.c. 200 mM).

4. 400 μl of Human insulin (30 I.E.).

5. 1% Sodium pyruvate (f.c. 100 mM).

6. 1% MEM NEAA (nonessential amino acids, 100×, without L-glutamine).

7. 1.5% of Hepes (1 M).

8. 8 μl of Hydrocortisone (50 mg/ml).

3 Methods

All the steps marked with "S" should be performed following recommended guidelines for working with biosafety level 2 organisms.

3.1 Transfection of HEK293FT Cells

1. For cultivating HEK293FT cells, add 500 μg/ml of G148 (Geneticin) to the DMEM culture medium with components (*see* Subheading 2.3) (*see* **Note 1**).

2. Three days prior to transfection, plate cells at a density of approximately 3.5×10^6 cells/per 1 T175 flask in 30 ml of medium with components and G148 to achieve optimal phase of cellular growth.

3. A schematic workflow of the procedure is shown in Fig. 1. Prepare the transfection mix by mixing 250 μl of packaging mix (corresponding to 25 μg) and 18 μg of expression plasmid DNA and add serum-free DMEM medium to the final volume of 4.5 ml in a 15 ml conical tube (solution 1). Add 105 μl of Turbofect in a final volume of 4.5 ml serum-free DMEM medium in a fresh tube (solution 2). Incubate both mixtures for 5 min at room temperature (*see* **Note 2**).

4. Mix both solutions (1 and 2), invert the tube 3–4 times, and incubate the final transfection mix for 15–20 min at room temperature.

5. ("S") Meanwhile trypsinize HEK293FT cells from Subheading 3.1 and dilute the cells to a final concentration of 1.8×10^7 cells in 21 ml DMEM full medium without G418 (*see* **Note 3**).

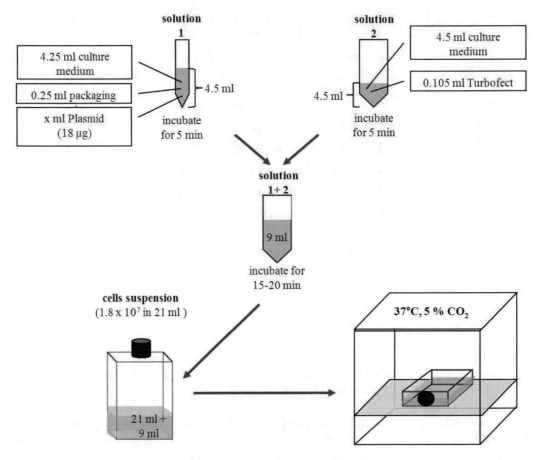

Fig. 1 Schematic workflow of the cell transfection steps. Prepare solution 1 by mixing 250 µl of packaging mix (corresponding to 25 µg), 18 µg of expression plasmid DNA, and serum-free culture medium to the final volume of 4.5 ml. Prepare solution 2 by mixing 105 µl of Turbofect in 4.5 ml serum-free culture medium and incubate both mixtures for 5 min at room temperature. Mix both solutions (1 and 2), invert the tube 3–4 times, and incubate the final transfection mix for 15–20 min at room temperature. Meanwhile dilute the cells to a final concentration of 1.8×10^7 cells in 21 ml full culture medium without G418. Add 9 ml of transfection mix, mix gently, and incubate the cells at 37 °C, 5 % CO_2

6. Transfer cells into fresh T175 flask; add 9 ml of transfection mix from Subheading 3.1, **step 3**; mix gently; and incubate the cells at 37 °C, 5 % CO_2 (*see* **Note 4**).

3.2 First Harvesting Step of Supernatant (48 h After Transfection) ("S") (See Note 5)

1. For collection, transfer the culture medium which contains lentiviral particles carrying shRNA/microRNA/antagomiRs sequences (ca. 30 ml) into a 50 ml tube. Add 30 ml of fresh medium to the cells for further incubation at 37 °C.

2. Centrifuge the transferred medium at $1750 \times g$ for 5 min at 4 °C to pellet cells or cellular debris.

3. Filter the supernatant through 0.45 µm PVDF filter using 50 ml syringes into ultracentrifuge tubes and centrifuge supernatant at $50,000 \times g$ for 90 min at 4 °C.

Table 1
Comparison of protocols using ultracentrifuge (option A) and PEG-it™ precipitation solution (option B)

	"Ultracentrifuge" protocol A	**"PEG-it" protocol B**
Time consumption	6 working days	7 working days
Lentiviral recovery/titer (TU/ml)	$\sim4\times10^7$	$\sim1\times10^7$
MOI to be used for successful transduction of primary cells	MOI 3	MOI 5
Handling	Simple	Simple
Costs	Onetime costs for ultracentrifuge	Repeated costs for acquisition of PEG-it

A. First option: using ultracentrifuge (refer to "Comparison of two methods in Table 1").

4A. After centrifugation, discard the supernatant and dry the pellet at room temperature for 3 min; dissolve the pellet in 50 μl of 1% BSA/PBS by keeping the tubes in a vertical position at 4 °C at least overnight (*see* **Note 6**).

B. Alternative option: polyethylene glycol precipitation using PEG-it™.

4B. Add 6 ml of $5\times$PEG-it™ solution to the filtered supernatant from Subheading 3.2, **step 3**, and mix by gently inverting the tube. Keep the tube at 4 °C at least overnight to precipitate lentiviral particles.

5B. Centrifuge the precipitated supernatants at $1750\times g$ for 30 min at 4 °C and dissolve the pellet in 50 μl of 1% BSA/PBS by keeping the tubes in a vertical position at 4 °C at least overnight (*see* **Note 6**).

6B. Harvest again the supernatant (72 h after transfection) ("S"). Repeat Subheading 3.2, **steps 1–4, 5** (A or B); the flasks with the cells can now be discarded following the safety standards for working with lentiviruses.

7B. Pool and aliquot lentiviral suspensions ("S"). The dissolved lentiviral pellets from the fist and second harvesting step can be pooled (*see* **Note 7**).

3.3 Titer Determination ("S")

1. For titer determination we use HT1080 cells (human sarcoma cell line) (*see* **Note 8**). Plate cells at density of 1×10^5 per well in a 12-well plate 1 day or at least 4 h prior to transduction.

2. Dilute the stock solution of polybrene in 300 μl full medium to achieve a final concentration of 6 μg/ml per well. Add 300 μl polybrene solution to each well (*see* **Note 9**).

3. For the transduction of the cells three different lentiviral dilutions have to be prepared. Therefore mix 0.5, 1, and 2 µl lentiviral solutions from step 3.5 with medium to achieve a final volume of 200 µl per well. Add 200 µl of lentiviral suspensions to each well to get a final total volume of 500 µl (300 µl polybrene solution + 200 µl lentiviral solution). Incubate cells at 37 °C and 5 % CO_2 for 2 days.

4. Three days after transduction trypsinize the cells by adding 150 µl of 0.05 % trypsin solution per well, incubate for 5–10 min, and dilute with 850 µl of medium.

5. Proceed to FACS measurement, counting 10,000 events per probe. The number of transfection unit (TU) per ml is calculated using the following equation (*see* **Note 10**):

$$TU / ml = [F \times C / V] \times 1000$$

where:

F = frequency of GFP-positive cells (percentage obtained by FACS measurement divided by 100).

C = total number of cells in the well at the time of transduction.

V = volume of inoculum in µl.

3.4 Transduction of Primary Human Hepatocytes ("S")

1. There are several options to obtain primary human hepatocytes. We obtain them in suspension, optimally 3 days after operative procedure. The full protocol and detailed description of cell isolation and cultivation have been reported [9]. Upon arrival, we centrifuge the cells at $1200 \times g/5$ min, and resuspend them in an appropriate amount of "full" Williams E Medium (*see* Subheading 2.3). Based on our experience, we recommend to use 12-well plate format coated with collagen (*see* Subheading 2.1) in a density of 4×10^5 cells/well. The plated cells should be further incubated at 37 °C, 5 % CO_2, for at least 2–3 h prior to transduction.

2. For transduction, aspirate the culture medium and replace it with the medium containing appropriate amounts of polybrene (6 µg/ml final concentration) and different MOI amounts of lentiviral vector (*see* **Note 11**). We recommend to start with MOI 2 per well, thereby gradually increasing the amount in additional wells. Based on our experience, primary hepatocytes show differential susceptibility towards transduction efficiency depending on disease status of the donor. Therefore it is advisable to test different MOI. In most cases, an average MOI of 4–5 allows reaching the transduction efficiency to over 95 %.

3. Exchange the medium 24 h after transductions (*see* **Note 12**).

4. On the basis of our experience, substantial effects can be detected on days 4–5 after transduction.

4   Notes

1. The cells should be passaged at least 1–2 times after thawing to adapt to the culture conditions.

2. All numbers and calculations correspond to the transfection of cells in one T175 flask.

3. It is strongly recommended that no G418 be added during transfections or any time during lentiviral vector production since it can result in an unacceptable cell mortality.

4. If the expression vector contains fluorescent gene marker, the transfection efficiency could be checked as soon as 24 h after transfection via fluorescence microscope. Expression of the VSV-G glycoprotein causes 293FT cells to fuse, resulting in the appearance of multinucleated syncytia. This morphological change is normal and does not affect production of lentivirus. If syncytia are not observed, virus production is likely to be impaired.

5. This step can be performed using option A or option B depending on the equipment available.

6. Do not resuspend via vortexing or vigorous pipetting, since lentiviral particles are labile.

7. For long-term storage, we recommend to aliquot viruses in 20–50 μl aliquots and to keep them at –80 °C. Important: Reserve 10 μl of each virus production for titer determination and keep it also at –80 °C for comparability with respect to freezing/thawing. According to Invitrogen benchmarks, lentivirus can lose up to 5 % of its titer with each freeze/thaw cycle. When stored properly, lentiviral stocks should be suitable for at least 1 year.

8. COS-1 cells (monkey kidney cells) are also widely used.

9. To facilitate docking of lentiviral particles on the cell surface, we routinely apply the cationic polymer, polybrene, which increases the efficiency of cell transduction with lentiviral vectors.

10. For example, lentiviral recovery in a well previously infected with 2 μl of lentiviral suspension, resulting in 48 % of GFP-positive cells, is calculated like:

    $TU/ml = [0.48 \times 100{,}000/2] \times 1000 = 2.4 \times 10^7$. The average of three measurements in duplicates should be taken as a final TU/ml value. According to our experience, it is more reliable to consider only results of FACS measurements that are under 50 %, since it reflects the amount of GFP-positive cells (transduced with one lentiviral particle per cell) in linear scale more precisely. FACS analysis of GFP-Lenti-transduced cells has been described in detail by Sastry et al. [10].

11. According to our experience, an application of MOI 3 (i.e., $3 \times 400{,}000 = 1.2 \times 10^6$ TU) is sufficient to infect cells with high efficiency.

12. Analysis of target genes on the mRNA level should be carried out on 4–5 days after transductions, but effects on protein level may require longer.

Acknowledgements

The EGFP-expressing lentiviral vector pLenti6-GFP was kindly provided by Dr. Martin Kriebel, NMI, Reutlingen. We also thank Igor Liebermann and Britta Klumpp, Stuttgart, for expert technical assistance. This study was supported by the German Federal Ministry of Education and Research (Virtual Liver Network Grant 0315755) and by the Robert Bosch Foundation, Stuttgart, Germany.

References

1. Feidt DM, Klein K, Nussler A et al (2009) RNA-interference approach to study functions of NADPH: cytochrome P450 oxidoreductase in human hepatocytes. Chem Biodivers 6:2084–2091

2. Thomas M, Burk O, Klumpp B et al (2013) Direct transcriptional regulation of human hepatic cytochrome P450 3A4 by peroxisome proliferator-activated receptor alpha. Mol Pharmacol 83:709–718

3. Zanger UM, Klein K, Thomas M et al (2014) Genetics, epigenetics, and regulation of drug-metabolizing cytochrome p450 enzymes. Clin Pharmacol Ther 95:258–261

4. Burns JC, Friedmann T, Driever W et al (1993) Vesicular stomatitis virus G glycoprotein pseudotyped retroviral vectors: concentration to very high titer and efficient gene transfer into mammalian and nonmammalian cells. Proc Natl Acad Sci U S A 90:8033–8037

5. Ilan Y, Saito H, Thummala NR et al (1999) Adenovirus-mediated gene therapy of liver diseases. Semin Liver Dis 19:49–59

6. Jover R, Bort R, Gomez-Lechon MJ et al (2001) Cytochrome P450 regulation by hepatocyte nuclear factor 4 in human hepatocytes: a study using adenovirus-mediated antisense targeting. Hepatology 33:668–675

7. Oehmig A, Klotzbücher A, Thomas M et al (2008) A novel reverse transduction adenoviral array for the functional analysis of shRNA libraries. BMC Genomics 9:4411

8. Zamule SM, Strom SC, Omiecinski CJ (2008) Preservation of hepatic phenotype in lentiviral-transduced primary human hepatocytes. Chem Biol Interact 173:179–186

9. Godoy P, Hewitt NJ, Albrecht U et al (2013) Recent advances in 2D and 3D in vitro systems using primary hepatocytes, alternative hepatocyte sources and non-parenchymal liver cells and their use in investigating mechanisms of hepatotoxicity, cell signaling and ADME. Arch Toxicol 87(8):1315–1530

10. Sastry L, Johnson T, Hobson MJ et al (2002) Titering lentiviral vectors: comparison of DNA, RNA and marker expression methods. Gene Ther 9:1155–1162

Chapter 7

Production and Concentration of Lentivirus for Transduction of Primary Human T Cells

Alan Kennedy and Adam P. Cribbs

Abstract

Lentiviral vectors have emerged as efficient tools for investigating T cell biology through their ability to efficiently deliver transgene expression into both dividing and nondividing cells. Such lentiviral vectors have the potential to infect a wide variety of cell types. However, despite this advantage, the ability to transduce primary human T cells remains challenging and methods to achieve efficient gene transfer are often time consuming and expensive. We describe a method for generating lentivirus that is simple to perform and does not require the purchase of non-standard equipment to transduce primary human T cells. Therefore, we provide an optimized protocol that is easy to implement and allow transduction with high efficiency and reproducibility.

Key words Lentivirus, Primary, CD4+ T cells, CD45RA+, Titer, Human T cell, Lentiviral vector

1 Introduction

T cells are lymphocytes that play an essential role in the adaptive immune response by interacting with many cells of the immune system such as B cells, monocytes, and dendritic cells. Compromised T cell responses can result in immunodeficiencies such as severe combined immunodeficiency (SCID). Strategies aimed at restoring defective T cell function are seen as a potential therapeutic strategy for diseases like SCID. As such, replication-deficient pseudotyped lentiviral vectors have the potential to be used as therapeutic agents because they can stably introduce a transgene into a target cell, without the requirement for repeated treatment [1, 2]. This stable integration is a feature that has also been utilized as a basic research tool to investigate ex vivo CD4+ T cell function [3]. Efficient lentiviral transduction has been used to successfully introduce a gene product to either overexpress a particular gene or to reduce the expression of a specific gene through the use of short-hairpin RNA (shRNA). However despite the versatility of

Maurizio Federico (ed.), *Lentiviral Vectors and Exosomes as Gene and Protein Delivery Tools*, Methods in Molecular Biology, vol. 1448, DOI 10.1007/978-1-4939-3753-0_7, © Springer Science+Business Media New York 2016

lentivirus technology, primary T cells are refractory to transduction by lentivirus, with quiescent cells being particularly challenging to transduce [4, 5].

Production of HIV-derived lentiviral vectors is performed by transfecting plasmids harboring self-inactivating long terminal repeat (LTR) regions together with the transgene on one vector into a packaging cell line such as HEK293T cells. Additional transcripts required for packaging (Gag/Pro/Pol) and encapsulation (Env) of the viral vectors are encoded on separate plasmids [6]. The commonly used second-generation packaging systems have all packaging genes encoded by one vector that is transfected along with the transfer vector and encapsulation vector to generate virions. A third-generation packaging system has the Rev gene encoded on a separate plasmid, which results in increased biosafety; however it reduces lentivirus titer and transduction efficiency [7, 8]. Efficient lentiviral transduction of numerous cell lines has been demonstrated previously [9]; however primary human T cells are refractory to transduction by lentivirus, with quiescent cells being the most difficult to transduce [4, 5, 8]. Here we present a detailed and optimized protocol for establishing the generation of high-titer lentivirus, which can transduce primary human T cells with a superior efficiency [8].

2   Materials

2.1   Lentivirus Production by Calcium-Phosphate Transfection

Prepare all solutions using ultrapure water unless otherwise stated (prepared by purifying deionized water to obtain a sensitivity of 18 MΩ at 25 °C, then filtering through a 0.2 μM filter to ensure sterility).

1. Lentiviral packaging constructs are shown in Fig. 1.

2. The pCCL transfer construct is shown in Fig. 2.

3. Phosphate-buffered saline (PBS): Made by dilution of a 10× stock solution with water.

4. Poly-L-lysine: 0.01% Dissolved in PBS.

5. Complete DMEM medium supplemented with 10% fetal calf serum (FCS), 1% L-glutamine, 1% Na pyruvate, and 1% non-essential amino acid (NEAA).

6. HEK293T cells (ATCC, Manassa, VA).

7. 2.5 M Calcium chloride ($CaCl_2$): Weigh 36.74 g of $CaCl_2$ and transfer to a glass beaker containing 100 mL of water. Filter-sterilize using a 0.2 μM filter flask. The solution can be stored in 10 mL aliquots at −20 °C and can be freeze-thawed without loss of efficacy.

8. 2× HEPES-buffered saline (HBS), pH 7.05: Weigh 1.6 g of NaCl, 1.19 g of HEPES, and 21 mg of Na_2HPO_4, transfer to

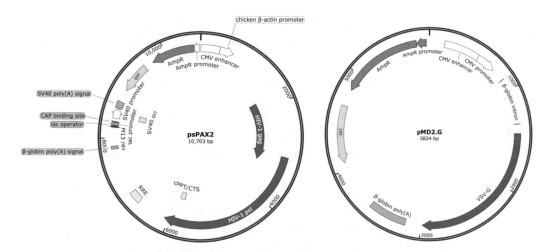

Fig. 1 Vector maps of the packaging constructs used in the production of lentivirus. The system uses two basic vectors, the envelope construct pMD2.G and the packaging construct psPAX2. Plasmid maps were generated using DNA dynamo

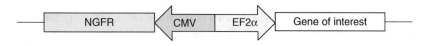

Fig. 2 Illustration of the lentivirus vector constructs

a glass beaker containing 100 mL of water, then adjust to pH 7 with 5 M of NaOH, and then filter-sterilize using a 0.2 μM filter flask (*see* **Note 1**). Store in 5 mL aliquots at −20 °C.

9. Sodium butyrate: 500 mM Dissolved in PBS.

10. 0.45 μm PVDF syringe filter.

11. 50 mL Syringe.

12. Sorvall™ WX ultracentrifuge with Ultra AH-629 rotor.

13. 38.5 mL Polyallomer ultracentrifuge tubes (Beckman Coulter, Pasadena, CA).

2.2 Titer Determination

1. Jurkat cells (ATCC, Manassa, VA).

2. RPMI 1640.

3. FACS wash buffer: PBS containing 2 % FCS and 0.09 % NaN₃.

4. Fixation solution: FACS buffer containing 1 % formaldehyde.

5. Flow cytometry tubes.

6. Human Fc receptor binding inhibitor (eBioscience, San Diego, USA).

7. Alexa Fluor@ 647-CD271 (ΔNGFR) antibody (BD Pharmingen, San Diego, USA).

2.3 Isolation of Peripheral Blood Mononuclear Cells

1. 10 mL Tube BD Vacutainer with K2EDTA.

2. Lympholyte®-H solution (density 1.077 g/L), Cedarlane (Burlington, Canada).

3. Hanks' balanced salt solution (HBSS).

2.4 Isolation of Primary CD45RA⁺ T Cells

1. Naïve T cell isolation kit for isolation of CD45RA⁺ T cells (Miltenyi, Cologne, Germany).

2. Magnetic separation stand and magnet (Miltenyi, Cologne, Germany).

3. MACS buffer: PBS supplemented with 0.5 % FCS and 2 mM of ethylenediaminetetraacetic acid (EDTA).

4. 12-Well and 48-well plates.

5. X-VIVO 15 medium (Lonza, Basel, Switzerland).

6. Recombinant human IL-2 and IL-7 (Peprotech, UK): Prepare IL-2 (100 ng/mL) and IL-7 (15 ng/mL) in sterile PBS with 0.1 % BSA and store in 20 μL aliquots at –80 °C.

7. Human serum (BioSera, Kansas City, USA) (*see* **Note 2**).

2.5 Transduction of CD45RA⁺ T Cells

1. CD3/CD28 activation beads (Invitrogen, Life Technologies, USA) for T cell activation.

2. Polybrene.

3 Methods

All incubations at 37 °C are in an incubator containing 5 % CO_2 unless otherwise stated.

3.1 Lentivirus Production by Calcium-Phosphate Transfection

For the efficient transfection of primary human T cells, lentivirus must be concentrated using ultracentrifugation to remove impurities. Many institutions require correct training for this type of work. Guidelines vary between institutions, so consult your local health and safety officer. At a minimum, work should be performed in biological safety cabinets with personnel wearing lab coats, eye protection, and gloves.

1. Prepare the high-purity vector plasmids including the packaging construct (psPAX2), envelope construct (pMD2.G), and expression construct (pCCL) (*see* **Note 4**).

2. Day 1: Pre-coat a T-175 flask with 5 mL of poly-L-lysine (0.01 %) and incubate at room temperature for 2 h.

3. Day 1: Remove the excess poly-L-lysine liquid from the flask and seed 25×10^6 293T cells on the pre-coated flask in 15–20 mL of complete DMEM medium 16–24 h prior to calcium transfection. Transfection should begin when the cells are 70–80 % confluent.

4. Day 2: Replace the growth medium with fresh complete DMEM medium 2 h prior to transfection.

5. Day 2: Prepare DNA for transfection by diluting 40 μg of pCCL, 10 μg of psPAX2, and 30 μg of pMD2.G plasmids in sterile water to a total volume of 1350 μL. Add 150 μL of $CaCl_2$ and mix gently. Insert a 2 mL pipette into a 15 mL Falcon tube containing 1500 μL of 2× HEPES-buffered saline (HBS). Bubble through the HBS solution and add the DNA mix dropwise.

6. Day 2: Vortex the DNA/HBS suspension and leave at room temperature for 30 min. Remove the cells from the incubator and add 1500 μL of DNA/HBS suspension to the flask (*see* **Note 5**). Alternative transfection methods can be used.

7. Day 2: Incubate transfected cells at 37 °C (3% CO_2) for 4 h and then remove the media. Wash the cells gently in 20 mL of PBS, then add 15 mL of fresh DMEM complete medium supplemented with 1 mM of sodium butyrate, and incubate at 37 °C (3% CO_2) for 16 h (*see* **Note 6**).

8. Day 3: Remove DMEM complete medium and replace with 15 mL of RPMI 1640 medium supplemented with 5% FCS and 1 mM of sodium butyrate.

9. Day 4: Collect 15 mL of the medium, add to a 50 mL Falcon tube, and store at 4 °C. Replace medium with 15 mL of RPMI supplemented with 5% FCS and 1 mM of sodium butyrate.

10. Day 5: Collect 15 mL of medium and combine with the 15 mL of media harvested on day 4 (*see* **Note 7**). Centrifuge Falcon tube at $400 \times g$ for 10 min and filter through 0.45 μm PVDF syringe filter to remove cell debris.

11. For concentration, use an ultracentrifuge such as Sorval Discovery 100SE centrifuge using an AH-629 swing rotor, with Beckman 36 mL pollyallomer conical tubes.

12. 30 mL of filtered virus supernatant is added to each tube and centrifugation was performed for 90 min at $20,000 \times g$ (*see* **Note 8**).

13. The supernatant was removed and the virus pellet was resuspended in 300 μL of PBS overnight at 4 °C and then stored at −80 °C until use (*see* **Note 9**).

3.2 Titer Determination

1. Day 0: Seed Jurkat cells at a density of 1×10^6 cells/mL in RPMI 1640 supplemented with 5% FCS and dispense 100 μL per well in a 96-well plate.

2. Day 0: Serial dilutions of the lentivirus are prepared at 1/100, 1/1000, 1/10,000, and 1/100,000.

3. Day 0: Neat and diluted lentivirus is added to well and cells are spun for 2 h at $860 \times g$ and then incubated at 37 °C for 24 h.

4. Day 1: Medium is replaced with fresh RPMI 1640 supplemented with 5 % FCS and incubated at 37 °C for 72 h.

5. Day 3: Cells are harvested and transferred to FACS tubes. The cells are resuspended in 300 μL of FACS wash buffer and incubated for 25 min at 4 °C with antibody to reporter gene (anti-CD271 for pCCL) (*see* **Note 10**).

6. The cells are washed in FACS wash buffer to remove any unbound antibody and the percentage of transgene (CD271 (ΔNGFR)-positive cells) is determined by flow cytometry.

3.3 Calculating Transduction Efficiency and Titer

1. The transduction efficiency is determined as the percentage positive CD271 (ΔNGFR) following transfection of 1×10^5 cells.

2. *Infectious titers*: Are specified as transducing units (TU)/mL and can be calculated using the formula titer = % CD271 expressing cells × number of cells (1×10^5) × dilution factor/mL of virus (inoculation factor).

3. *Multiplicities of infection (MOI)*: The MOI is described as the ratio between infectious particles and target cells and should be determined empirically. For example, to transduce primary human cells we use an MOI of 50.

3.4 Isolation of Peripheral Blood Mononuclear Cells

Blood should be collected in compliance with local ethical guidelines. Waste blood products should be disposed of in accordance with local rules.

1. Isolate 50 mL of blood into a 10 mL vacutainer tubes containing K2EDTA.

2. Centrifuge the blood at $400 \times g$ for 10 min and remove the plasma.

3. Transfer the blood into a 50 mL Falcon tube and dilute with HBSS to make the final volume up to 50 mL.

4. The blood/HBSS mixture is gently layered over two 50 mL Falcon tubes containing 20 mL of Lympholyte-H solution and centrifuged at $860 \times g$ for 30 min.

5. Remove the upper layer that contains the plasma and platelets and transfer the PBMC layer to a new 50 mL Falcon tube; wash twice with 40 mL of HBSS and centrifuge at $400 \times g$ for 5 min.

6. Resuspend the cells in RPMI medium and determine cell number and viability by trypan blue exclusion (*see* **Note 11**).

3.5 Isolation of Primary CD45RA+ T Cells

1. Add 40 μL of MACS buffer per 1×10^7 cells, add 10 μL of naïve CD4+ T cell biotin-antibody cocktail II per 1×10^7 cells, and incubate for 5 min at 4 °C s(*see* **Note 3**).

2. Add 30 µL of MACS buffer per 1×10^7 cells, add 20 µL of naïve CD4$^+$ T cell MicroBead cocktail II per 1×10^7 cells, and incubate for 10 min at 4 °C.

3. Place an LS column into a midiMACS separator and wash with 3 mL of MACS buffer.

4. Add the PBMCs containing antibody to the column and wash with 3 mL of MACS buffer.

5. Collect the flow-through containing unlabeled cells (*see* **Note 12**).

6. The cells were resuspended in X-VIVO 15 medium supplemented with 10% HS, IL-2 (100 ng/mL), and IL-7 (25 ng/mL) to a concentration of 1×10^6 cells/mL.

3.6 Transduction of CD45RA$^+$ T Cells

1. Day 1: Plate 1 mL of the CD4$^+$CD45RA$^+$ cells into a 12-well plate, add CD3/CD28 activation beads at a 1:1 bead:cell ratio, and then incubate for 24 h at 37 °C (*see* **Note 13**).

2. Day 2: Remove the cells from the 12-well plate and centrifuge at $400 \times g$ for 5 min.

3. Day 2: Resuspend the cells in IL-2 (100 ng/mL), IL-7 (25 ng/mL), and polybrene (6 µg/mL) and plate out in a fresh 12-well plate.

4. Add lentivirus at a multiplicity of infection (MOI) of 50 and centrifuge cells for 2 h at $400 \times g$ 37 °C (*see* **Note 14**).

5. Incubate the cells for a further 24 h at 37 °C and determine the level of transgene expression (*see* **Note 15**).

3.7 Evaluating the Transduction in Primary Human T Cells

1. The transduced T cells were divided into aliquots in FACS wash buffer and stained with antibody to reporter gene (anti-CD271 for pCCL). Incubation is performed at 4 °C for 25 min at concentrations indicated by the manufacturer.

2. The cells are washed once in FACS wash buffer and then incubated in FACS fix at 4 °C for 20 min (*see* **Note 16**).

3. The cells are washed once in FACS wash buffer and then resuspended in 300 µL of FACS wash buffer and transgene (CD127 expression) is evaluated by flow cytometric analysis.

4 Notes

1. The pH of this solution is critical to the successful formation of $CaPO_4$/DNA precipitates and therefore transfection efficiency. The optimal pH range is 7.05–7.12. To test the 2× HEPES-buffered saline, mix 250 µL of 2× HBS with 250 µL of $CaCl_2$ and vortex. An optimal solution develops a fine precipitate that is readily visible under a microscope.

2. It is important that the human serum used has been batch tested to ensure that it provides optimal conditions for the proliferation of the T cells.

3. It is important to follow the manufacturer's recommended incubation times precisely for the isolation of highly pure CD45RA$^+$ T cell populations.

4. To ensure that plasmids are endotoxin free we recommend that the vector plasmids are isolated using an EndoFree plasmid maxi kit.

5. Ensure that the DNA/HBS suspension is evenly dispersed across all of the cells in the flask.

6. Sodium butyrate was added to the medium to enhance the production of lentivirus.

7. Harvested lentivirus supernatant can be kept in the fridge for up to 1 week following final harvest with minimal effect on titer. Do not freeze prior to concentration as repeated freeze–thaw cycles can affect virion viability.

8. Ultracentrifugation at $20,000 \times g$ is a critical step for generation of high-titer lentivirus that is capable of transducing primary T cells to a high efficiency. Centrifugation using higher speeds can result in reduced virion viability.

9. During the first 4 h the pellet was dispersed by pipetting the PBS every half hour and then left in the fridge for the following 20 h. This step is to ensure that the maximum amount of lentivirus is recovered following concentration.

10. A common alternative reporter gene is green fluorescent protein (GFP) that can be detected in the FITC channel using flow cytometry. If the GFP signal is low then the signal can be amplified using an anti-GFP antibody.

11. Washing will remove the majority of platelets; however if there is high platelet contamination then centrifuge at $300 \times g$ for 15 min. If there is a high level of dead cell contamination then resuspend in 50 mL of HBSS and layer over two 25 mL of lympholyte-H.

12. The purity of naïve T cell subsets is routinely 90–98 %.

13. The cells can alternatively be activated using plate-bound anti-CD3 (5 µg/mL) and soluble anti-CD28 (1 µg/mL). However, optimal expression of the transgene is observed when T cells are activated with CD3/CD28 activation beads.

14. Centrifuging at 37 °C is favored; however if a heated centrifuge is unavailable then this step can be performed at room temperature.

15. Typically the transgene can be readily detectable following 24 h of culture; however further culture for 48 h may be needed to detect fluorescent transgenes, such as GFP.

16. Fixing the cells is required for increased biosafety when running the samples through the flow cytometer.

Acknowledgments

This work was supported by the Kennedy Trust for Rheumatology Research. We would like to acknowledge the intellectual contributions of Dr. B. Gregory and the late Prof. F. Brennan to these studies. We thank Prof. M. Levings for pCCL and Prof. D. Trono for pMD2.G and psPAX vectors.

References

1. Young LS, Searle PF, Onion D et al (2006) Viral gene therapy strategies: from basic science to clinical application. J Pathol 208:299–318

2. Biffi A, Naldini L (2005) Gene therapy of storage disorders by retroviral and lentiviral vectors. Hum Gene Ther 16:1133–1142

3. Geng X, Doitsh G, Yang Z et al (2014) Efficient delivery of lentiviral vectors into resting human CD4 T cells. Gene Ther 21:444–449

4. Verhoeyen E, Costa C, Cosset FL (2009) Lentiviral vector gene transfer into human T cells. Methods Mol Biol 506:97–114

5. Zack JA, Kim SG, Vatakis DN (2013) HIV restriction in quiescent CD4(+) T cells. Retrovirology 10:37

6. Naldini L, Blomer U, Gallay P et al (1996) In vivo gene delivery and stable transduction of nondividing cells by a lentiviral vector. Science 272:263–267

7. Dull T, Zufferey R, Kelly M et al (1998) A third-generation lentivirus vector with a conditional packaging system. J Virol 72:8463–8471

8. Cribbs AP, Kennedy A, Gregory B et al (2013) Simplified production and concentration of lentiviral vectors to achieve high transduction in primary human T cells. BMC Biotechnol 13:98

9. Swainson L, Mongellaz C, Adjali O et al (2008) Lentiviral transduction of immune cells. Methods Mol Biol 415:301–320

Chapter 8

Generating Transgenic Mice by Lentiviral Transduction of Spermatozoa Followed by In Vitro Fertilization and Embryo Transfer

Anil Chandrashekran, Colin Casimir, Nick Dibb, Carol Readhead, and Robert Winston

Abstract

Most transgenic technologies rely on the oocyte as a substrate for genetic modification. Transgenics animals are usually generated by the injection of the gene constructs (including lentiviruses encoding gene constructs or modified embryonic stem cells) into the pronucleus of a fertilized egg followed by the transfer of the injected embryos into the uterus of a foster mother. Male germ cells also have potential as templates for transgenic development. We have previously shown that mature sperm can be utilized as template for lentiviral transduction and as such used to generate transgenic mice efficiently with germ line capabilities. We provide here a detailed protocol that is relatively simple, to establish transgenic mice using lentivirally transduced spermatozoa. This protocol employs a well-established lentiviral gene delivery system (usual for somatic cells) delivering a variety of transgenes to be directly used with sperm, and the subsequent use of these modified sperm in in vitro fertilization studies and embryo transfer into foster female mice, for the establishment of transgenic mice.

Key words Lentiviral vectors, Spermatozoa, Transgenics, Germ line, Gene transfer, Pseudotyping, Transgenes

1 Introduction

The standard method for generating transgenic animals, i.e., animals incorporating foreign DNA, was developed by Gordon and Ruddle in 1980. This was done by microinjection of the gene of interest into the nucleus of a fertilized egg and the subsequent transfer of the injected embryos into a foster mother. About 0.1–1.0% of these injected eggs result in a transgenic animal [1]. This method is routine in mice as can be seen by the thousands of existing transgenic lines. In contrast, large transgenic animals are difficult to generate using this classic technique due to the inherent inefficiency of the technique, the small number of fertilized eggs

Maurizio Federico (ed.), *Lentiviral Vectors and Exosomes as Gene and Protein Delivery Tools*, Methods in Molecular Biology, vol. 1448, DOI 10.1007/978-1-4939-3753-0_8, © Springer Science+Business Media New York 2016

that can be harvested from large animals even after superovulation, and underdeveloped artificial reproductive technologies (ART) in many species.

Larger animals would be much more suitable than small animals to study the effects and treatment of most human diseases because of their greater similarity to humans in many aspects such as physiology, and also the size of their organs [2]. Now that transgenic animals with the potential for human xenotransplantation are being developed, larger animals, of a size comparable to man, will be required. Transgenic technology will allow that such donor animals will be immunocompatible with the human recipient. Consequently, generating large animals with current techniques is prohibitively expensive and remains technically challenging [3].

Alternative transgenic strategies have focused on transfecting male germ stem cells. Modifying the male germ line has a number of material advantages over the female, not least that male germ cells have much greater accessibility and numbers reducing the need for delicate micromanipulation. This is usually done by retrieval of male germ cells (that will subsequently become mature sperm) followed by in vitro genetic modification (retroviral transduction/transfection-electroporation) [4, 5] and subsequent transplantation of these modified immature germ cells into a suitably prepared recipient testis. It has also been shown that direct testicular injections/transduction in vivo (of suitable prepared or pre-pubescent testis) [6] can also generate transgenic animals following ART, with varying transgenic efficiencies albeit the associated technical complexity required (Winston and colleagues, unpublished observations). Mature spermatozoa can also be modified by direct incubation of foreign/naked DNA or RNA constructs [7], followed by ART to generate transgenic animals; however this method has low efficiency and poor levels of germ line gene transmission potential.

The ability to genetically modify somatic cells in culture for gene therapy or in whole organisms (transgenics) has been due to extensive research in disabling infectious viruses such as the Moloney murine leukaemia virus (MLV) and the human immunodeficiency virus (HIV/lentivirus), so that they become effective vector systems for gene delivery into host/target cells [8]. Reporter genes or the genetic payload such as short interfering RNAs [9, 10], cDNA, or micro RNA [11] can be engineered into these vectors. With the advent of gene editing strategies involving nucleases such as the CRSPR/Cas9 system, these protocols can easily be adapted within the retroviral vector payload as well commonly referred to as guide RNA (gRNA), thereby generating efficient gene knockout strategies. Commonly utilized promoters driving the reporter genes or genetic payload include phosphoglycerate kinase promoter (PGK), elongation factor 1 alpha promoters (EF-1), and cytomegalovirus promoter (CMV). The use of methylation-resistant promoters such as ubiquitous chromatin opening element promoter (lacking in enhancer activity) (UCOE) has been successfully utilized in gene transfer protocols while maintaining relative expression levels of reporter and increasing the safety profile of the vectors. The resulting self-inactivating lentiviral vectors can also be readily pseudotyped with diverse variety of viral envelope proteins, thus altering the natural tropism of the vectors for various cell types. The envelope most commonly utilized in lentiviral transduction protocols is the G-glycoprotein that originates from the vesicular stomatitis virus (VSV-G). VSV-G-pseudotyped lentiviral vectors have been shown to transduce a wide variety of somatic cells, and can be used to generate transgenic animals by microinjection into the perivitelline space of oocytes or of developing embryos, followed by transfer into pseudopregnant foster mothers.

We have recently shown that spermatozoa can be transduced with pseudotyped lentiviral vectors [12] and these transduced spermatozoa can be used to deliver a transgene (green fluorescent protein, GFP) to ovulated eggs for the efficient generation of transgenic mice with germ line capabilities [13]. As such we describe here a protocol that can be utilized with relative ease to obtain transgenic mice with germ line capabilities efficiently.

2   Materials

2.1   Lentivirus Preparation

2.1.1   Packaging Cells

1. 293T M-mbSCF [13–15].

2.1.2   Lentiviral Vector [16]

1. pgk-gfp-SIN18.
2. pgk-H2Bgfp-SIN18.
3. pgk-H2BCherry-SIN18.

2.1.3   Helper Construct [17]

1. pCMVΔ8.91.

2.1.4   Envelope Constructs [18]

1. pMD.VSV-G.

2.1.5   Reagents

1. Calcium phosphate transfection kit (Invitrogen).
2. Chloroquine (50 mM stock).
3. D10 (DMEM with glutamax and hepes, penicillin and streptomycin, and 10% heat-inactivated FCS).
4. Polybrene (chemically referred to as hexadimethrine bromide).
5. Chondroitin sulfate.

**2.2 Lentivirus
Infection
of Spermatozoa
and In Vitro Fertilization**

1. Four-well embryo culture plate.
2. Forceps.
3. Scissors.
4. 70 % Alcohol.
5. Sterile swabs.
6. 27 G Needle.
7. 1.5 ml Eppendorf tubes.
8. Krebs Ringer solution supplemented fresh with 0.2 mM calcium chloride, 3 mg/ml BSA, and 25 mM sodium bicarbonate.
9. Pregnant mare serum gonadotropin (PMSG).
10. Human chorionic gonadotropin (HCG).
11. Embryo/cell culture-tested mineral oil.
12. Human tubule fluid (HTF).
13. Sequential simplex optimization method (SOM).
14. Amino acid-supplemented (and higher Na^+ and K^+ concentration) SOM (AA-KSOM).
15. B6CBF1 female mice (19 to 21 days old).

**2.3 Analysis
of Transgenic Animals**

1. Mouse tail DNA extraction kit.
2. PCR master mix.
3. GFP Primers.
    (a) GFP-F 5′-AGCTGACCCTGAAGTTCATCTG-3′.
    (b) GFP-R 5′-GACGTTGTGGCTGTTGTAGTTGTA-3′.
4. 4 % Paraformaldehyde.
5. Optimum cutting temperature (OCT) compound.

3   Methods

**3.1 Lentiviral Vector
Preparation**

1. Day 1 (PM): Seed 1.5×10^6 packaging cells (in D10) per 10 cm tissue culture plate (total volume of 15 ml).
2. Day 2 (AM): Aspirate media from above and replenish with 12 ml of fresh D10.
3. Day 2 (PM): Perform transfection. The DNA ratio used is as follows: (3 Lenti vector:2 Packaging construct:1 VSV-G). So 15 µg:10 µg:5 µg, respectively.
    • Prepare DNA mixtures + water + $CaCl_2$ to a total of 500 µl.
    • Add dropwise (a) to 500 µl 2 × HBS while aspirating bubbles (using a 1 ml pipette).
    • Incubate at room temperature for 30 min.
    • Add chloroquine to reach a final concentration of 25 µM 10 cm plate-packaging cells (*see* **Notes 1** and **2**).

- Add dropwise to (d) calcium phosphate-DNA mixture (b).
- Incubate overnight at 37 °C, 5 % CO_2.

4. Day 3 (AM): about 18 h post-transfection. Remove media containing transfection mixture.

5. Wash plates 2× D10.

6. Add 8 ml D10 and incubate for 24 h.

7. Day 4: Harvest supernatant containing viral vectors, spin supernatant at $450 \times g$ for 5 min, filter the supernatant using a 0.45 μ sterile disposable filter, and store at −80 °C.

8. Day 5: Repeat **steps 5** and **6** and recollect supernatant (*see* **Note 3**).

3.2 Concentration and Cleanup of Lentivectors [19]

1. Add 60 μl (20 mg/ml stock) polybrene, quickly followed by 60 μl (20 mg/ml stock) chondroitin sulfate, to the viral supernatant collected from above and vortex briefly.

2. Incubate the sample at 37 °C in CO_2 incubator for 20 min.

3. Transfer the sample to a 15 ml tubes and centrifuge at $10,000 \times g$, RT, for 20 min.

4. A small visible pellet should form at the bottom of the tube. Carefully discard the supernatant and suspend the pellet in 1.4 ml (usually 100th the original volume of supernatant harvested) fresh IVF media, by gently pipetting up and down until the pellet is dissolved.

5. Aliquot 50 μl into fresh cryo tubes.

6. Store tubes at −80 °C.

3.3 Titrering for GFP Expression-Infectious Particles/ml

1. Plate 5×10^4 293T cells/well in a 24-well plate.

2. Day 1: Make a serial dilution of the concentrated virus (1:1, 1:10, 1:100, 1:1000) in D10.

3. Use 20 μl of the above viral dilution in a total volume of 1 ml containing 8 μg/ml polybrene, and incubate the cells at 37 °C, in CO_2, incubator for at least 12 h.

4. Day 2: Remove the supernatant, replace with fresh media, and incubate for another 48 h.

5. Day 4 : FACS analyze the cells for GFP expression:

$$\text{Titre}\,(\text{TU}/\text{ml}) = (F \times \text{Co}/V) \times D$$

F: Frequency of GFP-positive cells.

Co: Total number of target cell infected (10^4).

V: Volume of the inoculum (20 μl).

D: Viral dilution factor.

Take average of titer values at vector dilution corresponding to 20% of GFP-positive cells. Twenty microliters of concentrated supernatant (1:1) tends to give about 80–95% EGFP+ cells; that is why it is necessary to dilute the concentrated stock.

Example: Titer$= (0.2(20\%\ \text{GFP+ cells}) \times 50,000/0.02) \times 100$ (1:100 dilution):

$$\text{Titre} = 5 \times 10^7 \text{ TU}/\text{ml} = 5 \times 10^4 \text{ TU}/.1.$$

3.4 Lentiviral Transduction of Spermatozoa and In Vitro Fertilization

1. Sacrifice an adult male mouse of proven fertility (used as a stud but not older than 1 year) by cervical dislocation (*see* **Note 4**).

2. Spray the abdomen thoroughly with 70% alcohol.

3. Make a small incision in the inguinal region and fat pad carefully pulled out carrying with it the testis.

4. Excise the cauda epididymis and proximal end of the vas deferens (of both sides) and place it in one well of a four-well embryo culture plate containing 200 µl Krebs ringer solution supplemented fresh with 0.2 mM calcium chloride, 3 mg/ml BSA, and 25 mM sodium bicarbonate.

5. Use a 27 G needle to puncture various parts of the epididymis and along the vas deferens to allow sperm to swim out.

6. Add 200 µl of lentiviral vector preparation to the plate as well and incubate for 0–3 h at 32 °C and 5% CO_2 in atmosphere.

7. Perform control experiments in the same way except that lentiviral vector preparation should be omitted and replaced with a further 200 µl Krebs ringer solution.

8. Centrifuge control and transduced swim up population of sperm at $300 \times g$ for 5 min, discard the supernatant, wash it once in Krebs ringer solution, centrifuge again at $300 \times g$ for 5 min, and discard the supernatant. Suspend the sperm pellet in 100 µl fresh Krebs ringer solution.

9. Transduced sperm should then either FACS analyzed (3-h incubation) or used in IVF and IVF-embryo transfer studies (1-h virus-sperm incubation) (*see* **Note 5**).

3.5 In Vitro Fertilization

1. Day 1: Inject 0.1 U PMSG into 20 4-week-old female B6CBF1 per animal usually at 9 pm.

2. Day 3: Inject 0.1 U HCG per animal into day 1-injected animals (48 h post-PMSG,) usually at 8.30 pm.

3. Dish setup (Fig. 1): Fresh sperm: 35 mm dish for each strain with 1 ml of IVF media (HTF). Prepare dishes:

   • Fertilization dishes, 35 mm: one 500 µl drop of HTF media.

   • Wash dish, 60 mm: five 250 µl drops of HTF media.

   • Culture dish, 60 mm: five 250 µl drops of AA KSOM media.

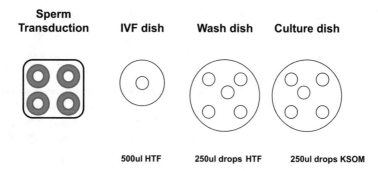

Fig. 1 In vitro fertilization dish setup

4. Cover with mineral oil and equilibrate with gas mixture (5 % CO_2, 5 % O_2, balance N_2). Insert 1 ml glass-pipette into oil container and let bubble for 30–40 s.

5. Place the plates in 37 °C incubator chamber.

6. Day 4: In vitro fertilization (IVF) (*see* **Note 6**).

   - Prepare one oocyte collection dish per IVF (2 ml HTF in small petri dish).

   - Cover dish and place in heated chamber at 37 °C.

   - Collect oocytes in separate wash dishes previously prepared.

   - Add transduced sperm (above) to IVF drops using a wide-mouth pipette tip.

   - Pipette oocytes into IVF drops containing transduced sperm (*see* **Note 7**).

   - Place IVF dishes into incubator for 4–5 h, depending on mobility of sperm.

   - Four to five hours later, wash oocytes to remove excess sperm.

   - Place putative embryos in a separate drop of HTF.

   - Place dishes in incubator.

   - Two-cell developing embryos the following day can either be imaged daily (but cultured in AA-KSOM) or transferred into pseudopregnant females for the generation of transgenic animals (below).

7. Day 5: Transfer embryos.

   - Pick up embryos from wash dishes.

   - Place into another clean KSOM drop.

   - Score resulting two-cell embryos and non-developed/uncleaved eggs.

   - Surgically transfer 10–15 two-cell embryos into the fallopian tubes of each pseudopregnant female.

   - Monitor pregnancies.

3.6 Analysis of Transgenic Animals

3.6.1 PCR Analysis of GFP Transgene

- Extract DNA from tail biopsies of 3-week-old founders or placenta from E12.5 embryos (Fig. 2).

- Use 100 ng DNA as template for PCR detection of the GFP reporter transgene encoded within the lentiviral vector.

- The cycling conditions are as follows: an initial denaturation step at 94 °C for 2 min, followed by 34 cycles at 94 °C for 1 min, 59 °C for 1 min, and 72 °C for 1 min. Carry out a final cycle with the extension step of 72 °C extended to 10 min.

- Resolve 20 % of PCR products on a 2 % agarose gel. A 328 bp product indicates the successfully amplified GFP DNA. HPRT gene can be used as a housekeeping gene for PCR and DNA quality (850 bp).

3.6.2 Inverse PCR (IV-PCR), Integration Analysis

- Digest 5 μg of genomic DNA should be digested with Eco R1 for 4 h.

- Purify the digested products using commercially available kits.

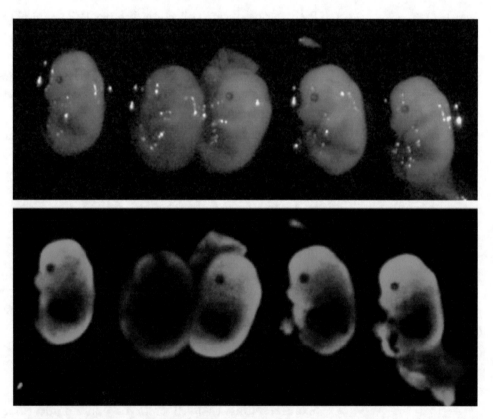

Fig. 2 Transgenic (and one non-transgenic) embryos from E12 stage from one IVF derived pregnancy. Imaging performed on a gel documentation system normally used to image agarose gel electrophoresis. *Top panel:* Transmitted light turned on. *Bottom panel:* Transmitted light Off and UV light on

- Self-ligate the eluted DNA using ligase enzyme at 4 °C overnight.

  - PCR-amplify the resulting circular DNA using primers: LTR-4 (AGTAGTGTGTGCCCGTCTGT) and LTR-8 (TGAGGCTTAAGCAGTGGGTTC).

  - Resolve the PCR products on a 2 % agarose gel.

  - Excise PCR products from the gel and purified them.

  - Clone purified PCR products into a PCR Cloning-Sequencing vector.

  - Sequence the cloning plasmid constructs containing the PCR products.

  - Align the sequences obtained (following detection of both LTR primer sequences and the Eco R1 site) and analyze them for integration spots using BLAST alignment software.

  - Carry out stringency of analysis at >90 %.

3.6.3 Confocal Microscopy and Histology

IVF Optimization Experiment

- Live-image two-cell embryos each day until the blastocyst stage.

- Transfer embryos to a 15 µl drop of KSOM in a two-well chamber slide (Tissue Tek) and cover the drop with mineral oil.

- Image the embryos on a Zeiss 510 inverted confocal microscope using a 40× W lens, DIC, and the 488 nm (GFP) and 561 nm (Cherry) lasers. In some cases Z stacks were taken of the embryos.

- Fit the microscope with an incubation chamber and heat stage so that the embryos are kept at 37 °C, 5 % CO_2, in atmosphere while they were being imaged.

- Keep the embryos in their original KSOM culture drops in the incubator in between imaging.

Histology-Confocal Microscopy

- Fix whole embryos or dissected tissues in 4 % PFA overnight at 4 °C.

- Wash fixed tissue three times in 10 % sucrose in phosphate-buffered saline buffer pH 7.4 (PBS) for 1 h each at 4 °C.

- Immerse tissue in 30 % sucrose until the tissue no longer floats (usually overnight).

- Embed the tissue in OCT and frozen slowly at –20 °C in an insulated box.

- Make 8 µm cryosections using a microtome and place them on a clean glass slide. Mount these sections with fluorophore mounting medium and image them on a Zeiss 510 confocal microscope at 488 nm (GFP expression).

Histology-Light Microscopy

- Analyze images using Imaris (Bitplane).
- Fix tissue biopsy material in 4 % PFA overnight at 4 °C.
- Process fixed tissue in an automated tissue processor.
- Embed processed tissue in paraffin.
- Obtain 4–8 micro thick tissue sections using a microtome and place on a clean glass slide.
- Deparaffinize tissue sections using histoclear.
- Dehydrate deparaffinized tissue sections in a series of ethanol.
- Carry out antigen retrieval with citrate buffer by microwaving section at high temperature for 20 min.
- Carry out primary antibody to GFP overnight at 4 °C or 1 h in a humidified chamber at 37 °C.
- Wash slides at least three times in PBS at room temperature.
- Detect the antibody staining using a secondary HRP-conjugated rabbit antibody, Histofine Simple Stain Mouse Max PO.
- Wash again slides thoroughly three times at room temperature.
- Detect the reaction by DAB and counterstain sections with hematoxylin according to the manufacturer's instruction.

4 Notes

1. The confluence of packaging cells on the day of transfection, following seeding of these cells, should not exceed 60 %. This is particularly important as the cells need to have time and space to grow. This is in contrast to using lipid-based transfections. As such, it may be useful to have duplicates/triplicates of plates.

2. Chloroquine prevents acidification of endosomes and as such reduces lysosomal degradation of calcium chloride-DNA transfection complex. However, toxicity to packaging cells has been observed, so the transfection mixture and exposure to chloroquine should not exceed 18 h. In addition, packaging cells must be washed at least twice in complete media to remove the transfection complex, prior to viral harvest.

3. Unpurified filtered viral laden supernatants may be frozen at –80 °C, thawed when convenient, pooled, and precipitated. This may be best practise as the precipitation steps may take the better part of the day (including labeling, aliquoting).

4. This is crucial step/criteria to ensure that the sperm are of good quality. These mice should not be too old (1 year maximum) and overweight either and have proven ability to sire offspring—usually previously used as studs. Sperm motility should be visually inspected using a dissecting microscope.

5. A critical parameter here is that for transfer into pseudopregnant mothers, sperm and virus should be exactly for 60 min and no longer as IVF efficiencies tend to decrease significantly with prolonged viral-sperm exposure. Dispose all tips and material in contact with viral supernatants in strong detergent solution followed by autoclaving according to GM rules.

6. This step should ideally be done no longer than 12 h following HCG injections. Timing is crucial in obtaining good-quality eggs. As such planning of sperm transduction should be anticipated. This usually means very early start of experiments.

7. When using a mouth pipetting device, a 0.2 μM filter should be fitted between the pipette and rubber tubing. Alternately, this step is not necessary if using specialized pipettes used in human IVF.

References

1. Gordon JW, Ruddle FH (1982) Germ line transmission in transgenic mice. Prog Clin Biol Res 85(Pt B):111–124

2. Paris MC, Snow M, Cox SL, Shaw JM (2004) Xenotransplantation: a tool for reproductive biology and animal conservation? Theriogenology 61:277–291

3. Prather RS (2007) Targeted genetic modification: xenotransplantation and beyond. Cloning Stem Cells 9:17–20

4. Nagano M, Brinster CJ, Orwig KE et al (2001) Transgenic mice produced by retroviral transduction of male germ-line stem cells. Proc Natl Acad Sci U S A 98:13090–13095

5. Dhup S, Majumdar SS (2008) Transgenesis via permanent integration of genes in repopulating spermatogonial cells in vivo. Nat Methods 5:601–603

6. Sehgal L, Thorat R, Khapare N et al (2011) Lentiviral mediated transgenesis by in vivo manipulation of spermatogonial stem cells. PLoS One 6:e21975

7. Lavitrano M, Busnelli M, Cerrito MG et al (2006) Sperm-mediated gene transfer. Reprod Fertil Dev 18:19–23

8. Howe SJ, Chandrashekran A (2012) Vector systems for prenatal gene therapy: principles of retrovirus vector design and production. Methods Mol Biol 891:85–107. doi:10.1007/978-1-61779-873-3_5

9. Lavial F, Bessonnard S, Ohnishi Y et al (2012) Bmi1 facilitates primitive endoderm formation by stabilizing Gata6 during early mouse development. Genes Dev 26:1445–1458. doi:10.1101/gad.188193.112, gad.188193.112 [pii]

10. Witney TH, Carroll L, Alam IS et al (2014) A novel radiotracer to image glycogen metabolism in tumors by positron emission tomography. Cancer Res 74:1319–1328. doi:10.1158/0008-5472.CAN-13-2768, 74/5/1319 [pii]

11. Tan GC, Chan E, Molnar A et al (2014) 5′ isomiR variation is of functional and evolutionary importance. Nucleic Acids Res 42:9424–9435. doi:10.1093/nar/gku656, gku656 [pii]

12. Chandrashekran A, Isa I, Dudhia J, Thrasher AJ et al (2014) Lentiviral vector transduction of spermatozoa as a tool for the study of early development. FEBS Open Bio 4:266–275. doi:10.1016/j.fob.2014.02.008, S2211-5463(14)00019-9 [pii]

13. Chandrashekran A, Sarkar R, Thrasher A et al (2014) Efficient generation of transgenic mice by lentivirus-mediated modification of spermatozoa. FASEB J 28:569–576. doi:10.1096/fj.13-233999, fj.13-233999 [pii]

14. Chandrashekran A, Gordon MY, Casimir C (2004) Targeted retroviral transduction of c-kit + hematopoietic cells using novel ligand display technology. Blood 104:2697–2703

15. Chandrashekran A, Gordon MY, Darling D, Farzaneh F, Casimir C (2004) Growth factor displayed on the surface of retroviral particles without manipulation of envelope proteins is biologically active and can enhance transduction. J Gene Med 6:1189–1196

16. Zufferey R, Dull T, Mandel RJ et al (1998) Self-inactivating lentivirus vector for safe and efficient in vivo gene delivery. J Virol 72: 9873–9880

17. Ailles LE, Naldini L (2002) HIV-1-derived lentiviral vectors. Curr Top Microbiol Immunol 261:31–52

18. Pan D, Gunther R, Duan W et al (2002) Biodistribution and toxicity studies of VSVG-pseudotyped lentiviral vector after intravenous administration in mice with the observation of in vivo transduction of bone marrow. Mol Ther 6:19–29

19. Landazuri N, Le Doux JM (2006) Complexation with chondroitin sulfate C and Polybrene rapidly purifies retrovirus from inhibitors of transduction and substantially enhances gene transfer. Biotechnol Bioeng 93:146–158

Chapter 9

The LAM-PCR Method to Sequence LV Integration Sites

Wei Wang, Cynthia C. Bartholomae, Richard Gabriel, Annette Deichmann, and Manfred Schmidt

Abstract

Integrating viral gene transfer vectors are commonly used gene delivery tools in clinical gene therapy trials providing stable integration and continuous gene expression of the transgene in the treated host cell. However, integration of the reverse-transcribed vector DNA into the host genome is a potentially mutagenic event that may directly contribute to unwanted side effects. A comprehensive and accurate analysis of the integration site (IS) repertoire is indispensable to study clonality in transduced cells obtained from patients undergoing gene therapy and to identify potential in vivo selection of affected cell clones. To date, next-generation sequencing (NGS) of vector-genome junctions allows sophisticated studies on the integration repertoire in vitro and in vivo. We have explored the use of the Illumina MiSeq Personal Sequencer platform to sequence vector ISs amplified by non-restrictive linear amplification-mediated PCR (nrLAM-PCR) and LAM-PCR. MiSeq-based high-quality IS sequence retrieval is accomplished by the introduction of a double-barcode strategy that substantially minimizes the frequency of IS sequence collisions compared to the conventionally used single-barcode protocol. Here, we present an updated protocol of (nr)LAM-PCR for the analysis of lentiviral IS using a double-barcode system and followed by deep sequencing using the MiSeq device.

Key words Gene therapy, Lentiviral vector, (nr)LAM-PCR, Clonality, Integration sites, Safety, Next-generation sequencing (NGS), Double-barcoding strategy

1 Introduction

Gene therapy using integrating vector systems has been successfully applied for the treatment of monogenetic diseases in several clinical trials [1, 2]. The occurrence of severe adverse event in few clinical trials using gamma-retroviral vectors due to vector-induced overexpression of nearby cellular proto-oncogenes highlighted the necessity to comprehensively analyze the integration site (IS) repertoire of gene therapy-treated patients [3–6]. Concomitantly, investigators focused on the development of new vector systems supposed to offer advantageous biosafety features. These factors

Maurizio Federico (ed.), *Lentiviral Vectors and Exosomes as Gene and Protein Delivery Tools*, Methods in Molecular Biology, vol. 1448, DOI 10.1007/978-1-4939-3753-0_9, © Springer Science+Business Media New York 2016

have led to the broad exchange of full long terminal repeat (LTR)-driven gamma-retroviral vectors by self-inactivating LTR lentiviral vectors in translational and clinical studies [7–9].

To identify IS in gene therapy-treated patients and/or to study integration profiles of different vector systems various PCR-based technologies are available. Among these, numerous variants of linker-mediated (LM)-PCR [10] and linear amplification-mediated (LAM)-PCR [11] are currently the most widely used methods. The resulting PCR amplicons can be sequenced to localize the vector ISs by aligning the individually trimmed sequence reads to the host genome. The development of next-generation sequencing technologies enabled researchers to sequence numerous thousands to millions sequences of individual PCR amplicons. To date, the MiSeq sequencing technology provides much higher sequence read numbers (up to 15 million) compared to Sanger sequencing (shotgun 96 reads) or 454 pyrosequencing technology (up to 1 million reads) [12], thus enabling a more profound representation of the IS repertoire. However, the huge increase in individual sequences bares an increased risk to detect false-positive ISs, i.e., contaminating IS which are shared between different samples.

Given the large size of the mammalian genome it is widely accepted that the likelihood to identify identical IS in individually transduced samples is close to zero. Thus, the same IS detected in multiple samples that are independent from the initially transduced target cell population (e.g., samples derived from different patients) have to be considered as collisions and to be removed from further analysis. To minimize the frequency of IS sequence collisions, the use of a double-barcoding strategy is indispensable. For (nr)LAM-PCR, we added the first barcode during ligation of the linker sequence (linker barcode) prior to any exponential amplification. The second barcode was introduced during preparation of LAM-PCR amplicons for sequencing by the MiSeq system (vector barcode). For downstream analyses only sequences that matched the unique combination of linker barcode and vector barcode are considered. Our data revealed that deep sequencing of LAM-PCR amplicons by this double-barcoding strategy designed for the MiSeq device is feasible and reaches high-quality accurate IS sequence retrieval.

2　Materials

2.1　DNA Extraction and Quantification

1. DNA Isolation Kit for Cells and Tissues/Mammalian Blood (Roche Diagnostics, Germany).

2. PCR grade water.

3. Qubit 2.0 Fluorometer and Qubit dsDNA Assay Kit (Life Technologies, USA).

2.2 Linear PCR

1. Taq DNA Polymerase (Genaxxon Bioscience, Germany).
2. 10× PCR buffer (Qiagen, Germany).
3. dNTPs (Genaxxon Bioscience, Germany).
4. PCR grade water.
5. Human Genomic DNA (Negative Control, Roche Diagnostics, Germany).
6. Linear PCR Primers (Eurofins MWG Biotech, Germany).
   LV3LTR1bio: (B) 5′-AGCTTGCCTTGAGTGCTTCA-3′.
   (B): This primer is biotinylated at the 5′-end.

2.3 Magnetic Capture

1. Dynabeads M-280 Streptavidin (Life Technologies, USA).
2. Magnetic separation units for 1.5 ml tubes and 96-well plate (Life Technologies, USA).
3. Phosphate-buffered saline (PBS, pH 7.4).
4. Bovine serum albumin.
5. Lithium chloride.
6. 3 M/6 M Lithium chloride (LiCl) solution: Dissolve 6.36 g (3 M) or 12.72 g (6 M) of LiCl in 0.5 ml 1 M Tris–HCl (pH 7.5) and 0.1 ml 0.5 M EDTA (pH 8.0) and adjust the volume with PCR grade water to 50 ml. Filtrate the solution using a 0.45 μm filter. Solutions can be stored at room temperature for several months.
7. PBS/0.1 % BSA: Dissolve 1 g of BSA in 1 L PBS, and aliquot into 1 ml sterile microfuge tube. Solution can be stored at −20 °C for up to 3 months.

2.4 Linker Cassette Construction

1. 250 mM Tris–HCl, pH 7.5.
2. 100 μM MaCl$_2$.
3. Barcoded oligonucleotides (Eurofins MWG Biotech, Germany).
   Oligo1: 5′-GACCCGGGAGATCTGAATTCAGTGGCACA GCAGTTAGG(N)$_{12bp}$CTA-3′.
   Oligo2: 5′-TATAG(N)$_{12bp}$CCTAACTGCTGTGCCACTGA ATTCAGATC-3′.
   (N)$_{12bp}$: Barcode composed by 12 random nucleotides.
4. Microcon-30 (Millipore, USA).

2.5 DNA Double-Strand Synthesis (Hexanucleotide Priming)

1. Klenow Polymerase (Roche Diagnostics, Germany).
2. Hexanucleotide mixture (Roche Diagnostics, Germany).

2.6 Restriction Digest

1. Enzyme MluCI and MseI. (NEB, Germany).

2.7 Ligation of Linker Cassette

1. Fast-link DNA ligation Kit (Epicentre Biotechnologies, USA).

2.8 Denaturation

1. 1 N NaOH.

2.9 Ligation of Single-Stranded Oligonucleotide

1. 10× Ligation buffer (Biozym, Germany).
2. Single-stranded oligonucleotide (Eurofins MWG Biotech, Germany).

   OligonrLAM: 5′-TAG(N)$_{12bp}$CCTAACTGCTGTGCCACT GAATTCAGATCTCCCGGGT-3′.

   (N)$_{12bp}$: Barcode composed by 12 random nucleotides.

   Modifications: Phosphate modification at the 5′-end and dideoxynucleotide modification at the 3′-end.
3. Mangan chloride MnCl$_2$.
4. CircLigase ssDNA Ligase (Biozym, Germany).

2.10 Exponential PCRs

1. Taq DNA polymerase.
2. dNTPs.
3. Primers (Eurofins MWG Biotech, Germany).

   First exponential PCR:

   LV3LTR2bio: (B) 5′-AGTAGTGTGTGCCCGTCTGT-3′.

   LCI: 5′-GACCCGGGAGATCTGAATTC-3′.

   (B): This primer is biotinylated at the 5′-end.

   Second exponential PCR:

   LV3LTR3: 5′-GTGTGACTCTGGTAACTAGAG-3′.

   LCII: 5′-GATCTGAATTCAGTGGCACAG-3′.

2.11 Visualization of the (nr)LAM-PCR Product with Spreadex High-Resolution Gel- Electrophoresis

1. Spreadex high-resolution agarose gel. Serva, Germany
2. Gel electrophoresis apparatus.
3. 40× TAE buffer.
4. 5× Blue run loading buffer.
5. Ethidium bromide.
6. 100 bp DNA ladder.

2.12 Sample Preparation for Miseq Platform

1. Agencout AMPure XP Beads (Beckman Coulter, USA).
2. Absolute ethanol.
3. Taq DNA polymerase.
4. dNTPs.

5. Primers (Eurofins MWG Biotech, Germany).
MegaLinker: 5′-GCCTTGCCAGCCCGCTCAGAGTGGCACA
GCAGTTAGG-3′.
BarcodedMega: 5′-GCCTCCCTCGCGCCATCAG(N)$_{10bp}$ACGA
GTTTTAATGACTCCAAC-3′.
(N)$_{10bp}$: Barcode composed by ten random nucleotides.

6. Agilent Tapstation/Bioanalyzer 2100.

7. Agilent High Sensitivity DNA kit.

3 Methods

3.1 DNA Extraction and Quantification

The procedure described here starts with the analysis of extracted DNA. A comparison of common DNA extraction procedures (organic, anion-exchange, or silica-based methods) did not reveal any differences on the qualitative outcome of the LAM-PCR technique. DNA samples extracted using commercial kits have consistently provided high-quality results, because the associated reagents have been subjected to quality control before use and are not likely to introduce problems. High-quality analytes ensure the best and most robust performance of following procedures and can provide reliable results. Perform DNA extraction and any following step of sample processing, e.g., dilution and quantification, in a dedicated hood for molecular biology in order to avoid any contamination.

3.2 Linear PCR

The first step of LAM-PCR is a linear amplification of the vector-genome junctions, accomplished with a 5′-biotinylated vector-specific primer(s) hybridizing to the U3- and/or U5 region of the vector long terminal repeat (LTR). The primer sequences are given in Subheading 2.2.

1. Mix the following components in a sterile nuclease-free PCR tube:

   Input 100–500 ng genomic DNA.

   1.67 nM 5′ Biotinylated primer.

   10× PCR buffer.

   200 μM dNTPs each.

   0.5 μl (2.5 U) Taq polymerase.

   Fill the reaction up with PCR grade water to a final volume of 50 μl.

2. Mix by pipetting followed by a quick spin to collect all liquid from the sides of the tube.

3. Place the PCR tube in a thermocycler, with the heated lid set to 105 °C, and run the following program:

$$2\text{min @ 95 °C Initial denaturation}$$

$$\left.\begin{array}{l} 45\text{s @ 95 °C Denaturation} \\ 45\text{s @ 60 °C Annealing} \\ 60\text{s @ 72°C Extension} \end{array}\right\} 50 \text{ cycles}$$

$$5\text{min @ 72°C Final extension}$$

$$\text{Hold @ 4°C}$$

4. After completion of the PCR add another 0.5 μl (2.5 U) Taq polymerase to each PCR reaction and repeat the 50-cycle PCR.

3.3 Magnetic Capture (See Note 1)

The magnetic capture allows enriching the amplified linear products through biotin-streptavidin binding.

1. Expose 20 μl magnetic beads to a magnetic separation unit (MSU). Incubate for 5 min at room temperature until the solution becomes clear.

2. Carefully remove and discard the supernatant, remove the tube from the MSU, and resuspend the magnetic beads with 40 μl PBS/0.1 % BSA.

3. Wash the magnetic beads again with 40 μl PBS/0.1 % BSA and carefully remove and discard the supernatant while the tube is on the MSU.

4. Remove the tube from the MSU, resuspend the magnetic beads with 20 μl 3 M lithium chloride solution (*see* **Note 2**), and carefully remove and discard the supernatant while the tube is on the MSU.

5. Remove the tube from the MSU, and resuspend the magnetic beads with 50 μl 6 M lithium chloride solution.

6. Add 50 μl of prepared magnetic beads to the linear PCR product (1:1 ratio, *see* **Note 3**).

7. Incubate the DNA/bead complexes on a horizontal shaker at 300 rpm overnight at room temperature (*see* **Note 4**).

3.4 Generation of a Linker Cassette

The oligonucleotide sequences are given in Subheading 2.4.

1. Mix the following components in a sterile microfuge tube:

40 μl 100 pmol/μl Oligonucleotide oligo1.

40 μl 100 pmol/μl Oligonucleotide oligo2.

110 μl 250 mM Tris–HCl (pH 7.5).

10 μl 100 mM $MgCl_2$.

2. Mix by pipetting followed by a quick spin to collect all liquid from the sides of the tube.

3. Incubate in a thermal heat block for 5 min at 95 °C.

4. Switch the heat block off and let the sample cool down slowly overnight within the heat block.

5. Add 300 μl of PCR grade water into the tube and transfer the sample on a Microcon-30 column.

6. Centrifuge the sample for 10 min at room temperature and $14,000 \times g$.

7. Place the column reversed onto a fresh tube and centrifuge the sample for 2 min at room temperature and $1000 \times g$.

8. Fill the concentrated sample up with distilled water to a final volume of 80 μl.

9. Aliquot the linker cassette and store it at −20 °C (*see* **Note 5**).

3.5 Hexanucleotide Priming

1. Prepare hexanucleotide priming mixture in a sterile microfuge tube:

   1× Concentrated hexanucleotide mixture.

   200 μM dNTPs each.

   1 U Klenow polymerase.

   Fill the mixture up with PCR grade water to a final volume of 10 μl.

2. Mix by pipetting followed by a quick spin to collect all liquid from the sides of the tube.

3. Expose the DNA/bead complexes on the MSU for 60 s after overnight incubation.

4. Remove and discard the supernatant while the tube is on the MSU. Be careful not to disturb the beads that contain the DNA targets.

5. Wash the magnetic beads with 100 μl PCR grade water, and carefully remove and discard the supernatant while the tube is on the MSU.

6. Remove the tube from the MSU, and resuspend the magnetic beads with 10 μl premade hexanucleotide mixture.

7. Incubate in a thermal cycler for exactly 1 h at 37 °C.

8. Add 90 μl of PCR grade water into the reaction, and expose the mixture on the MSU for 60 s.

9. Remove and discard the supernatant while the tube is on the MSU, and wash the magnetic beads with 100 μl PCR grade water.

3.6 Restriction Digest (See Note 6)

1. Prepare restriction digest mixture in a sterile microfuge tube:

   1 μl 10× Restriction buffer.

   2 U MseI.

   Fill the reaction mixture up with PCR grade water to a final volume of 10 μl.

2. Mix by pipetting followed by a quick spin to collect all liquid from the sides of the tube.

3. Carefully remove and discard the supernatant while the tube is on the MSU, remove the tube from the MSU, and resuspend the magnetic beads with 10 µl premade restriction digest mixture.

4. Incubate in a thermal cycler for exactly 1 h at temperature recommended by the manufacturer (*see* **Note 7**).

5. Add 90 µl of PCR grade water into the reaction, and expose the mixture on the MSU for 60 s.

6. Remove and discard the supernatant while the tube is on the MSU, and wash the magnetic beads with 100 µl PCR grade water.

3.7 Linker Cassette Ligation

1. Prepare ligation mixture in a sterile microfuge tube:

   2 µl of restriction enzyme linker cassette.

   1× Concentrated fast-link ligation buffer.

   10 mM ATP.

   2 U Fast-link ligase.

   Fill the reaction mixture up with PCR grade water to a final volume of 10 µl.

2. Mix by pipetting followed by a quick spin to collect all liquid from the sides of the tube.

3. Carefully remove and discard the supernatant while the tube is on the MSU, remove the tube from the MSU, and resuspend the magnetic beads with 10 µl premade ligation mixture.

4. Incubate for 5 min at room temperature.

5. Add 90 µl of PCR grade water into the reaction, and expose the mixture on the MSU for 60 s.

6. Remove and discard the supernatant while the tube is on the MSU, and wash the magnetic beads with 100 µl PCR grade water.

3.8 Alkaline Denaturation

1. Prepare 1 ml of 0.1 N NaOH in a sterile microfuge tube:

   PCR grade water (900 µl).

   Stock 1.0 N NaOH (100 µl).

   Invert the tube several times to mix.

2. Carefully remove and discard the supernatant while the tube is on the MSU, remove the tube from the MSU, and resuspend the magnetic beads with 5 µl freshly prepared 0.1 N NaOH solution.

3. Incubate the magnetic beads at room temperature on a shaker (300 rpm) for 10 min.

4. Expose the denatured sample on the MSU for 60 s, and collect the supernatant into a fresh microfuge tube (*see* **Note 8**).

3.9 Ligation of a Single-Stranded Oligonucleotide (See Note 9)

This step leads to the ligation of a single-stranded oligonucleotide to the unknown part of the DNA amplicons. As both ends after the ligation consist of known sequences, a subsequent exponential amplification of the PCR products is then possible. The sequence of the oligonucleotide and the modifications are shown in Subheading 2.9.

1. Prepare ligation mixture in a sterile microfuge tube:

   1 μl 10× Ligation buffer.

   1 μl OligonrLAM (10 pmol/μl).

   0.5 μl $MnCl_2$ (10 mM).

   0.5 μl ATP (10 mM).

   0.5 μl Circligase ssDNA ligase.

   Fill the reaction mixture up with PCR grade water to a final volume of 10 μl.

2. Mix by pipetting followed by a quick spin to collect all liquid from the sides of the tube.

3. Expose the DNA/bead complex (Subheading 3.3, **step 7**) to the MSU, and incubate for 5 min at room temperature until the solution becomes clear.

4. Carefully remove and discard the supernatant, remove the tube from the MSU, and resuspend the magnetic beads with 10 μl of prepared ligation reaction.

5. Incubate the reaction for at least 16 h and not longer than 24 h at 300 rpm on a horizontal shaker, at room temperature.

6. Add 90 μl of PCR grade water into the reaction, and expose the mixture on the MSU for 60 s.

7. Remove and discard the supernatant while the tube is on the MSU, and wash the magnetic beads with 100 μl PCR grade water.

8. Carefully remove and discard the supernatant, remove the tube from the MSU, resuspend the magnetic beads with 10 μl PCR grade water, and transfer it to a fresh 0.5 ml microfuge tube.

3.10 Exponential PCRs and Magnetic Capture

Primer sequences for the first and second exponential PCR are listed in Subheading 2.10.

1. Mix the following components in a sterile nuclease-free PCR tube:

   1 μl of the denaturation product/2 μl ligation product of nrLAM-PCR as template.

   8.3 μM of each primer.

   10× PCR buffer.

   200 μM dNTPs each.

   0.25 μl (1.25 U) Taq polymerase.

Fill the reaction up with PCR grade water to a final volume of 25 µl.

2. Place the PCR tube in a thermocycler, with the heated lid set to 105 °C, and run the following program:

$$2\,min\ @\ 95\ °C\ Initial\ denaturation$$

$$\left.\begin{array}{l}45s\ @\ 95\ °C\ Denaturation\\45s\ @\ 60\ °C\ Annealing\\60s\ @\ 72°C\ Extension\end{array}\right\}\ 36\ cycles$$

$$5\,min\ @\ 72°C\ Final\ extension$$

$$Hold\ @\ 4°C$$

3. An additional magnetic capture step after the first exponential PCR is optional. For the detailed protocol please see Subheading 3.3 (*see* **Note 10**).

4. Mix the following components for second exponential PCR in a sterile microfuge tube:

1 µl of the denaturation product of first exponential PCR as template.

8.3 µM of each primer.

10× PCR buffer.

200 µM dNTPs each.

0.5 µl (2.5 U) Taq polymerase.

Fill the reaction up with PCR grade water to a final volume of 50 µl.

5. Carry out the PCR reaction using the same condition as the first exponential PCR.

3.11 Visualization of the (nr)LAM-PCR Product with Spreadex High-Resolution Gel Electrophoresis

1. Fill the electrophoresis tank with 1.9 L of 1×concentrated TAE buffer, fix a Spreadex gel within the electrophoresis tank using an appropriate catamaran.

2. Load 10 µl of each (nr)LAM-PCR product with 2 µl of 5×concentrated blue run loading buffer.

3. Add 1 kb plus DNA ladder for molecular weight reference.

4. Let the gel run at 10 V/cm electrode gap.

5. Switch the buffer pump 5 min later after the electrophoresis starts.

6. After the electrophoresis, stain the gel for 20 min in ethidium bromide solution (~0.5 µg ethidium bromide/ml PCR grade water) on a shaker at 50 rpm and room temperature.

7. Visualize the DNA on a gel documentation system.

3.12 Library Preparation of (nr) LAM-PCR Samples for High-Throughput Sequencing Using MiSeq Platform

The (nr)LAM-PCR samples are further prepared for high-throughput sequencing to identify the precise localization of the ISs in the host genome. In the following, we will give a guideline for how to proceed optimally with the (nr)LAM-PCR samples to allow subsequent high-throughput sequencing. In brief, 40 ng of purified (nr)LAM-PCR products are used to perform a third exponential PCR. This PCR step allows adding the Illumina-specific amplification and sequencing adaptors on both sides of the (nr)LAM-PCR amplicons. By incorporating a 10–12 bp barcode into customized sequencing adaptors and linker cassette, different samples can be finally pooled for multiplexing sequencing on MiSeq platform.

1. Vortex AMPure XP beads to resuspend.

2. Add 44 μl (1.1×) of resuspended AMPure XP Beads to the second exponential PCR product (~40 μl), mix well, and incubate for 5 min at room temperature.

3. Place the tube on an appropriate MSU to separate beads from supernatant. After the solution is clear (about 5 min), carefully remove and discard the supernatant. Be careful not to disturb the beads that contain the DNA targets.

4. Add 200 μl of 80% freshly prepared ethanol to the sample while in the MSU. Incubate at room temperature for 30 s, and then carefully remove and discard the supernatant.

5. Repeat **step 4** once.

6. Air-dry beads for 5 min while the tube is on the MSU with the lid open (*see* **Note 11**).

7. Remove the tube from the MSU. Elute the DNA target by adding 24 μl of PCR grade water to the beads.

8. Mix well on a vortex mixer or by pipetting up and down and incubate for 2 min at room temperature.

9. Put the tube in the MSU until the solution is clear. Transfer 22 μl of supernatant (or desired volume) to a new tube, and proceed to third exponential PCR.

10. Mix the following components for third exponential PCR in a sterile microfuge tube (for primer sequences for the third exponential PCR please see Subheading 2.12).

    40 ng of the Ampure bead-purified second exponential PCR product.

    0.5 μl of each primer (10 pmol/μl).

    5 μl 10× PCR buffer.

    1 μl dNTPs each (10 mM).

    0.5 μl (2.5 U) Taq polymerase.

    Fill the reaction up with PCR grade water to a final volume of 50 μl.

11. Place the PCR tube in a thermocycler, with the heated lid set to 105 °C, and run the following program:

> 2 min @ 95 °C Initial denaturation
> 45 s @ 95 °C Denaturation ⎫
> 45 s @ 60 °C Annealing   ⎬ 15 cycles
> 60 s @ 72°C Extension   ⎭
> 5 min @ 72°C Final extension
> Hold @ 4°C

12. Purify the third exponential PCR products with Ampure XP beads as **steps 1–9**.

13. Measure the purified DNA concentration by using a Qubit fluorometer.

14. Pool the desired DNA samples according to their multiplexes, and analyze the peak distribution using 1 μl pooled library by Agilent Bioanalyzer 2100/Tap station using DNA High Sensitivity Kit (*see* **Note 12**). The amount of DNA of each sample within the pool is proportional to the number of retrieved sequencing reads.

15. Store the pooled library at –20 °C, or directly continue for MiSeq sequencing.

3.13 Bioinformatics/ Sequence Analyses

Public available bioinformatics tools like Seqmap 2.0 [13], QuickMap [14], or our own developed HISAP pipelines, such as noted in Ref. 15, can process the retrieved sequences.

4   Notes

1. If non-restrictive LAM-PCR is being performed, please go directly to Subheading 3.9 after this step.

2. Alternatively binding solution provided by the manufacturer of the magnetic beads can also be used. LiCl solution in our hand performs in a comparable way and is cost effective.

3. The ratio of PCR product and LiCl solution must always be 1:1.

4. This capturing step needs to be carried out at least for 8 h.

5. After thawing the aliquot of linker cassette, do not refreeze it.

6. This protocol provides the detail procedure for restriction enzyme MseI; please adjust the components for this step if other restriction enzyme is used.

7. Choose the restriction enzyme in a way that no restriction site is located within the known sequence of interest and the ampli-

fied part of the vector. Incubate the restriction digest mixture at the temperature recommended by the manufacturer to achieve maximum enzyme activity for 1 h in a thermocycler.

8. Store the denatured LAM product at –20 °C.

9. This step should be followed after **subheading 3.3** if nrLAM-PCR is performed.

10. This magnetic capture step should be performed to increase the sensitivity and specificity.

    Minor changes to the magnetic capture protocol are described in Subheading 3.3.

    – Resuspend the magnetic beads in 25 μl 6 M LiCl instead of 50 μl.

    – After adding the magnetic beads to each first exponential PCR product (1:1 ratio), incubate the DNA/bead complexes for at least 1 h on a shaker at 300 rpm and room temperature.

    – Denature the DNA from DNA/bead complexes with 20 μl of freshly prepared 0.1 N NaOH solution.

11. Do not overdry the beads. This may result in lower recovery of DNA target.

12. To obtain the precise and reproducible results of NGS, high-quality analytes with Poisson distribution and precisely estimated DNA concentration are crucial.

References

1. Hacein-Bey-Abina S, Le Deist F, Carlier F et al (2002) Sustained correction of X-linked severe combined immunodeficiency by ex vivo gene therapy. N Engl J Med 346:1185–1193

2. Boztug K, Schmidt M, Schwarzer A et al (2010) Stem-cell gene therapy for the Wiskott-Aldrich syndrome. N Engl J Med 363:1918–1927. doi:10.1056/NEJMoa1003548

3. Hacein-Bey Abina S, von Kalle C, Schmidt M et al (2003) A serious adverse event after successful gene therapy for X-linked severe combined immunodeficiency. N Engl J Med 348:255–256

4. Braun CJ, Boztug K, Paruzynski A et al (2014) Gene therapy for Wiskott-Aldrich syndrome—long-term efficacy and genotoxicity. Sci Transl Med 6:227ra33. doi:10.1126/scitranslmed.3007280

5. Schwarzwaelder K, Howe SJ, Schmidt M et al (2007) Gammaretrovirus-mediated correction of SCID-X1 is associated with skewed vector integration site distribution in vivo. J Clin Invest 117:2241–2249. doi:10.1172/JCI31661

6. Deichmann A, Hacein-Bey-Abina S, Schmidt M et al (2007) Vector integration is nonrandom and clustered and influences the fate of lymphopoiesis in SCID-X1 gene therapy. J Clin Invest 117:2225–2232

7. Bartholomae CC, Arens A, Balaggan KS et al (2011) Lentiviral vector integration profiles differ in rodent postmitotic tissues. Mol Ther 19:703–710

8. Cartier N, Hacein-bey-abina S, Bartholomae CC et al (2009) Hematopoietic stem cell gene therapy with a lentiviral vector in X-linked adrenoleukodystrophy. Science 326:818–823

9. Aiuti A, Biasco L, Scaramuzza S et al (2013) Lentiviral hematopoietic stem cell gene therapy in patients with Wiskott-Aldrich syndrome. Science 341:1233151

10. Mueller PR, Wold B (1989) In vivo footprinting of a muscle specific enhancer by ligation mediated PCR. Science 246:780–786

11. Schmidt M, Schwarzwaelder K, Bartholomae C et al (2007) High-resolution insertion-site analysis by linear amplification-mediated PCR (LAM-PCR). Nat Methods 4:1051–1057

12. Paruzynski A, Arens A, Gabriel R et al (2010) Genome-wide high-throughput integrome analyses by nrLAM-PCR and next-generation sequencing. Nat Protoc 5:1379–1395

13. Hawkins TB, Dantzer J, Peters B et al (2011) Identifying viral integration sites using SeqMap 2.0. Bioinformatics 27:720–722

14. Appelt J-U, Giordano FA, Ecker M et al (2009) QuickMap: a public tool for large-scale gene therapy vector insertion site mapping and analysis. Gene Ther 16:885–893

15. Arens A, Appelt J-U, Bartholomae CC et al (2012) Bioinformatic clonality analysis of next-generation sequencing-derived viral vector integration sites. Hum Gene Ther Methods 23:111–118. doi:10.1089/hgtb.2011.219

Chapter 10

Conditional RNAi Using the Lentiviral GLTR System

Elisabeth Pfeiffenberger, Reinhard Sigl, and Stephan Geley

Abstract

RNA interference (RNAi) has become an essential technology for functional gene analysis. Its success depends on the effective expression of target gene-specific RNAi-inducing small double-stranded interfering RNA molecules (siRNAs). Here, were describe the use of a recently developed lentiviral RNAi system that allows the rapid generation of stable cell lines with inducible RNAi based on conditional expression of double-stranded short hairpin RNA (shRNA). These lentiviral vectors can be generated rapidly using the GATEWAY recombination cloning technology. Conditional cell lines can be established by using either a two-vector system in which the regulator is encoded by a separate vector or by a one-vector system. The available different lentiviral vectors for conditional shRNA expression cassette delivery co-express additional genes that allow (1) the use of fluorescent proteins for color-coded combinatorial RNAi or monitoring RNAi induction (pGLTR-FP), (2) selection of transduced cells (pGLTR-S), and (3) the generation of conditional cell lines using a one-vector system (pGLTR-X).

Key words RNAi, shRNA, Tetracycline, Inducible, Lentivirus, Knockdown, Human cell line, GATEWAY

1 Introduction

RNA interference (RNAi) has become the most important and most widely used technology for functional gene analysis. Although RNAi dominance has been challenged by genome editing technologies, it will remain an important tool provided that it is applied properly [1]. Genome-wide loss-of-function screening to identify and further characterize essential genes will remain an important application for this technology [2]. It exploits a conserved gene regulatory mechanism activated by double-stranded RNA (dsRNA) molecules that are processed into small interfering RNA (siRNA) molecules by the type III endoribonuclease DICER. Individual siRNA strands are then incorporated into the multi-subunit RNA-induced silencing complex (RISC) to serve as guide RNAs for the identification, binding, and subsequent RISC endonuclease-dependent cleavage of complementary target mRNAs, which leads to their rapid degradation and subsequent decline in protein levels [3].

Maurizio Federico (ed.), *Lentiviral Vectors and Exosomes as Gene and Protein Delivery Tools*, Methods in Molecular Biology, vol. 1448, DOI 10.1007/978-1-4939-3753-0_10, © Springer Science+Business Media New York 2016

RNAi can be induced by several means. (1) Chemically synthesized double-stranded RNA (dsRNA) molecules, so-called small interfering RNAs (siRNA), can be used for transient RNAi upon transfection. (2) siRNAs can also be generated from cellularly expressed short hairpin RNA (shRNA) molecules. Since these shRNAs are expressed from specific RNA polymerase-III-dependent promoters, such as U6- or H1-RNA promoter, this approach allows longer lasting gene knockdown [4, 5]. (3) Alternatively, the dsRNA precursors can be expressed within the context of micro-RNA (miRNA) molecules [6], expressed from RNA polymerase-II-dependent promoters. These dsRNA precursors are first processed by nuclear DROSHA, another member of the RNase-III family, to release the pre-miRNA from the primary RNA transcript and then by DICER to generate siRNAs in the cytoplasm [7].

For our stable and conditional RNAi system, we use a modified RNA polymerase-III-dependent H1 promoter and exploit the "tetracycline system" [8] to drive shRNA expression in a tetracycline (Tet)-dependent manner. Our "THT" promoter carries a heptamerized Tet-operator (TetO) sequence upstream of the H1 promoter and a single TetO element between the TATA-box and the transcription start site. These modifications render the "THT" promoter repressible by TetR or TetR-fusion proteins. Although TetR alone is sufficient for the tight control of shRNA expression by steric hindrance, we also use the TetR-KRAB [9] fusion protein for silencing of shRNA gene expression. The transcriptional silencing domain KRAB of Kox1 silences RNA polymerase-II- and -III-dependent gene expression, facilitating a "tighter" control of shRNA expression. Moreover, the silencing effect tends to spread from the TetR-KRAB-binding locus and can, thus, co-regulate (reporter) genes in its proximity [10].

We have designed GATEWAY "ENTR" vectors that harbor either the wild-type H1-RNA gene promoter (pENTR-H1) or the conditional THT promoter to construct shRNA expression cassettes between attL recombination sequences [11]. These vectors can be used by themselves to induce RNAi by transient transfection or they can be utilized in GATEWAY transfer reactions to construct lentiviral RNAi vectors for more efficient delivery.

Lentiviral transduction is a powerful means to achieve permanent gene transfer in a high percentage of target cells. Due to its active nuclear import mechanism, a lentivirus can also stably transduce nondividing primary or differentiated, i.e., postmitotic, cells. For experimental and therapeutic applications lentiviral vector systems have been developed to minimize the risk of self-propagation of these infectious particles. Thus, these vectors are (1) replication incompetent, (2) lack an LTR-based promoter, and (3) require trans-complementation and pseudotyping in packaging cells for production of infectious particles [12].

In the current protocol a "second-generation" three-plasmid system is used to produce recombinant virus particles in human embryonic kidney (HEK)-derived 293T cells. Trans-complementation is achieved by expression of viral genes from the packaging plasmid psPAX2 (AddGene, a kind gift of D. Trono, Lausanne, Switzerland), which expresses gag, pol, rev, and tat under the control of a modified human cytomegalovirus early promoter (CAG). For pseudotyping, we use the glycoprotein G from vesicular stomatitis virus (VSV-G), which is also expressed from an hCMV promoter (pGM-D plasmid, kindly provided by Didier Trono). VSV-G pseudotyping generates a polytropic particle that can infect many different cell types and enhances the mechanical stability of the virus [13]. Finally, the RNA molecule to be packaged is encoded by one of the "GLTR" DEST-vectors (GATEWAY-compatible *l*entiviral *t*etracycline-regulated *R*NAi) pGLTR-FP, pGLTR-S, pGLTR-X-FP, or pGLTR-X-S.

The GLTR expression vectors are constructed by GATEWAY-mediated recombination between any of the available GLTR-DEST vectors and one of the ENTR-H1 or -THT plasmids. For selection or monitoring of lentiviral transduction, we used the SFFV promoter to express the reporter genes: green fluorescent protein (GFP) or red fluorescent protein (RFP) in pGLTR-FP or pGLTR-X-FP and puromycin resistance gene in pGLTR-S or pGLTR-X-S. For our "one-step system" we have designed the vectors pGLTR-X-FP (GFP reporter) and pGLTR-X-S (puromycin resistance reporter), which stably integrate the shRNA expression cassette, a reporter gene, and TetR for control of the shRNA expression. TetR and GFP or puromycin are encoded by a fusion gene but separated by a "2A peptide" [14], which allows "bicistronic" expression due to "ribosomal skipping" [15]. In our vectors we use the T2A (*Thosea asigna* virus) and P2A (porcine teschovirus-1) sequences in pGLTR-X-FP and pGLTR-X-S, respectively.

The use of TetR-KRAB in combination with the pGLTR-FP vectors allows monitoring shRNA expression upon tetracycline administration due to the co-regulation of the cis-encoded fluorescent reporters. TetR-KRAB is efficient to silence the transgene, but requires the generation of TetR-KRAB-expressing cell lines, e.g., by transducing cells with the retroviral vector pLib-TetR-KRAB-IRES-BlaS.

1.1 Safety Guidelines   Despite the use of second-generation packaging systems described here HIV-based vectors fall within NIH Biosafety Level 2 criteria. Although the risk for recombination with endogenous viral sequences is low, the risk of forming self-replicating virus cannot be completely eliminated. Similarly, retro- and lentiviral vectors are insertional mutagens that have to be considered potential health hazards.

For information *see* http://www.cdc.gov/od/ohs/biosfty/
bmbl4/bmbl4s3.htm and your local national and institu-
tional guidelines on using retro- and lentiviral vectors.

Use standard microbiological practices:

Work in certified laboratories, self-protective clothing
(gloves, lab coat) during all procedure containing infectious material. Clearly indicate and document if BSL2
work is carried out:

Label all work areas, instruments, and waste that may contain
infectious material.

Only work in a BSL II-certified laminar flow hood.

Work carefully to avoid spilling and aerosol formation.

Collect waste and decontaminate before disposal.

Decontaminate work surfaces.

2   Material

2.1 Laboratory Equipment

1. Cell culture: Biosafety Level 2 (BSL-2) facility (depending on legislation and local guidelines) containing a cell incubator at 37 °C with 5 % CO_2, saturated humidity, sterile work bench, water baths, centrifuges for pelleting cells.

2. DNA technology: Molecular biology/cloning: standard molecular biology laboratory equipment biosafety level 1.

3. Immunoblot analysis: Vertical electrophoresis system, blotting/transfer system, power supply, nitrocellulose membrane, chemiluminescence substrate, film developer, or digital chemiluminescence visualization system.

4. Others: Tabletop centrifuge for pelleting cells under BSL-2 conditions; flow cytometer for analysis of transduced cells, inverted epifluorescence microscope, Sorvall RC5B centrifuge (or equivalent) for viral particle pelleting under BSL-2 conditions.

2.2 Cell Lines, Cultivation, and Transfection

1. Cell line for lentivirus production: HEK 293T (embryonic kidney epithelial cell line, ATCC CRL11268) (*see* **Note 1**).

2. Cell line for retrovirus production: Phoenix (ATCC CRL-3214TM) (*see* **Note 2**).

3. Target cell line for efficiency testing: Any desired/available cell line such as Hela (cervix epithelial cell line, ATCC CCL-2), U2OS (osteosarcoma epithelial cell line, ATCC HTB-96) (*see* **Note 3**).

4. Experimental target cell line: To be chosen depending on the experiment.

5. "Standard growth medium" for Hela, U2OS, and HEK 293T cells: DMEM supplemented with 10% FBS, 100 µg/ml streptomycin, and 100 U/ml penicillin.

6. Appropriate "growth medium" for experimental target cells.

7. Selection medium is based on "standard medium" or "growth medium" (depending on target cells) and contains the appropriate selection antibiotic (puromycin or blasticidin S).

8. For transient transfection with shRNA-expressing ENTR plasmid: Metafectene, alternatively any other transfection regent can be used such as Lipofectamine 2000.

9. Opti-MEM.

10. Cell incubator with saturated humidity at 37 °C, 5% CO_2, for standard growth conditions.

2.3 Virus Particle Production, Concentration, and Target Cell Infection

1. HEK 293T producer cells.

2. Target cells, e.g., Hela or U2OS.

3. Second-generation lentiviral packaging system plasmids (*see* Subheading 2.4): pSPAX2, pGM.D, lentiviral vector (*see* **Note 4**).

4. Cell transfection reagent: Metafectene or similar lipid-based reagents as well as any other effective transfection reagent or protocol (*see* **Notes 5–7**).

5. Opti-MEM.

6. 5 ml Syringes.

7. Syringe filters 0.2 µm or 0.45 µm.

8. 1000× Polybrene: 8 mg/ml in sterile water (*see* **Note 8**).

2.4 Plasmids

The plasmids used in this method [11] are available at "Addgene" (http://www.addgene.org).

1. ENTR plasmids: pENTR-THT or pENTR-THT-III.

2. DEST plasmids: pGLTR-FP-GFP, pGLTR-FP-RFP, pGLTR-S-PURO, pGLRT-X-GFP, pGLTR-X-Puro.

3. Second-generation lentiviral packaging system plasmids: pGLTR shRNA expression vector plasmid, pSPAX2 (http://www.addgene.org/12260), or any other second-generation packaging plasmid, pMD.G (http://www.addgene.org/12259/), or any other envelope plasmid expressing VSV-G envelope protein for pseudotyping.

4. pLib-TetR-KRAB-IRES-BlaS: Retroviral bicistronic expression vector for stable TetR-KRAB expression. Promoter: MMLV-LTR. Selection marker in transduced cells: Blasticidin S.

5. pHR-SFFV-TetR-KRAB-IRES-PURO: Lentiviral bicistronic expression vector for TetR-KRAB. Promoter: SFFV. Selection marker in transduced cells: Puromycin. pLENTI6/TR

(Invitrogen): lentiviral expression vector for TetR. Promoter: CMV. The selection marker gene blasticidin S deaminase (bsr) is expressed from the SV40 promoter.

2.5 Oligonucleotides, PCR, and Sequencing

Primers for insert amplification and sequencing: ENTR-THT fwd: 5′ TGT AAA ACG ACG GCC AGT; ENTR-THT rev: 5′ CTG CAG GAA TTC GAA CGC TGA CG.

2.6 Cloning, Plasmid Preparation, and DNA Analysis

1. 1× TE buffer: 10 mM Tris–HCl pH 8.0, 1 mM EDTA.

2. 50× TAE buffer 1 L: 242 g Tris, 57.5 ml acetic acid (100%), 100 ml EDTA (0.5 M), adjust the solution to 1 L with distilled water.

3. Agarose gel: 1% Agarose (w/v) in 1× TAE, heat up to dissolve agarose, 0.5 μg/ml ethidium bromide.

4. 10× Agarose loading buffer: 20% Ficoll 400, 1 mM EDTA, 1% SDS, 0.25% bromophenol blue, 0.25% xylene cyanol.

5. DNA molecular weight size marker.

6. Restriction enzymes for ENTR cloning: BglII, HindIII.

7. Restriction enzymes for DEST plasmid verification: EcoRI, HindIII.

8. DNA ligation kit.

9. Plasmid purification kit.

10. DNA purification kit.

2.7 GATEWAY-Cloning

GATEWAY reagents are available from Invitrogen/Life Technologies: BP Clonase, LR Clonase, Proteinase K solution.

2.8 Bacteria Transformation, Culture, and Selection

1. *E. coli* strains: DB3.1 chemically transformation competent, DH5α chemically transformation competent (*see* **Note 9**).

2. SOC medium, 1 L: 20.0 g tryptone, 5.0 g yeast extract, 0.6 g NaCl, 0.2 g KCl, 2.0 g MgCl2, 2.5 g MgSO4, 3.6 g glucose; sterile filtered.

3. LB medium, 1 L: 10 g Bacto tryptone, 5 g yeast extract, 10 g NaCl, autoclaved.

4. LB agar plates: LB medium, 15 g agar, autoclaved.

5. 1000× antibiotic stocks: Ampicillin 100 mg/ml (Amp), chloramphenicol 50 mg/ml (Cm), gentamycin 50 mg/ml (Gent), kanamycin 50 mg/ml (Kan).

2.9 Immunoblot Analysis

1. SDS sample buffer: 2% SDS, 80 mM Tris–HCl pH 6.8, 10% glycerol, bromophenol blue.

2. Antibodies: TetR, GFP, target protein of interest, secondary HRP-conjugated antibodies.

3   Methods

3.1   shRNA Sequence Design and Oligonucleotide Generation

1. Select target sequences by identifying 19 nucleotides followed by an AA motif using consensus criteria described in [16].

2. The shRNA-encoding DNA sequences are designed as sense-loop-antisense molecules with ttcaagaga as the loop sequence. The top and bottom strand shRNA-encoding sequences are flanked by a Bgl II- and Hind III-compatible 3′ overhang, respectively. The top strand sequence of an shRNA-encoding oligonucleotide thus is 5′ GATCCCC-NN19sense-ttcaagaga-NN19 antisense-TTTTTGGAAA. The 5′ thymidine stretch serves as the transcription termination signal for RNA polymerase III.

3.2   Cloning shRNA Sequence into pENTR Vectors

3.2.1   Vector Preparation

1. Digest 5 μg of the chosen ENTR vector with 10 U Bgl II and Hind III for 1 h at 37 °C in a reaction volume of 50 μl in the appropriate restriction enzyme buffer.

2. Analyze 2 μl of the restriction enzyme digest by agarose gel electrophoresis. Complete restriction enzyme digestion results in the release of a 1.39 kb stuffer fragment that is subsequently removed by gel purification (see below).

3. Dephosphorylate the vector by adding 5 μl 10× dephosphorylation buffer and 5 μl (5 U) of alkaline (calf intestinal) phosphatase for 30 min at 37 °C.

4. Purify the vector DNA by preparative 1% agarose gel electrophoresis. The ~3.1 kb band is carefully excised using a UV-light transilluminator, purified, and quantified by measuring OD_{260} in a spectrophotometer.

3.2.2   Insert Preparation

1. Mix 1 μl of each shRNA-encoding DNA oligonucleotide (10 μM) in the presence of 1 mM ATP and T4-polynucleotide kinase in a 10 μl nucleotide phosphorylation reaction for 30 min at 37 °C.

2. Heat inactivate and denature at 95 °C for 2 min, spin the sample briefly, and incubate at 37 °C for up to 2 h to allow double-strand DNA formation.

3. Dilute the annealed oligonucleotides 1:10 in nuclease-free water.

3.2.3   Ligation and Transformation

1. Ligate 50–100 ng of the purified dephosphorylated vector with 1–3 μl of double-stranded phosphorylated oligonucleotides in a volume of 10 μl using T4-DNA ligase using a 2× ligation buffer (132 mM Tris–HCl, 20 mM $MgCl_2$, 2 mM DTT, 2 mM ATP, 15% PEG 6000, pH 7.6) for 15 min at room temperature.

2. Mix the ligation reaction with 50 μl of competent bacteria, incubate for 30 min on ice, heat shock for 1 min at 42 °C, place on ice for 2 min before adding 200 μl SOC medium, and further incubate for 30 min at 37 °C.

3. Plate the entire transformation reaction on selection agar plates by spreading with sterile 3 mm glass beads.

3.2.4 Plasmid Verification

1. Prepare plasmid DNA from 3 ml liquid overnight saturation cultures inoculated with single colonies.

2. Verify successful cloning by PCR using primers ENTR-THT-fwd and ENTR-THT-rev or by restriction enzyme digest using EcoRI and HindIII, which results in a 0.28 and ~3 kb fragment that can be analyzed by agarose gel electrophoresis.

3. For DNA sequencing, amplify the DNA fragment using primers ENTR-THT-fwd and ENTR-THT-rev, gel purify the 0.28 kb fragment, and subject it to DNA sequencing using either PCR primer (*see* **Note 10**).

3.3 Functional Evaluation of ENTR-shRNA Constructs

1. Test the sequence-verified ENTR-shRNA constructs for RNAi efficacy by transient transfection into target cell lines using any high-efficiency transfection procedure. RNAi efficacy can also be determined by co-transfecting the target gene of interest (*see* **Note 11**).

2. Verify target gene knockdown 48–96 h after transfection using a suitable reporter assay or immunoblotting.

3.4 GATEWAY-Based Generation of Lentiviral shRNA Expression Vectors

1. Amplify GLTR-DEST vectors in *E. coli* strain DB3.1 and verify by restriction enzyme digestion.

2. Combine 0.5 μl (150 ng) of the DEST vector with 0.5 μl of the ENTR-shRNA vector in the presence of 1 μl LR clonase II for 1 h up to overnight at room temperature.

3. Add 0.5 μl proteinase K (10 mg/ml) and incubate for 15 min at 37 °C.

4. Transform competent bacteria (e.g., DH5α) with entire LR reaction mix and plate on selection agar plates.

5. Isolate plasmid DNA from bacterial saturation cultures obtained by inoculating 3 ml of bacterial broth with a single colony.

6. Verify successful recombination using restriction enzymes EcoRI and BamHI, which release fragments of 0.9 and ~9.6 in the case of pGLTR-S and pGLTR-FP vectors and in 0.7, 0.9, and ~9.3 kb fragments in the case of the pGLTR-X vectors.

Table 1
Metafectene transfection protocol for generating lentiviral vectors

	24-Well	6-Well	10 cm dish
293T cell number	0.18×10^6	0.8×10^6	5×10^6
Vol. culture medium [ml]	0.5	3	10
Target cell number	0.8×10^4	0.4×10^5	0.25×10^6
Vol. of infection medium + standard medium [ml]	0.75 + 0.75	1.5 + 1.5	10 + 10
pGLTR vector [μg]	0.5	2	10
psPAX2 vector [μg]	0.25	1	5
pMD-G vector [μg]	0.25	1	5
Optimem [μl]	25 + 25	100 + 100	250 + 250
Metafectene [μl]	3	12	60

3.5 Lentiviral Particle Production and Target Cell Infection

1. The day before transfection (day 0) seed 1×10^6 HEK 293T cells in a 6-well plate/3 cm diameter dish (5×10^6 cells in 10 cm dish) in standard growth medium.

2. For transfection (day 1) (Table 1) dilute plasmids in 100 μl Opti-MEM (2 μg lentiviral vector plasmid, 1 μg pSPAX2, and 1 μg pMD.G). For a 10 cm plate transfection use 250 μl Opti-MEM, 10 μg lentiviral vector, 5 μg pSPAX2, and 5 μg pMD.G. In a separate reaction tube dilute 12 μl Metafectene in 100 μl Opti-MEM ("10 cm plate format": 250 μl Opti-MEM with 60 μl Metafectene) (*see* **Note 12**).

3. Combine and mix both solutions and incubate for 20 min at room temperature.

4. Exchange media of HEK 293T producer cells with 2 ml of standard growth medium ("10 cm plate format": 10 ml), add the lipid/DNA mix drop-wise, and gently tilt the plate to mix but avoid swirling. *From now on, BSL-2 working conditions are mandatory.*

5. On the following day (day 2) exchange media for fresh growth medium appropriate for the target cells (*see* **Note 13**). If virus particle concentration (*see* **Note 14**) is planned standard growth medium can be used. When using a lentiviral vector with a fluorescent reporter protein, expression and transfection efficiency can be monitored with an epifluorescence microscope.

6. Seed target cells at ~50% confluency in a 6-well plate (*see* **Note 15**).

7. Harvest lentiviral particle-containing supernatant from the transfected HEK293T cells on day 3 (48 h-post transfection

(hpt)) with a syringe and pass it through a 0.45 μm filter (48 h SN). Add 2 ml ("10 cm plate format": 10 ml) of fresh growth medium to HEK293T cells and cultivate for an additional day.

8. For transduction, add filtered 48hSN complemented with 4 μg/ml polybrene (*see* **Note 16**) to the target cells. In case the target cells are adherently growing, medium is removed and exchanged for the virus-containing media. Cells cultivated in suspension are pelleted and resuspended in polybrene-supplemented 48hSN (see **Note 17**). If not used immediately, the 48hSN can be concentrated (see below) or snap-frozen in liquid N_2 and stored at –80 °C (*see* **Note 18**).

9. After 6 h of growth in 48hSN add 1 ml standard growth medium to the 6-well ("10 cm plate format": 7 ml).

10. On day 4 (72hpt), collect supernatant (72hSN) from the transfected HEK293T cells, filter it, and either use for transduction, virus concentration, or storage.

11. On day 5 remove the 72hSN from the target cells and grow the target cells for 1 or 2 more days (until day 6 or 7).

12. On day 6 or 7, start the selection procedure appropriate for the viral vector. After passaging, cells can be further cultivated under standard safety conditions. In Table 2, a lentiviral vector production workflow is depicted.

3.6 Retroviral Particle Production and Generation of TetR or TetR-KRAB Transgenic Cell Lines

Retroviral particle generation is carried out as described for lentiviral particles, except that the HEK293-derived Phoenix cell line is used as a packaging cell line. This cell line is transgenic for the retroviral gag and pol genes, so only the VSV-G pseudotyping plasmid needs to be co-transfected along with the retroviral plasmid. All other steps are essentially carried out as described above.

3.7 TetR or TetR-KRAB Transgenic Cell Lines

1. To establish TetR- or TetR-KRAB-expressing cell lines, retro- or lentiviral vectors can be used. Upon transduction, clones should be established by limiting dilution cloning and characterized for transgene expression using immunoblotting or reporter gene expression.

2. The choice of using TetR or TetR-KRAB depends on the downstream application. If antibiotics selection is used to enrich for transduced target cell, TetR has to be used as regulator. If co-induction of fluorescent proteins is required to monitor RNAi induction in transduced cells, then TetR-KRAB is the regulator of choice.

3.8 Target Cell Enrichment

The GLTR vectors allow several different cell enrichment procedures to rapidly isolate transduced cells. The selectable vectors (GLTR-S and GLTR-X-Puro) can be selected using antibiotics, while the color-encoding viruses (GLTR-FP) can be enriched using flow cytometry.

Table 2
Lentiviral vector production workflow

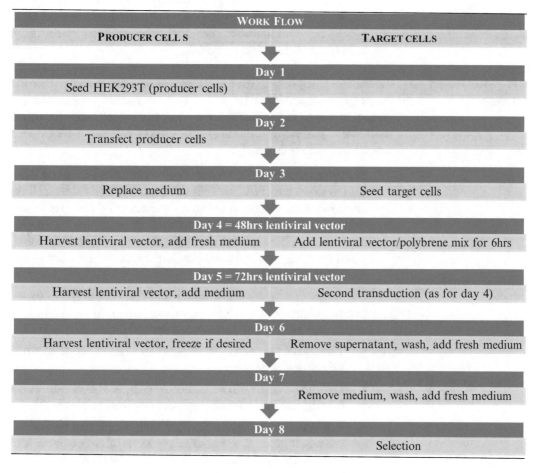

WORK FLOW	
PRODUCER CELL S	**TARGET CELLS**
Day 1	
Seed HEK293T (producer cells)	
Day 2	
Transfect producer cells	
Day 3	
Replace medium	Seed target cells
Day 4 = 48hrs lentiviral vector	
Harvest lentiviral vector, add fresh medium	Add lentiviral vector/polybrene mix for 6hrs
Day 5 = 72hrs lentiviral vector	
Harvest lentiviral vector, add medium	Second transduction (as for day 4)
Day 6	
Harvest lentiviral vector, freeze if desired	Remove supernatant, wash, add fresh medium
Day 7	
	Remove medium, wash, add fresh medium
Day 8	
	Selection

1. Antibiotic selection of transduced cells: On day 6 or 7 after infection, replate transduced cells to ~25 % confluency before addition of the selection antibiotics: 1–5 μg/ml puromycin, 0.5–1 mg/mlG418.

2. For color selection: On day 6 or 7 harvest green or red fluorescent cells and subject them to flow cytometry sorting using standard excitation and emission settings for GFP and dTomato (*see* **Note 19**).

3.9 RNAi Induction and Knockdown Analysis

To evaluate RNAi in transduced target cells seed 0.5×10^6 cells in 6-well plates. The following day start a time course and doxycycline dose-response experiment.

1. Time course experiment: Induce expression of the shRNA by adding 1 μg/ml doxycycline to the cells for 0–6 days (*see* **Notes 20** and **21**). Prepare whole-cell lysates every day by adding 100 μl of SDS sample buffer to the cells or the cell pellet.

Analyze target gene expression by immunoblotting or, if no suitable antibody is available, by qPCR on total RNA.

2. Dose-response curve: Add increasing amounts of doxycycline (0, 20, 40, 80, 160, and 320 ng/ml) to the cells for 96 h (*see* **Note 21**) and harvest cells for immunoblotting or target mRNA quantification by qPCR.

3.10 RNAi Control Experiments

RNAi is an important tool for loss-of-function analysis. In most cases gene knockdown by RNAi can be readily established but stringent controls are mandatory. The most significant drawbacks of RNAi experiments are nonspecific effects, off-target effects, and insufficient knockdown.

1. Nonspecific effects can be induced by the transfection or infection to deliver siRNAs, by cellular responses to dsRNA, cellular effects due to extended in vitro cultivation of cells, or inhibition of endogenous dsRNA processing pathways by shRNA expression. These nonspecific effects can be effectively monitored by using control shRNAs that target "irrelevant" genes, such as firefly luciferase.

2. Off-target effects are unavoidable and plentiful in RNAi experiments. Controls for RNAi experiments should be established at the start of the experiment and should include:

    • The use of at least two independent shRNA sequences that target the same gene.

    • Phenotype analysis in bulk infected cells, or, if clones are established, in at least three independent clones (*see* **Note 22**).

    • RNAi rescue experiments using siRNA-resistant versions of the target gene. RNAi-resistant versions often require at least three silent mutations introduced into the siRNA target site. Care needs to be paid also to the expression levels of the transgene to avoid overexpression artifacts (*see* **Note 23**).

---

4 Notes

1. Lentiviral packaging cell lines: Several lentiviral packaging cell lines are available, most of which are based on HEK293 cells, because these cells can be readily transfected and some, such as HEK293T cells, express SV40-T, which allows episomal replication of plasmids containing the SV40 origin of DNA replication. Other cell lines, including ones that allow stable production of lentiviral particles, have been described [17].

2. Retroviral packaging cell line: Phoenix cells [18] are transgenic for retroviral gag, pol, and optional env genes; express human

CD8 for monitoring; and are resistant to hygromycin B (250 µg/ml) and diphtheria toxin (1 µg/ml). Co-transfection of VSV-G-encoding plasmids allows the generation of polytropic virus.

3. Using pseudotyping a wide variety of cell types can be transduced by lentiviral particles. Some cell types, such as PBMCs, HSCs, and differentiated cardiomyocytes, seem to be difficult to transduce.

4. The lentiviral production protocol described here is based on a second-generation packaging system. Please note that the GLTR lentiviral vectors cannot be used with third-generation packaging systems.

5. Any highly efficient transfection protocols for HEK293 cells can be used. Calcium phosphate coprecipitation or PEI-mediated transfection is cheap yet still a highly efficient method.

6. Calcium phosphate coprecipitation:

Materials:

- 2.5 M $CaCl_2$ (sterile).
- 2× HBS.

  - 50 mM HEPES, 280 mM NaCl, 1.5 mM Na_2HPO_4.
  - Adjust pH exactly to 7.10.
  - Filter sterilize.
  - Aliquot and store at –20 °C.
- 0.1× TE Buffer

  - 0.1 mM Tris–HCl pH 8.
  - 0.01 mM EDTA.

Procedure:

- Seed the HEK293T cells so that they will be 70–80 % confluent at the time of transfection (cell division is necessary for successful transfection). Works better if cells are at a low passage.
- Transfection: on same day (next day also possible).
- All solutions must have room temperature when performing the transfection (put the HBS and $CaCl_2$ on the heating block to bring them to 24 °C)!
- Change the medium 2 h before transfection.
- Dilute the plasmid DNA with 0.1× TE buffer to the given volume.

Format	DNA µg	DNA Vol. µl	2.5 M CaCl₂ µl	2× HBS µl
6 Well (per well)	3.4	68.5	7.6	76.1
10 cm dish	20.8	418.3	46.5	464.7

- Add 2.5 M $CaCl_2$ and incubate for 5 min at room temperature.
- Vortex the tube containing the $DNA/CaCl_2$ solution (slowest setting) while adding the 2× HBS dropwise.
- Close tube and vortex shortly on highest setting and add within 1–2 min to cells. Try to cover the growing area as well as possible.
- Leave on the cells o/n, and change medium after 24 h.
- The following day exchange with fresh medium.
- Proceed with virus collection and target cell infection as described for the lentiviral protocol.

7. PEI-based transfection protocol:

Material:

Polyethylenimine (branched PEI) (e.g., Sigma-Aldrich (#408727)) is diluted in 10 ml H_2O to 1 mg/ml, neutralized with HCl, filter sterilized, aliquoted, and stored at –80 °C.

Procedure:

- The ratio DNA:PEI has to be 1:3.
- For transfection use media without antibiotics (e.g., OptiMEM).
- At the time of transfection, cells should be 60–80% confluent.
- For a 6-well transfection:
- Mix 1 µg DNA in 100 µl OptiMEM.
- Mix 3 µl PEI in 100 µl OptiMEM.
- Mix DNA and PEI, vortex for 5 s and incubate at room temperature for 15 min.
- Add reaction dropwise to the cells.
- Exchange media after 24 h.
- Proceed with virus harvesting as described in the lentiviral protocol.

8. The stock solution of polybrene is made by dissolving hexadimethrine bromide in sterile water to 8 mg/ml. Final concentration during infection: 4–8 µg/ml.

9. Generation of transformation-competent bacteria:

- A single colony of freshly streaked *E. coli* is grown in 250 ml SOB media (20 g tryptone, 5 g yeast extract, 0.6 g NaCl, 0.2 g KCl, 2 g MgCl$_2$, 2.5 g MgSO$_4$) until OD600 = 0.6.

- Harvest cells by centrifugation (2,800 × g on a tabletop centrifuge, 4 °C, 10 min) and resuspend carefully in cold 80 ml transformation buffer TB (10 mM Pipes, 15 mM CaCl$_2$, 250 mM KCl, 55 mM MnCl$_2$, pH 6.7).

- Pellet as described above and resuspend in 20 ml TB.

- Add 1.5 ml DMSO.

- Aliquot on ice and snap freeze in liquid N$_2$.

10. In our hands, DNA sequencing of the hairpin sequence is facilitated by first amplifying the THT-shRNA cassette by PCR, followed by DNA sequencing using one of the PCR primers.

11. The success of evaluating RNAi efficiency by transient transfection of ENTR-THT-shRNA plasmids into target cells followed by immunoblotting depends on three factors: (1) the quality of the selected target sequence, (2) the transfection efficiency, and (3) the half-life of the protein. Because in many cases none of these parameters is established at the beginning of an experiment, we recommend to co-transfect the gene of interest fused to a fluorescent protein. This approach eliminates dependency of high transfection efficiency and does not much depend on protein half-life because in this approach the expression of the fusion protein is inhibited from the beginning. Using this approach the quality of the target sequence can rapidly be established.

12. To obtain high virus yield, optimization of the transfection protocol is critical. In many cases the ratio of DNA to transfection reagent needs to be optimized.

13. For target cell transduction, the supernatant of the transfected HEK293 cells is simply transferred to the target cells. Thus, the media need to be adapted to those of the target cells. HEK293 cells tolerate a wide range of growth media. For example if the target cells grow in RPMI1640, exchange the standard growth media (DMEM) with RPMI1640 so that virus is produced in media appropriate for the target cells.

14. Some cell types need high virus titers for efficient transduction. To concentrate the virus, two protocols can be used: virus precipitation and concentration by ultrafiltration.

Virus precipitation:

- Add PEG 6000 to 8.5 % and NaCl to 0.4 M final concentration.

- Store at 4 °C for 1.5 h, mixing every 15–30 min.

- Pellet at $7000 \times g$ using a precooled fixed-angle rotor for 15 min, 4 °C.
- Carefully remove supernatant (BSL2!).
- Resuspend pellet in a small volume of 50 mM Tris–HCl, pH 7.4 or PBS.
- Aliquot concentrated virus into cryotubes, freeze on dry ice, and store at −80 °C (or keep at 4 °C for short-term storage).

Virus ultrafiltration:
- Add virus-containing supernatant to an ultrafiltration device (cutoff: 100 kDa).
- Concentrate by centrifugation.

15. Target cell density is more critical for transduction by retroviral vectors which depend on mitosis to get access to the DNA for integration. Thus, cells have to be able to replicate for lentiviral vector integration. Although this is not critical for lentiviral transduction, cells should be proliferative to obtain most efficient transduction.

16. Polybrene facilitates the fusion of the virion with the target cell plasma membrane and thereby strongly enhances transduction efficiency. In most cell types polybrene can be used safely from 4–8 μg/ml.

17. Some cells types, e.g., Hct116 cells, are not readily transduced by the standard procedure. In the case of Hct116 cells, highly efficient transduction can be obtained by first trypsinizing and washing the cells before resuspending them in lentiviral vector-containing medium.

18. Lentiviral vector-containing supernatant can be kept at 4 °C for several days without significant loss of viral titer or up to months frozen at −80 °C. Freezing results in a ~50% drop of titer.

19. The excitation/emission maxima for GFP and dTomato are 488/509 and 554/581.

20. The induction kinetics of shRNA induction are usually very fast and for proteins with high cell turnover, e.g., cell cycle-regulated proteins, one can observe knockdown of protein expression already at 12 h after induction. A time period of 96 h at maximum induction should always yield a noticeable knockdown if the protein of interest has a half-life of less than 24 h.

21. The THT promoter is very sensitive to low amounts of tetracyclines. In many instances the promoter can already be activated by 10 ng/ml doxycycline. Due to the potentially toxic effects of tetracyclines on mitochondria, the lowest amount of doxycycline required to induce maximum RNAi needs to be determined.

22. Single-cell cloning is achieved by limiting dilution cloning. To this end, cells are counted and seeded in 96-well plates at a concentration of 0.5, 1, and 2 cells per well. After seeding, cells can be selected using antibiotics or analyzed for fluorescence protein expression using epifluorescence microscopy. If transduction efficiency is low, fluorescent protein can first be enriched by FACS, prior to limiting dilution cloning.

23. RNAi rescue experiments are essential to establish the specificity of the observed RNAi effect. In many cases such rescue experiments are, however, difficult to perform, e.g., because the overexpression levels of the proteins cannot be well controlled which might lead to overexpression artifacts. One solution to this problem is the use of tetracycline-inducible expression systems, which are compatible with the GLTR system. The RNAi-resistant target gene can be cloned downstream of the CMV-TO promoter such that addition of doxycycline not only induces RNAi towards the endogenous gene but also simultaneously induces the expression of the transgene.

For the rapid evaluation of rescue transgenes (wild type or mutants, tagged or untagged) it is recommended to select for an shRNA sequence in the non-translated regions. If overexpression rescue cannot be achieved due to toxicity or other issues it is possible to mutate the shRNA target sequence by CRISPR-based genome editing. In this case two efficient shRNAs can be compared for their phenotypes.

References

1. Boettcher M, McManus MT (2015) Choosing the right tool for the job: RNAi, TALEN, or CRISPR. Mol Cell 58:575–585

2. Mohr SE, Smith JA, Shamu CE, Neumuller RA, Perrimon N (2014) RNAi screening comes of age: improved techniques and complementary approaches. Nat Rev Mol Cell Biol 15:591–600

3. Ipsaro JJ, Joshua-Tor L (2015) From guide to target: molecular insights into eukaryotic RNA-interference machinery. Nat Struct Mol Biol 22:20–28

4. Brummelkamp TR, Bernards R, Agami R (2002) Stable suppression of tumorigenicity by virus-mediated RNA interference. Cancer Cell 2:243–247

5. Paddison PJ, Caudy AA, Bernstein E, Hannon GJ, Conklin DS (2002) Short hairpin RNAs (shRNAs) induce sequence-specific silencing in mammalian cells. Genes Dev 16:948–958

6. Fellmann C, Hoffmann T, Sridhar V, Hopfgartner B, Muhar M, Roth M, Lai DY, Barbosa IA, Kwon JS, Guan Y et al (2013) An optimized microRNA backbone for effective single-copy RNAi. Cell Rep 5:1704–1713

7. Bartel DP (2004) MicroRNAs: genomics, biogenesis, mechanism, and function. Cell 116:281–297

8. Gossen M, Bujard H (1992) Tight control of gene expression in mammalian cells by tetracycline- responsive promoters. Proc Natl Acad Sci U S A 89:5547–5551

9. Deuschle U, Meyer WK, Thiesen HJ (1995) Tetracycline-reversible silencing of eukaryotic promoters. Mol Cell Biol 15:1907–1914

10. Groner AC, Meylan S, Ciuffi A, Zangger N, Ambrosini G, Denervaud N, Bucher P, Trono

D (2010) KRAB-zinc finger proteins and KAP1 can mediate long-range transcriptional repression through heterochromatin spreading. PLoS Genet 6:e1000869

11. Sigl R, Ploner C, Shivalingaiah G, Kofler R, Geley S (2014) Development of a multipurpose GATEWAY-based lentiviral tetracycline-regulated conditional RNAi system (GLTR). PLoS One 9:e97764

12. Sakuma T, Barry MA, Ikeda Y (2012) Lentiviral vectors: basic to translational. Biochem J 443:603–618

13. Bartz SR, Vodicka MA (1997) Production of high-titer human immunodeficiency virus type 1 pseudotyped with vesicular stomatitis virus glycoprotein. Methods 12:337–342

14. Donnelly ML, Hughes LE, Luke G, Mendoza H, ten DE, Gani D, Ryan MD (2001) The 'cleavage' activities of foot-and-mouth disease virus 2A site-directed mutants and naturally occurring '2A-like' sequences. J Gen Virol 82:1027–1041

15. Kim JH, Lee SR, Li LH, Park HJ, Park JH, Lee KY, Kim MK, Shin BA, Choi SY (2011) High cleavage efficiency of a 2A peptide derived from porcine teschovirus-1 in human cell lines, zebrafish and mice. PLoS One 6:e18556

16. Pei Y, Tuschl T (2006) On the art of identifying effective and specific siRNAs. Nat Methods 3:670–676

17. Ikeda Y, Takeuchi Y, Martin F, Cosset FL, Mitrophanous K, Collins M (2003) Continuous high-titer HIV-1 vector production. Nat Biotechnol 21:569–572

18. Swift S, Lorens J, Achacoso P, Nolan GP (2001) Rapid production of retroviruses for efficient gene delivery to mammalian cells using 293T cell-based systems. Curr Protoc Immunol. Chapter 10

Chapter 11

Lentiviral Vectors for the Engineering of Implantable Cells Secreting Recombinant Antibodies

Aurélien Lathuilière and Bernard L. Schneider

Abstract

The implantation of genetically modified cells is considered for the chronic delivery of therapeutic recombinant proteins in vivo. In the context of gene therapy, the genetic engineering of cells faces two main challenges. First, it is critical to generate expandable cell sources, which can maintain stable high productivity of the recombinant protein of interest over time, both in culture and after transplantation. In addition, gene transfer techniques need to be developed to engineer cells synthetizing complex polypeptides, such as recombinant monoclonal antibodies, to broaden the range of potential therapeutic applications. Here, we provide a workflow for the use of lentiviral vectors as a flexible tool to generate antibody-producing cells. In particular, lentiviral vectors can be used to genetically engineer the cell types compatible with encapsulation devices protecting the implanted cells from the host immune system. Detailed methods are provided for the design and production of lentiviral vectors, optimization of cell transduction, as well as for the quantification and quality control of the produced recombinant antibody.

Key words Recombinant antibodies, Chronic delivery, Ex vivo gene therapy, Cell transplantation, Cell encapsulation

1 Introduction

1.1 Gene Therapy for Antibody Delivery

Gene therapy is a promising alternative for the continuous delivery of recombinant proteins, particularly when the protein has to be chronically administered over a long period of time, or in poorly accessible sites such as the central nervous system (CNS). However, recombinant proteins can be made of complex macromolecular assemblies. This raises specific challenges for technologies used to deliver genes in mammalian cells, in particular in the context of gene therapy. The use of lentiviral vectors for the genetic engineering of dividing cell sources provides a means to address some of these challenges.

As an example of such complex recombinant proteins, monoclonal antibodies (mAb) are considered as a very successful class of biopharmaceuticals. Since the first marketed antibody in 1986,

Maurizio Federico (ed.), *Lentiviral Vectors and Exosomes as Gene and Protein Delivery Tools*, Methods in Molecular Biology, vol. 1448, DOI 10.1007/978-1-4939-3753-0_11, © Springer Science+Business Media New York 2016

about 50 different mAbs have been approved in Europe or the USA [1]. This extraordinary success has mainly relied on incremental technical breakthroughs that have allowed to engineer molecules with lower immunogenicity, better safety profiles and improved pharmacokinetic properties [2]. Recombinant antibodies have very high affinity and specificity for their targets, which allows to selectively interfere with various pathologic pathways implicated in cancer, autoimmunity, or neurodegenerative disorders. Most mAb-based treatments require repeated high dosage administration, often via bolus intravenous injection. The long-term mAb treatments proposed for chronic conditions have significant limitations, which include the need for medical intervention. Significant direct and indirect costs may also dramatically increase the economic burden on healthcare systems, particularly for Alzheimer's disease, a highly prevalent chronic disorder that may require years of mAb treatment. In addition, therapeutic efficacy may be limited in poorly accessible organs or tissue using current techniques for bolus mAb administration. Hence, the development of alternative delivery technologies appears as an attractive solution to extend the range of potential mAb-therapies, and facilitate the access to such treatments. The use of gene therapy, using either viral vectors for in vivo gene delivery, or cellular implants genetically modified ex vivo for mAb production, has recently gained more attention as an alternative for the continuous administration of mAb [3, 4]. Cellular implants genetically modified ex vivo for mAb production have the key advantage that the dose and the quality of the recombinant antibody can be controlled before the treatment is delivered to the patient. Therefore, we here focus on this approach, and describe detailed methods for genetic engineering of the cells using lentiviral vectors.

1.2 Encapsulated Cell Implantation

Because grafted cells from non-self origin are rapidly cleared by the host immune system in the absence of immunosuppression, the macro-encapsulation of cells within a permeable polymer membrane has been proposed. The permeable porous membrane provides a physical barrier that prevents any direct contact between the grafted cells secreting the therapeutic protein of interest (e.g., a mAb) and the host immune cells (reviewed in [3]). This technique can be used to (1) protect allogeneic cells from the host immune system and (2) confine the implanted cells in a device that can be surgically removed to halt the treatment. The allogeneic transplantation of cells using the encapsulated cell technology (ECT), is a promising approach for mAb delivery, the success of which mainly depends on two technical aspects: (1) the effective design of an encapsulation device allowing for the long-term survival of the grafted cells [5]; (2) the generation of stable cell lines which secrete high levels of recombinant protein and can survive long term in the capsule.

The present chapter is describing methods for generating antibody-secreting cell lines that are suitable for ECT. The need for long-term mAb delivery applicable to chronic diseases implies that engineered cells have to survive and maintain stable protein expression over at least several months. The technology is typically based on dividing cells than can be easily expanded and continue to proliferate inside the device, albeit at a lower rate. Phenotypic stability and strong contact inhibition are desired features for the cell of choice. As metabolic conditions inside the device are restrictive, only few cell types are compatible with ECT. In addition, it is important to generate a cell source, which has the capacity to stably express high levels of functional recombinant antibodies. Therefore, it is critical to develop effective techniques for genetic engineering applicable to ECT. Here, we describe the use of lentiviral vectors for cell transduction, in order to expand the repertoire of renewable cell lines that are compatible with ECT for the long-term production of therapeutic mAbs in vivo [6].

1.3 Lentiviral Vectors for Genetic Engineering of Renewable Cell Sources

Lentiviral vectors (LV) are widely used for genetic engineering because they are considered a very efficient system for stable integration of genetic material into cell lines, stem cells and primary cell cultures. One of the main features of classical lentiviral systems is their ability to integrate transgene copies into transcriptionally active regions of the cell genome, both in dividing and postmitotic cells [7, 8]. The packaging capacity of LV is close to 10 kb, which makes this vector suitable for most applications, including the transfer of genes encoding full IgG antibodies. The latest LV generations carry multiple targeted modifications that minimize the genomic content in viral sequences, and inactivate the replication capability of the virus [9]. Importantly, the vector does not lead to the expression of any viral gene in the host cell, which allows for long-term transgene expression in immunocompetent recipients. Overall, the biosafety profile of LV has been largely improved [10], allowing for their utilization in several clinical trials [11].

As LV lead to effective integration of DNA sequences in the host cell genome, transgene expression is very stable over cell divisions and during differentiation. Therefore, the use of LV has been widely developed to genetically modify various types of stem cells [12–14]. Moreover, LV-mediated gene transfer has also been reported for the genetic engineering of mammalian cell lines to stably produce recombinant proteins in bioreactors [15].

1.4 Lentiviral Vectors as a Tool to Generate Cell Lines for Recombinant Antibody Production

Immunoglobulin G (IgG) is the most common type of recombinant antibody produced by genetic engineering. IgGs are heterotetrameric polypeptides composed of two light chains (LC) and two heavy chains (HC), which are linked by disulfide bonds. Alternative antibody formats have been proposed for certain applications. These include antibody fragments such as scFv, Fab fragments or diabodies (reviewed in [16]), which can often be produced from a single polypeptidic chain. To be properly folded and assembled, full IgGs are processed in the endoplasmic reticulum (ER) of eukaryotic cells, via interaction with various protein chaperones [17]. LC and HC are normally in a 1:1 stoichiometric ratio. When not associated with the LC, the HC is sequestered inside the ER and induces unfolded protein response with subsequent toxic effects [18]. Therefore, the ratio HC to LC is a critical factor to optimize antibody production, and it was demonstrated that an excess of intracellular LC is advantageous for high yield secretion [19].

In order to optimize antibody production, it is therefore preferred to separately control the transduction of the sequences encoding the IgG LC and HC using two separate LV vectors, as described in the current protocol. By independently controlling the level of expression of each protein chain, it is possible to determine the LC:HC expression ratio leading to highest expression of the full antibody. However, one should take into account that each population of cells transduced with the mix of the two LV will contain individual cell clones with different LC:HC ratios. To further optimize productivity, optimal cell clones can be isolated in a second step. In some conditions, it might be preferred to use a single LV encoding both the LC and HC. Single vector designs allowing the expression of two proteins are discussed in **Note 1**.

In order to generate stable cell lines secreting high amount of the antibody of interest, the major steps of the workflow comprise LV cloning, production and titration, cell transduction, clone sorting, assessment of antibody secretion level as well as antibody quality control.

The sorting of clonal cell lines from the population of transduced cells is useful for several reasons. The culture of clonal cells that are genetically identical and phenotypically stable ensures long-term steady expression of the recombinant protein. Using clonal selection, it is also possible to identify individual cell clones, which may display high secretion rates of the recombinant protein, even higher than the average productivity measured in the original pool of transduced cells. Moreover, clonal cell lines can show specific features that are superior to the original pool of cells, such as increased survival when implanted using ECT. In the absence of any reporter system for transgene expression to guide the selection process, clonal cells can be simply isolated using the limiting dilution method.

The quality control of the genetically engineered cells may vary according to the intended application. In the context of generating cell lines for high-level antibody production by ECT, we propose to assess (1) the number of integrated transgene copies per cell, which is a direct measurement of LV transduction efficacy and (2) the stability of antibody expression over time.

The production of a complex assembly of polypeptide chains such as an IgG antibody, depends on many factors. Obviously, the number of inserted transgene copies in the LV-modified cells will first determine the transgene expression level, but the site of transgene integration in the cell genome will also have a major impact on the transgene transcriptional activity. Finally, as mentioned above, the stoichiometric ratio between the LC and HC, as well as the cell's ability to properly assemble the final IgG molecule and make the needed posttranslational modifications are as well critical. Therefore, the most appropriate method to assess cell clones is to measure cell productivity and verify the quality of the secreted antibody. In case the recombinant antibodies and the cell used to produce this antibody are from different species (e.g., a human IgG expressed by mouse cells), or when using cell sources that do not normally secrete functional antibodies (e.g., myoblast cells), it is recommended to perform a thorough quality control of the antibody produced by analyzing antibody glycosylation patterns using mass spectrometry (*see* ref. [6]). Indeed, this analysis will be useful to predict antibody efficacy, as it is recognized that the glycosylation pattern can affect antibody stability, functionality or immunogenicity [20–22]. A schematic workflow for generating antibody-secreting cell lines using LV is shown in Fig. 1.

2 Materials

2.1 Production of Lentiviral Vectors

1. Cells. HEK 293 T (American Type Culture Collection (ATCC®)).

2. Plasmids. pMD2.G: plasmid encoding the vesicular stomatitis virus G envelope (Addgene); pCMVΔR8.92: packaging plasmid encoding all the viral elements needed in trans; pRSV-Rev: plasmid encoding the Rev protein of HIV-1 (Addgene); pRRLSIN.cPPT.PGK-GFP.WPRE: transfer plasmid containing an internal cassette for the cloning of the gene of interest (Addgene). This third-generation lentiviral system has been described in [23].

3. Dishes for tissue culture. 24.5 × 24.5 cm (500 cm²) cell factories (Nunclon™Δ, NUNC A/S, Roskilde, Denmark).

4. Culture media. Dulbecco's Modified Eagle's Medium; fetal bovine serum (FBS); EpiSerf (Gibco®); penicillin–streptomycin 10,000 U/ml.

5. Trypsinization medium. Trypsin–EDTA in PBS 1:250 (0.05 %/0.02 %) without Ca^{++} and Mg^{++}; store at 4 °C.

6. Other reagents for LV production. Benzonase (Novagen, used at 1 U/ml final concentration); phosphate-buffered saline (PBS); Bovine serum albumin fraction V.

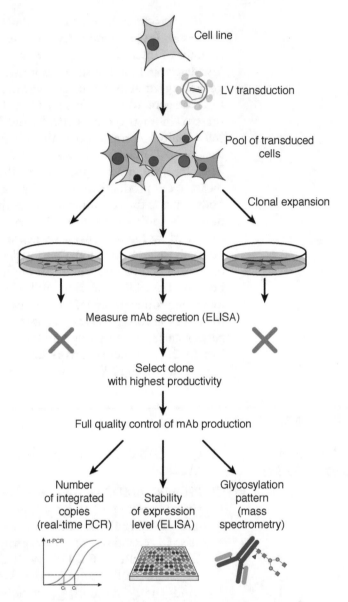

Fig. 1 Schematic workflow for the generation of antibody-secreting cell lines using lentiviral vectors. A selected cell line is transduced by LV encoding the antibody LC and HC. Individual clones with high secretion rate are isolated. The production of the recombinant antibody by the implantable cell line is assessed both quantitatively and qualitatively

7. Transfection mix. $CaCl_2$ 0.5 M (73.5 g $CaCl_2$ $2H_2O$; complete to 500 ml with H_2O); to prepare 2× HBS: 28 ml 5 M NaCl, 50 ml 1 M HEPES, 750 µl 1 M Na_2HPO_4, complete to 500 ml with H_2O, if needed adjust to pH 7.1 with NaOH; aliquot and store at −20 °C.

8. Vector concentration and storage. Polystyrene tubes; 0.22 μm filter; centrifuge tubes: 30 ml thinwall polyallomer *konical™* tubes (Beckman Coulter); ultracentrifuge L-90 K (Beckman Coulter), equipped with a SW28 swing-bucket rotor (Beckman Coulter); 1.7 ml low retention Eppendorf tubes for storage (Maximum Recovery, Axygen).

2.2   Cell Transduction and Antibody Production Quantification

1. Culture medium and reagents. Use culture medium recommended for the selected cell type. For C2C12 myoblasts, cells are grown in DMEM supplemented with 10% FBS and 1% penicillin–streptomycin. Hanks Balanced Salt Solution (HBSS). Trypsin–EDTA in PBS 1:250 (0.05%/0.02%) without Ca^{++} and Mg^{++}.

2. Petri dishes; 24-well, 12-well, 6-well plates; 25–300 cm^2 culture dishes.

3. Protamine sulfate; stock solution at 4 mg/ml in distilled water, 0.22 μm filtered. Store frozen.

4. Automated cell counter (Countess®, Invitrogen) or equivalent system such as Neubauer chambers.

2.3   Evaluation of the Number of Integrated Transgene Copies

1. Cell culture. 6-well petri dishes, HBSS.

2. Trypsinization medium. Trypsin–EDTA in PBS 1:250 (0.05%/ 0.02%) without Ca^{++} and Mg^{++}. Store at 4 °C.

3. RNAse A dissolved in water at 20 mg/ml.

4. Nucleospin Tissue kit (Macherey-Nagel # 740952.10).

5. Rotor-Gene Probe PCR kit (Qiagen # 204372).

6. Set of real-time PCR primers (forward and reverse primers, probe) for a transgene-specific sequence inside the vector genome (*see* **Note 2**).

7. Rotor-Gene Q cycler (Qiagen).

8. Strips of 4 four tubes for real-time PCR (Qiagen # 981103).

9. Linearized LV plasmid with known DNA concentration to be used as standard.

3   Methods

3.1   Lentiviral Vectors Production and Titration

1. Carefully select LV construct according to **Note 3** and clone cDNA encoding either LC or HC into LV according to available restriction sites.

2. One day before transfection, plate HEK 293 T cells at a density of 4^{E}7 cells in 500 cm^2 dish for tissue culture, in 100 ml DMEM supplemented with 10% FBS and 1% penicillin–streptomycin (*see* **Note 4**).

3. One day later, in order to transfect HEK 293 T cells using calcium phosphate precipitation, prepare DNA for each cell factory as follows. Add to a 50 ml polystyrene tube: 130 µg pCMVΔR8.92, 30 µg pRSV-Rev, 37.5 µg pMD2G, 130 µg pRRLSIN.cPPT.PGK-LC/HC.WPRE with 2.5 ml CaCl₂ 0.5 M.

4. Complete with sterile distilled water to a final volume of 5 ml.

5. Prepare a second tube with 5 ml of 2× HBS.

6. Add 2× HBS dropwise to the mix DNA + CaCl₂ + H₂O, while continuously shaking the recipient tube.

7. After 10 min, gently add the precipitate solution to the cells.

8. Transfer the cells in biosafety level 2 (BSL2) laboratory and incubate at 37 °C, 5 % CO₂ for 6 h.

9. Aspirate the media and replace by 70 ml EpiSerf media containing benzonase at a final concentration of 1 U/ml (the EpiSerf culture medium does not contain any antibiotic).

10. 48 h after transfection, harvest the cell supernatant containing the vector suspension in 50 ml polystyrene tubes.

11. Centrifuge the supernatant for 3 min at 1500 rpm ($425 \times g$) to eliminate cell debris, and pass the supernatant through a 0.22 µm filter.

12. In order to concentrate the lentiviral particles, ultracentrifuge the supernatant in two conical polyallomer tubes at $65,000 \times g$, 4 °C for 1 h 30′ in the SW28 rotor.

13. Aspirate the supernatant and add in each tube 1 ml of PBS/0.5 % BSA.

14. Let the pellet incubate for 1 h on ice.

15. Resuspend the virus by pipetting the liquid up and down.

16. Pool the vector suspension from both tubes, carefully rinse the tubes, and complete the suspension volume to 3 ml with PBS/0.5 % BSA.

17. Make 100 µl aliquots of the 10× concentrated vector suspension in low retention tubes. Avoid collecting clumps of vector that are not properly resuspended. Freeze rapidly the vector suspension in dry ice mixed with 70 % ethanol. The aliquots can be stored at −80 °C for several years without significant loss in LV infectivity. Freeze-thaw cycles should be avoided to prevent any decrease of LV efficacy.

18. Titrate LV according to the preferred method (*see* **Note 5**).

3.2 Lentiviral Transduction of Cells for Recombinant Antibody Production

The following protocol describes the use of LV vectors for the transduction of cell populations to induce the production of recombinant IgG antibodies [6].

1. Carefully select a cell line according to the type of application (*see* **Note 6**).

2. On day 0, plate the cells in 24-well plates. Cell density is adapted to obtain 70% confluence the following day. Prepare two extra wells to determine the number of cells present in the well at the time of LV infection.

3. On day 1, determine the number of cells present in the extra wells, in order to accordingly calculate the amount of LV to be added for effective transduction. LV suspensions encoding either the HC or LC are serially diluted to obtain incremental multiplicity of infection (MOI) values, which can be determined according to the number of cells per well (*see* **Note 7**).

4. Thaw LV stock suspensions, and mix them with conditioned culture medium. Adapt the volume of LV and conditioned medium to obtain the proper MOI. Add the LV suspension to the well and adjust the final volume of medium to 250 μl per 24-well (*see* **Note 8**).

5. Incubate cells at 37 °C/5% CO_2.

6. On day 2, add 250 μl of fresh culture medium in each well.

7. On day 3, aspirate the medium, wash cells with 1 ml HBSS and add fresh culture medium.

8. During the following days, continue to feed the cells. Trypsinize the cells when they reach confluence and progressively increase the size of the wells to finally transfer the cells into 10-cm petri dishes. When large amounts of cells are obtained, generate a cell bank including cells at low number of passages, which can be kept frozen in liquid nitrogen after suspension in culture medium supplemented with 10% dimethylsulfoxide (DMSO) (*see* **Note 9**).

3.3 Isolation of Cell Clones

1. Harvest the LV-transduced cells by trypsinization.

2. Count the cells using an automated cell counter.

3. Dilute cell suspension in culture medium at a concentration of 2 cells/ml.

4. Add 200 μl of cell suspension in each well of a cell culture-treated flat bottom 96-well plate (on average, there should be 0.4 cells per well).

5. Grow the cells in regular culture conditions (37 °C/5% CO_2). For cells that are difficult to maintain at low density, it is recommended to regularly add conditioned culture medium to each well.

6. 8 h after plating, observe each well using an inverted phase contrast microscope. Discard wells containing two or more cells.

7. Replace culture medium every 2–3 days. As soon as clonal cell populations are grown to confluence, transfer the cells into incrementally larger wells until the cells can be maintained by regular passaging in 10-cm petri dishes (*see* **Note 10**).

8. Once pools of transduced cells are sufficiently expanded, use a fraction of the cells for the characterization of integrated transgene copy numbers and IgG secretion rate.

3.4 Assessment of the Number of Integrated Transgene Copies

1. Grow the selected transduced cell clones in 6-well plates.

2. Once cells have reached confluence, wash with HBSS. Add 1 ml trypsinization medium and incubate for 5 min at room temperature.

3. Neutralize the trypsin with culture medium and collect the cells in a 1.5 ml tube.

4. Centrifuge 5 min at 2000 rpm ($400 \times g$). Aspirate supernatant.

5. Resuspend the cells in 40 µl PBS + 10 µl 20 mg/ml RNAse A and vortex to dissociate the cell pellet.

6. Perform genomic DNA extraction with Nucleospin Tissue kit according to manufacturer's instructions.

7. Determine DNA concentration by measuring absorbance at 260 nm.

8. Prepare standard reactions using DNA from linearized shuttle plasmids containing either the IgG LC or HC cDNA. Determine the number of double-stranded plasmid copies using the DNA concentration, according to the following formula: copies per g of plasmid = $1/([\text{size in bp}]*1.096^{\text{E}}\text{-}21 \text{ g/bp})$.

9. Prepare five 1:10 serial dilutions of linearized LV plasmid to obtain standard concentrations of 10^7, 10^6, 10^5, 10^4, and 10^3 plasmid copies/µl.

10. Prepare a genomic DNA standard extracted from the cells of interest. From the measured mass of genomic DNA, calculate the number of copies using the following formulae: number of haploid *human* genome copies = DNA mass/3.3 pg; number of haploid *mouse* genome copies = DNA mass/3.0 pg.

11. Prepare 3 serial dilutions of a genomic DNA sample (50–150 ng of genomic DNA per PCR reaction) to set the standard curve for determination of genomic DNA abundance.

12. Prepare real-time PCR reactions according to standard protocols. Here is an example with the Rotor-Gene Probe PCR kit. For each reaction: forward primer 1.6 µl (final concentration 800 nM), reverse primer 1.6 µl (final concentration 800 nM), probe 1.6 µl (final concentration 200 nM), Rotor Gene 2× master mix 8 µl, DNA sample 2 µl and 1.2 µl of water to reach a final volume of 16 µl.

13. Run samples on a Rotor Gene Q cycler with the following cycling conditions: 3 min 95 °C, 40 cycles of 3 s 95 °C, 10 s 60 °C.

14. Measure fluorescence in the adequate channel, according to the dye/quencher combination used for the TaqMan® probe.

15. For each reaction, determine the threshold cycle (Ct) and calculate the number of transgene and genome copies in the sample according to the standards measured in parallel reactions. The number of transgene copies per cell (n) is calculated using the formula $n = 2*$[number of LV transgene copies]/[cell gDNA copies].

3.5 Assessment of Antibody Secretion Rate

1. Plate LV-infected cells in a 6-well plate. For each cell line, perform the assay in triplicates.

2. Chose cell density to obtain 80–100 % confluence the following day.

3. One day after plating, aspirate the culture medium, wash the cells with HBSS and add 2.5 ml of fresh culture medium.

4. Incubate the cells for 1 h in regular culture conditions (37 °C/ 5 % CO_2).

5. Collect the conditioned culture media in low retention tubes, and place the tubes immediately on ice.

6. Count the cells in each well using an automated cell counter.

7. Quantify absolute IgG amounts present in the conditioned medium using an adequate ELISA assay based on the IgG's binding ability to its specific antigen (*see* **Note 11** and Fig. 3).

8. Calculate IgG production yield in [pg/cell/24 h]. Perform this measurement on populations of LV-infected cells as well as individual cell clones.

9. Repeat this assay several times over weeks or even months in culture to verify the stability of the IgG secretion rate (*see* **Note 12**).

4 Notes

1. When the simultaneous expression of two transgenes is required, different systems have been developed in order to drive the expression of the two genes from a single LV (bicistronic vectors). One strategy is to drive expression of the two different cDNAs using separate expression cassettes [24]. In this setting, it is preferred to have the two cassettes in opposite orientations (head-to-head). This orientation allows for LV production (which is blocked if poly A sequences are included in the vector), and avoids transcriptional interference between the two cassettes. Efforts have been made to generate bidirectional promoter systems that drive transgene expression in opposite

directions [25]. Another option is use a single expression cassette to transcribe a bicistronic element composed of two cDNAs separated by an internal ribosome entry sites (IRES). It should however be anticipated that the level of expression of the second sequence will be lower. Alternatively, it is also possible to encode a single transcript and translate a single polypeptide containing an internal viral 2A self-processing peptide sequence. This peptide will induce the immediate "cleavage" of the protein due to ribosome skipping. The later strategy allows for the 1:1 stoichiometric expression of the two separate IgG chains [26].

2. Design a set of real-time PCR primers (forward and reverse primers, probe) for a transgene-specific sequence inside the vector genome. Primers can be designed using dedicated online tools (see for instance URL http://eu.idtdna.com/primerquest/home/index). Probe-based TaqMan® assays are preferred for their higher specificity. Nevertheless, it is also possible to use SYBR green to detect the PCR product amplified using a pair of specific forward and reverse primers. When two vectors are used to transduce the cells (e.g., LV encoding the LC and HC), specific primer sets should be designed for each of them. Here is an example of a primer set specific to the woodchuck posttranscriptional regulatory element (WPRE), which is often included in LV constructs: forward 5'-CCG TTG TCA GGC AAC GTG-3'; reverse 5'-AGC TGA CAG GTG GTG GCA AT-3'; probe 5'-FAM-TGC TGA CGC AAC CCC CAC TGG T-TAMRA-3'.

   An additional primer set is designed to measure the abundance of a single-copy gene in the haploid genome and which will be used to assess the number of host cell genome copies. A primer set for human albumin is provided as an example: forward 5'-TGA AAC ATA CGT TCC CAA AGA GTT T-3'; reverse 5'-CTC TCC TTC TCA GAA AGT GTG CAT AT-3'; probe 5'-FAM-TGC TGA AAC ATT CAC CTT CCA TGC AGA-TAMRA-3'.

3. Various LV systems have been described in the literature and are currently available. The most important aspect to take into account when choosing a vector for cell engineering is the enhancer/promoter, which drives transgene expression. When considering LV for recombinant protein expression, the expression level and its stability over time are two critical variables to carefully monitor. The promoter will be selected according to the targeted cell type. The most effective constitutive promoters that drive strong expression in a given cell type can be identified by flow cytometry using a fluorescent reporter protein. Promoters derived from viral components can usually induce high expression levels. However, they are prone to expression shutdown probably due to cellular protection mechanisms [27,

28]. The use of the human phosphoglycerate kinase (PGK) constitutive promoter is of particular interest when developing cell lines for encapsulated transplantation because it is further activated under hypoxic conditions through interaction with hypoxia-inducible-factor-1α (HIF-1α) [29]. Here, methods using the pRRLSIN.cPPT.PGK-GFP.WPRE LV are described. The shuttle DNA constructs used to produce this vector are represented in Fig. 2.

4. On the day of transfection the cells should be 50–70% confluent. If cell density is too low, virus yield will be significantly decreased.

5. Various methods have been proposed to assess the efficacy of LV preparations and are now routinely performed (for review, *see* ref. [30]). The quantification of the concentration of the p24 viral capsid antigen using a commercial ELISA assay provides an estimate of the amount of vector particles in a given suspension volume, which is useful for the monitoring of LV production efficiency. However, p24 concentration overestimates the

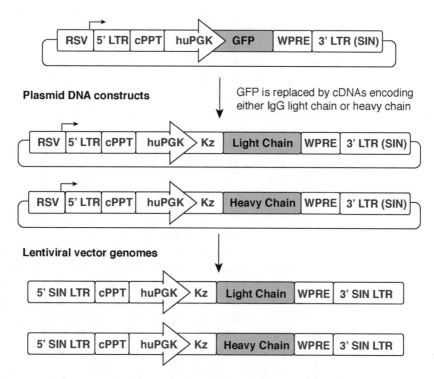

Fig. 2 Lentiviral vector constructs used for antibody production. The DNA constructs encoding the antibody LC and HC are derived from the pRRLSIN.cPPT.PGK-GFP.WPRE shuttle plasmid. The LV genome produced from this construct contains two self-inactivating long terminal repeats. Abbreviations: RSV Rous Sarcoma Virus promoter; LTR long terminal repeats; SIN self-inactivating; cPPT central polypurine tract; huPGK human phosphoglycerate kinase 1 promoter; Kz optimized Kozak sequence; WPRE woodchuck hepatitis posttranscriptional regulatory element

functional vector titer as it also measures free p24 or empty viral particles. Therefore, it is preferred to measure a biological titer reflecting the infectivity of the LV batch. The assessment of LV infectivity, often expressed as transducing units (TU), is obtained by real-time PCR to quantify the amount of integrated vector copies in the genome of a standard cell line (HeLa cells) which is permissive to LV infection (see detailed protocol in [31]).

6. The major role of ECT is to provide immunoprotection by preventing cell-to-cell contacts with host immune cells. Using this technology, genetically modified cells can be transplanted in immunocompetent allogeneic recipients without the need for any immunosuppressive treatment. Hence, cells from the same species as the recipient should be used for ECT implantation in tissues or organs that are not immune-privileged. The continuous delivery of mAb by ECT implies that engineered cells have to survive and maintain stable mAb expression over the whole period of implantation, which can last from several weeks to more than 1 year in rodents. Several factors must be considered when selecting a cell type for encapsulation, including the ease of genetic engineering. Adequate cells should be able to produce functional exogenous proteins with appropriate posttranslational modifications, and sustain prolonged secretion of the recombinant protein, even in the restrictive metabolic conditions that prevail inside the ECT device. Additionally, it is preferred to select cell sources that retain phenotypic characteristics over time. It is recommended to use cell lines with strong contact inhibition, as they will stop expanding inside the ECT device once it is fully colonized. Adherent cell lines necessitate the implementation of an artificial supporting matrix inside the encapsulation device. Adequate cell lines include for example the C2C12 mouse myoblast cell line (ATCC # CRL 1722) and the human retinal epithelial cell line ARPE-19 (ATCC # CRL 2302).

7. Multiplicity of infection (MOI) corresponds to the ratio of viral particles which can transduce a given cell type (TU) to the number of target cells present in the well. The probability of infection after LV transduction follows a Poisson distribution. At an MOI of 1, about 65% of cells are infected. In order to enhance the proportion of infected cells, or further increase the average amount of integrated transgene copies per cell, the cells can be exposed to higher MOIs. In order to maximize transgene expression, cells should be exposed to incremental doses of vector. The optimal dose will be selected by determining the highest possible amount of vector that does not cause any significant toxicity to the cells.

8. It is important to decrease the volume of medium in order to maximize cell exposure to the vector suspension. Depending upon the targeted cell type, the culture medium can be

supplemented with 5 µg/ml protamine sulfate, a cationic peptide which is used to enhance LV transduction efficiency. The addition of protamine sulfate into the culture medium enhances the LV transduction efficiency only in certain cell lines. For instance, we have observed that protamine sulfate substantially increases LV transduction efficiency on mouse C2C12 myoblasts.

9. Expand cells for at least 10 days after LV infection (>6.7 population doubling corresponding to 100-fold amplification) in order to ensure that non-integrated transgene copies are eliminated before performing any analysis. It is also critical to verify that there is no shedding of viral particles from the transduced cell populations before performing any routine experiment in BSL1 lab using LV-infected cell lines. It is therefore recommended to measure by ELISA the presence of the p24 antigen in the conditioned culture medium of LV-infected cells, several passages after exposure to the viral vector.

10. It is important to expand individual cell clones until the amount of cells is sufficient to perform assays for the quantification of the antibody secretion rate.

11. It is important to verify that the antibody produced by the LV-infected cells is functional, i.e., is able to bind the antigen. Therefore, we recommend to quantify the amount of antibody produced by LV-infected cells using a sandwich ELISA assay capturing the secreted mAb via its binding to the specific antigen. Possible formats are based either on wells directly coated with the antigen or via binding of the antigen to a primary antibody which does not recognize the same epitope as the antibody to be measured. Possible ELISA strategies are schematized in Fig. 3.

12. We have found that LV-infected C2C12 myoblasts can maintain stable expression of a recombinant IgG for >8 weeks under regular culture conditions, or >10 months when implanted in an ECT device.

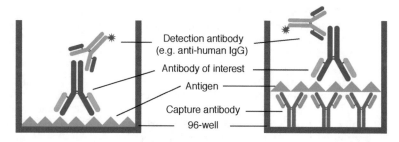

Fig. 3 Schematic representation of functional ELISA assays based on antigen binding used to quantify antibody concentration. Antigen is either directly coated on the well or bound to a capture antibody. Antigen binding is used to fix the recombinant antibody of interest, the concentration of which is later measured using an isotype-specific or species-specific secondary antibody for immunodetection

Acknowledgments

This work was supported by the Swiss Commission for Technology and Innovation (CTI, grant no. 14666.1 PFLS-LS). The authors thank Fabienne Pidoux for her expert help in establishing protocols for production of lentiviral vectors.

References

1. Ecker DM, Jones SD, Levine HL (2015) The therapeutic monoclonal antibody market. MAbs 7:9–14

2. Nelson AL, Dhimolea E, Reichert JM (2010) Development trends for human monoclonal antibody therapeutics. Nat Rev Drug Discov 9:767–774

3. Lathuiliere A, Mach N, Schneider BL (2015) Encapsulated cellular implants for recombinant protein delivery and therapeutic modulation of the immune system. Int J Mol Sci 16:10578–10600

4. Guijarro-Munoz I, Compte M, Alvarez-Vallina L et al (2013) Antibody gene therapy: getting closer to clinical application? Curr Gene Ther 13:282–290

5. Lathuiliere A, Cosson S, Lutolf MP et al (2014) A high-capacity cell macroencapsulation system supporting the long-term survival of genetically engineered allogeneic cells. Biomaterials 35:779–791

6. Lathuiliere A, Bohrmann B, Kopetzki E et al (2014) Genetic engineering of cell lines using lentiviral vectors to achieve antibody secretion following encapsulated implantation. Biomaterials 35:792–802

7. Naldini L, Blomer U, Gallay P et al (1996) In vivo gene delivery and stable transduction of nondividing cells by a lentiviral vector. Science 272:263–267

8. Schroder AR, Shinn P, Chen H et al (2002) HIV-1 integration in the human genome favors active genes and local hotspots. Cell 110:521–529

9. Zufferey R, Nagy D, Mandel RJ et al (1997) Multiply attenuated lentiviral vector achieves efficient gene delivery in vivo. Nat Biotechnol 15:871–875

10. Zufferey R, Dull T, Mandel RJ et al (1998) Self-inactivating lentivirus vector for safe and efficient in vivo gene delivery. J Virol 72:9873–9880

11. Escors D, Breckpot K (2010) Lentiviral vectors in gene therapy: their current status and future potential. Arch Immunol Ther Exp 58:107–119

12. Cherry SR, Biniszkiewicz D, van Parijs L et al (2000) Retroviral expression in embryonic stem cells and hematopoietic stem cells. Mol Cell Biol 20:7419–7426

13. Capowski EE, Schneider BL, Ebert AD et al (2007) Lentiviral vector-mediated genetic modification of human neural progenitor cells for ex vivo gene therapy. J Neurosci Methods 163:338–349

14. Matrai J, Chuah MK, VandenDriessche T (2010) Recent advances in lentiviral vector development and applications. Mol Ther 18:477–490

15. Oberbek A, Matasci M, Hacker DL et al (2011) Generation of stable, high-producing CHO cell lines by lentiviral vector-mediated gene transfer in serum-free suspension culture. Biotechnol Bioeng 108:600–610

16. Frenzel A, Hust M, Schirrmann T (2013) Expression of recombinant antibodies. Front Immunol 4:217

17. Melnick J, Dul JL, Argon Y (1994) Sequential interaction of the chaperones BiP and GRP94 with immunoglobulin chains in the endoplasmic reticulum. Nature 370:373–375

18. Zhou P, Ma X, Iyer L et al (2014) One siRNA pool targeting the lambda constant region stops lambda light-chain production and causes terminal endoplasmic reticulum stress. Blood 123:3440–3451

19. Schlatter S, Stansfield SH, Dinnis DM et al (2005) On the optimal ratio of heavy to light chain genes for efficient recombinant antibody production by CHO cells. Biotechnol Prog 21:122–133

20. Krapp S, Mimura Y, Jefferis R et al (2003) Structural analysis of human IgG-Fc glycoforms reveals a correlation between glycosylation and structural integrity. J Mol Biol 325:979–989

21. Mimura Y, Sondermann P, Ghirlando R et al (2001) Role of oligosaccharide residues of IgG1-Fc in Fc gamma RIIb binding. J Biol Chem 276:45539–45547

22. Chung CH, Mirakhur B, Chan E et al (2008) Cetuximab-induced anaphylaxis and IgE specific for galactose-alpha-1,3-galactose. N Engl J Med 358:1109–1117

23. Dull T, Zufferey R, Kelly M et al (1998) A third-generation lentivirus vector with a conditional packaging system. J Virol 72:8463–8471

24. Yu X, Zhan X, D'Costa J et al (2003) Lentiviral vectors with two independent internal promoters transfer high-level expression of multiple transgenes to human hematopoietic stem-progenitor cells. Mol Ther 7:827–838

25. Amendola M, Venneri MA, Biffi A et al (2005) Coordinate dual-gene transgenesis by lentiviral vectors carrying synthetic bidirectional promoters. Nat Biotechnol 23:108–116

26. Szymczak AL, Workman CJ, Wang Y et al (2004) Correction of multi-gene deficiency in vivo using a single 'self-cleaving' 2A peptide-based retroviral vector. Nat Biotechnol 22:589–594

27. Loser P, Jennings GS, Strauss M et al (1998) Reactivation of the previously silenced cytomegalovirus major immediate-early promoter in the mouse liver: involvement of NFkappaB. J Virol 72:180–190

28. Everett RS, Evans HK, Hodges BL et al (2004) Strain-specific rate of shutdown of CMV enhancer activity in murine liver confirmed by use of persistent [E1(-), E2b(-)] adenoviral vectors. Virology 325:96–105

29. Lam W, Leung CH, Bussom S et al (2007) The impact of hypoxic treatment on the expression of phosphoglycerate kinase and the cytotoxicity of troxacitabine and gemcitabine. Mol Pharmacol 72:536–544

30. Geraerts M, Willems S, Baekelandt V et al (2006) Comparison of lentiviral vector titration methods. BMC Biotechnol 6:34

31. Barde I, Salmon P, Trono D (2010) Production and titration of lentiviral vectors. Curr Protoc Neurosci 53:4.21.1–4.21.23

Part III

Integrase-Mutant LVs

Chapter 12

Transient Expression of Green Fluorescent Protein in Integrase-Defective Lentiviral Vector-Transduced 293T Cell Line

Fazlina Nordin, Zariyantey Abdul Hamid, Lucas Chan, Farzin Farzaneh, and M.K. Azaham A. Hamid

Abstract

Non-integrating lentiviral vectors or also known as integrase-defective lentiviral (IDLV) hold a great promise for gene therapy application. They retain high transduction efficiency for efficient gene transfer in various cell types both in vitro and in vivo. IDLV is produced via a combined mutations introduced on the HIV-based lentiviral to disable their integration potency. Therefore, IDLV is considered safer than the wild-type integrase-proficient lentiviral vector as they could avoid the potential insertional mutagenesis associated with the nonspecific integration of transgene into target cell genome afforded by the wild-type vectors.

Here we describe the system of IDLV which is produced through mutation in the integrase enzymes at the position of D64 located within the catalytic core domain. The efficiency of the IDLV in expressing the enhanced green fluorescent protein (GFP) reporter gene in transduced human monocyte (U937) cell lines was investigated. Expression of the transgene was driven by the spleen focus-forming virus (SFFV) LTRs. Transduction efficiency was studied using both the IDLV (ID-SFFV-GFP) and their wild-type counterparts (integrase-proficient SFFV-GFP). GFP expression was analyzed by fluorescence microscope and FACS analysis.

Based on the results, the number of the GFP-positive cells in ID-SFFV-GFP-transduced U937 cells decreased rapidly over time. The percentage of GFP-positive cells decreased from ~50 % to almost 0, up to 10 days post-transduction. In wild-type SFFV-GFP-transduced cells, GFP expression is remained consistently at about 100 %. These data confirmed that the transgene expression in the ID-SFFV-GFP-transduced cells is transient in dividing cells. The lack of an origin of replication due to mutation of integrase enzymes in the ID-SFFV-GFP virus vector has caused the progressive loss of the GFP expression in dividing cells.

Integrase-defective lentivirus will be a suitable choice for safer clinical applications. It preserves the advantages of the wild-type lentiviral vectors but with the benefit of transgene expression without stable integration into host genome, therefore reducing the potential risk of insertional mutagenesis.

Key words Integrase-defective lentiviral vector, D64 point mutation, Transduction efficiency, GFP reporter gene, U937 cell lines

Maurizio Federico (ed.), *Lentiviral Vectors and Exosomes as Gene and Protein Delivery Tools*, Methods in Molecular Biology, vol. 1448, DOI 10.1007/978-1-4939-3753-0_12, © Springer Science+Business Media New York 2016

1   Introduction

Viral vector systems based on lentiviruses have been extensively analyzed and used for gene therapy applications [1–3] due to their several advantageous properties [4, 5] over other viral vectors. Moreover, lentiviral vectors have been shown to be capable in transducing both dividing and nondividing cells, including stem cells which allow higher level of gene delivery to these cells [6–8].

Despite all of the advantages concerning the use of lentiviral vectors, a number of problems [9] have limited their use. These include the risk of insertional mutagenesis and subsequent malignant transformation of the transduced cells which is afforded by their stable integration to the genome of host cells [10, 11]. Thus, the integrase-defective lentiviral vectors (IDLVs) have been developed to overcome these limitations. IDLVs have been shown to mediate efficient gene expression both in vitro and in vivo with a lower risk of insertional mutagenesis, and thus offer an invaluable prospect in the field of gene therapy [5, 12–14].

IDLVs can be produced through combined mutations into enzyme integrase domains which are consisted of three functional protein domains as follows: (1) N-terminal domain, (2) the catalytic core domain, and (3) the C-terminal domain [15, 16]. The mutations were made to disable the viral RNA integration in the host genome while maintaining the transgene expression episomally in order to minimize the risk of insertional mutagenesis [17].

In this study, we describe the system of IDLV produced through D64 amino acid point mutations located within the catalytic core domain. This type of mutation is commonly used to establish IDLV [18, 19]. ID-SFFV-GFP and their wild-type counterparts (SFFV-GFP) were produced and transduced into U937 cells at multiplicity of infection (MOI) 5, and GFP expression was analyzed using fluorescence microscope and FACS analysis.

2   Materials

Prepare all solutions using deionized water or ultrapure water (prepared by purifying deionized water to attain a sensitivity of 18 MΩ cm at 25 °C) and analytical grade reagents. Prepare and store all reagents at room temperature unless indicated otherwise. Follow all safety regulations including waste disposal procedure when disposing waste materials. Pay close attention to hazardous materials and follow the SOP as provided in the laboratory.

2.1   Lysis Buffer (LyB)

10 mL LyB stock: 20 mM HEPES, 50 mM sodium chloride (NaCl$_2$), 10 mM sodium fluoride (NaF), 1 mM ethylene glycol tetraacetic acid (EGTA), 1 mM sodium orthovanadate, 1 mM phenylmethylsulfonyl fluoride (PMSF), 2.0 % Nonidet P40, 0.5 % sodium

deoxycholate, 0.5 % sodium dodecyl sulfate (SDS), and 10 µL protease inhibitor cocktail (*see* **Note 1**). Mix and add water. Aliquot into 1.5 mL tube. Store at –20 °C.

2.2 2× Laemmli Sample Buffer with β-Mercaptoethanol

10 mL of Laemmli Sample Buffer (LSB) stock: 100 mM Tris–HCl (pH 6.8), 2 % SDS, 20 % glycerol, and 4 % β-mercaptoethanol (added fresh). Mix well and make up to 10 mL water. Aliquot into 1.5 mL tube. Store at –20 °C.

2.3 Tris-Buffered Saline

10× of Tris-buffered saline (TBS) stock buffer: 1 M Trizma base, and 1.5 M $NaCl_2$. Mix and make up to 1 L water. Dilute 10× TBS with water at 1:9 to make 1× working solution. Store at room temperature.

2.4 Blocking Buffer (Bb)

Bb stock buffer: 1× TBS, 7.5 g skimmed milk powder (*see* **Note 2**), and 0.1 % Tween-20. Mix and make up to 150 mL water. Store at 4 °C, and use within 1 month from the date of preparation.

2.5 Antibody Buffer (Ab)

Ab stock buffer: 1× TBS, 1.0 g bovine serum albumin (faction V), and 0.01 % sodium azide (*see* **Note 3**). Mix and make up to 20 mL water. Store at 4 °C, and use within 1 month from the date of preparation.

2.6 2× HeBSS

2× HeBSS stock buffer: 50 mM BES (*N,N*-bis[2-hydroxyethyl]-2aminuteoethanesulfonic acid), 280 mM NaCl, and 1.5 mM Na_2HPO_4. Mix and adjust pH with HCL to 6.96 (*see* **Note 4**). Make up to 1 L water. Store at room temperature.

2.7 Resolving Gel Buffer 10 %

Mix all of these chemicals and reagents: 3 mL 30 % Bis-acrylamide, 2.5 mL 1.5 M Tris–HCl (pH 8.8), 100 µL 10 % APS, 100 µL 10 % SDS, and 4 µL TEMED. Add 4 mL of water. Pour the mixture slowly in the disposable cassette (*see* **Note 5**). Let it stand for 30 min or until the gel is solid.

2.8 Stacking Gel Buffer 5 %

Mix all of these chemicals and reagents: 0.67 mL 30 % Bis-acrylamide, 0.5 mL 1.5 M Tris–HCl (pH 6.8), 40 µL 10 % APS, 40 µL 10 % SDS, and 4 µL TEMED. Add 2.7 mL of water. Layer the mixture slowly onto the solid resolving gel in the disposable cassette (*see* **Note 6**). Carefully insert and fix the combs into the cassette. Let it stand for 30 min or until the gel is solid. Keep the pre-cast gel in the container with 1× running buffer (Rb) covering the whole cassette (*see* **Note 7**). Store at 4 °C.

2.9 Antibodies and Conjugates

1. Primary antibody: Rabbit polyclonal GFP antibody (Cell Signaling), and mouse monoclonal α-tubulin antibody (Sigma).

2. Secondary antibody: Goat anti-rabbit HRP antibody, and goat anti-mouse HRP antibody. Both are from Santa Cruz Biotech. Inc.

2.10 Commercial Kits

1. ECL plus detection kit (GE Healthcare Life Sciences) (*see* **Note 8**).

2. Lenti-X™ qRT-PCR Titration Kit; Clontech, USA.

3. RNA isolation kit (Macherey-Nagel).

2.11 Cell Lines

Human embryo kidney (HEK) 293T cell lines are adherent cells, and will be used as packaging cells to produce lentivirus. Human monocyte cell lines (U937) are suspension cells and will be used as target cells to determine virus titre.

2.12 Culture Media

293T cell lines: Dulbeccos's modified Eagle medium (DMEM) (Sigma Aldrich) supplemented with 10 % (v/v) heat-inactivated fetal calf serum (FCS) (PAA, Laboratories), 100 μg/mL penicillin-streptomycin (Sigma Aldrich). U937 cell lines: RPMI 1640 (Roswell Park Memorial Institute) (Sigma Aldrich) supplemented with 10 % heat-inactivated FCS, 100 μg/mL penicillin-streptomycin.

3   Methods

3.1 Vector Expression Plasmids

Briefly, clone the GFP cDNA into Rous Sarcoma lentivirus (RSV) vector backbone which contains two promoters: RSV promoter located upstream of the HIV-1 Rev Response Element (RRE) site, and the spleen-focus-forming virus (SFFV) promoter located downstream of the RRE site (Fig. 1). SFFV promoter, which is located at 5′LTR, drives the expression of the transgene. The lentiviral vector is produced by using combination of four helper plasmids (the four-plasmid system): MDG (envelope plasmid), Rev (packaging plasmid), integrase-defective or MDLg/pRR (packaging plasmid), and vector plasmid type (transfer plasmid). Hereafter the lentiviral vectors are referred to as SFFV-GFP (wild type), and ID-SFFV-GFP (integrase defective). Preparing of the vector expression plasmids is according to the standard molecular biology methods for cloning (*see* **Note 9**).

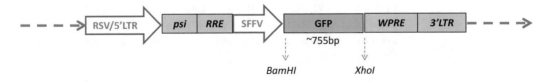

Full vector size: 7426 bp

Fig. 1 Schematic diagram of vector plasmid used as transfer plasmid to express transgene (GFP). GFP cDNA was cloned into *BamHI* and *XhoI* sites of RSV expression vector in-frame between SFFV (spleen focus-forming virus) promoter (5′LTR) and WPRE (3′LTR)

3.2 Calcium Phosphate (Ca-PO₄) Coprecipitation

Briefly, lentivirus is produced using the 293T cell line by seeding 4 million cells in 80 mL of complete media (DMEM supplemented with 10% heat-inactivated FBS (v/v), and 100 µg/mL penicillin-streptomycin) in 435 cm^2 triple-layer culture flask (*see* **Note 10**). The transfection of plasmids is performed using the standard calcium phosphate (Ca-PO₄) coprecipitation transfection protocol as described elsewhere with slight modification [20].

1. Perform the transfection according to the following recipes: 24 µg MDG plasmid, 40 µg MDLg/pRRE plasmid (either the wild type, or the integrase defective type), 20 µg Rev plasmid, and 80 µg vector plasmid.

2. Mix all plasmids in dH$_2$O to final volume of 1977.3 µL. Add the same volume (1:1) of CaCl$_2$ (0.5 M) to the plasmid mixtures to make the final concentration of 0.25 M. Vortex the mixture.

3. Add the mixtures dropwise slowly (one drop every other second) to 1:1 of 2× HeBSS (pH 6.7) while vortexing at moderate speed (*see* **Note 11**). Incubate the DNA Ca-PO₄ coprecipitation mixture at room temperature for 30 min to form a fine opalescent precipitation (*see* **Note 12**).

4. Add the DNA Ca-PO₄ coprecipitation mixture into 80 mL of complete fresh media. Gently mix the mixture evenly. Pour the mixture slowly onto the inside of the triple-layer flask's bottle neck (*see* **Note 13**).

5. Secure the cap and let the flask stand for a few minutes, or when the mixture has settled evenly within the three compartments of the flask (*see* **Note 14**). Quickly lay the flask horizontally (*see* **Note 15**). Incubate at 37 °C with 5% CO$_2$. Replenish fresh complete media within 5–7 h post-transfection (*see* **Note 16**).

6. Harvest the culture medium containing the lentiviral vector particles at 48 h (*see* **Note 17**), and 72 h post-transfection by centrifugation at $300 \times g$ for 10 min at 4 °C following filtration through 0.45 µM syringe filter. Mix both harvested lentiviral vector particles into one 250 mL centrifuge container.

3.3 Concentration of Lentiviral Vectors

1. Centrifuge the filtered culture medium containing the lentiviral vectors at $3900 \times g$ overnight at 4 °C.

2. Discard the supernatant. Remove as much as supernatant from the pellet (*see* **Note 18**).

3. Dissolve pellet (which contains the lentiviral vectors) in 1 mL of serum-free media (X-Vivo 15) and aliquot in 0.2 mL tubes (*see* **Note 19**).

4. Keep the lentiviral vector at −80 °C and determine the titer by flow cytometry analysis or qRT-PCR (*see* **Note 20**).

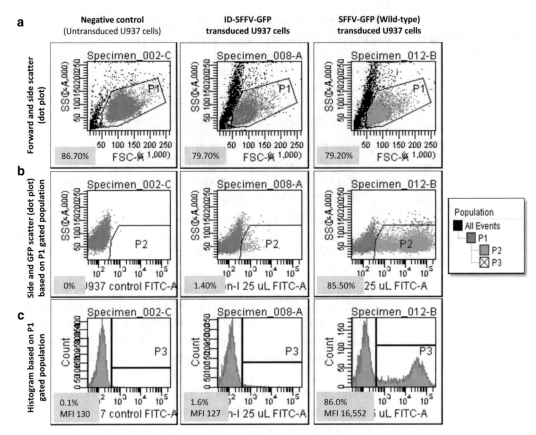

Fig. 2 FACS analysis of ID-SFFV-GFP- and SFFV-GFP-transduced U937 cells on day 3 post-transduction (0.5 μL virus). (**a**) P1-gated region in the dot plot indicates the viable U937 population. (**b**) GFP (FITC-A)-specific side scatter was plotted based on P1-gated population to distinguish the GFP. (**c**) Histogram based on P1-gated population. GFP-positive cells were shifted to the right as labeled in P3 region of the histogram. Percentage and MFI of GFP-positive cells were taken from histogram as displayed in row "**c**." Non-transduced U937 cells were used as a negative control. *MFI* mean fluorescence intensity

3.4 Determination of Lentiviral Vector Titer by Flow Cytometry Analysis

1. Perform this assay in triplicate for statistical analysis.

2. Transduce 200,000 U937 cells per mL with different volumes of concentrated virus in 10 μg/mL polybrene added prior to infection (*see* **Note 21**).

3. Incubate at 37 °C with 5 % CO_2.

4. Determine titer at day 3 post-transduction in culture with 5–20 % GFP-expressing cells (Fig. 2) (*see* **Note 22**).

5. Calculate lentiviral vector titer using this formula:

$$\frac{\text{Mean of GFP} - \text{expressing cells at day 3 post} - \text{transduction}\,(\%) \times \text{Total number of seeded cells} \times 1000\mu L}{{}^{*}\,\mu L \text{ of virus / vector}}$$

3.5 Qualitative Reverse Transcriptase Polymerase Chain Reaction (qRT-PCR)

1. Use the RNA isolation kit to extract the lentiviral's RNA.

2. Elute RNA pellet in RNase-free H_2O, to the final concentration ranged between 55 and 90 µg/mL, and keep at –80 °C.

3. Use Lenti-X™ qRT-PCR Titration Kit to perform qRT-PCR.

4. Treat RNA with DNase (containing 1× DNase I buffer, 20 U DNase I enzyme, and RNase-free H_2O).

5. Incubate the mixture at 37 °C for 30 min, and then at 70 °C for 5 min.

6. Keep samples on ice for qRT-PCR analysis.

7. Perform qRT-PCR amplification in duplicate by mixing the viral RNA with master reaction mix (MRM) (Table 1).

8. Prepare Lenti-X RNA control template dilutions to generate a standard curve for determination of viral RNA copy numbers.

9. Perform samples analysis in a qPCR instrument (G-Storm, Gene Technologies Ltd., UK) (*see* **Note 23**) using the recommended qRT-PCR reaction cycles (Table 2).

Table 1
Master reaction mix (MRM) for qRT-PCR

Regents	Volume/well (µL)
RNase-free water	8.0
Quant-X buffer (2×)	12.5
Lenti-X Forward primer (10 µM)	0.5
Lenti-X Reverse primer (10 µM)	0.5
ROX™ reference dye LSR	0.5
Quant-X enzyme	0.5
RT enzyme mix	0.5
Total	23.0

Table 2
qRT-PCR reaction cycles

Programs	Temperatures/duration
RT reaction	42 °C/5 min 95 °C/10 s
qPCR×40 cycles	95 °C/5 s 60 °C/30 s
Dissociation curve	95 °C/15 s 60 °C/30 s All (60–95 °C)

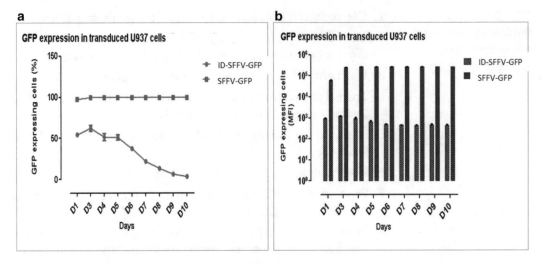

Fig. 3 GFP expression in ID-SFFV-GFP- and SFFV-GFP-transduced U937 cells. A total of 5×10^5 U937 cells/2 mL were transduced with the indicated vectors (MOI 5) and further incubated up to 10 days. GFP expression was determined by FACS. (**a**) Percentage of GFP-expressing cells in SFFV-GFP- and ID-SFFV-GFP-transduced cells. The ID-SFFV-GFP -transduced U937 cells showed reduced GFP expression while GFP expression was consistently higher in the SFFV-GFP-transduced U937 cells. (**b**) Mean fluorescence intensity (MFI) in the SFFV-GFP- and ID-SFFV-GFP-transduced cells. Data shown are the mean ± standard deviation (SD) of triplicate samples

3.6 Transduction of U937 with Lentiviral Vectors

1. Seed U937 cells at 500,000 cells per 2 mL in six-well plates and incubate overnight.

2. Day 0: Add 10 μg/mL of polybrene to each culture to increase transduction efficiency (*see* **Note 24**). Add either SFFV-GFP lentiviral (wild type) or ID-SFFV-GFP lentiviral at MOI 5 and further incubate for fluorescence microscopy, flow cytometry, and western blot analyses.

3. Days 1–10: Take 100 μL of U937-transduced lentiviral to determine the percentage of cell expressing GFP by flow cytometry analysis (Fig. 3).

4. Day 3: Make morphology observation of GFP expression using fluorescence microscopy (Fig. 4).

5. Day 3: Take 1 mL of U937-transduced lentiviral to detect GFP protein by western blot analysis (Fig. 5).

3.7 Preparation of Cell Lysates

1. Wash twice 3×10^6 of cell pellet in DPBS.

2. Dissolve the cell pellet in 100 μL of LyB.

3. Incubate sample for 10 min on ice, and centrifuge for 10 min at $10,000 \times g$ at 4 °C (*see* **Note 25**).

4. Store cell lysates at −20 °C.

3.8 SDS-PAGE Gel Electrophoresis

1. Perform the gel electrophoresis using 10 % SDS-polyacrylamide gradient gels (SDS-PAGE).

2. Mix protein with 2× LSB to 1:1.

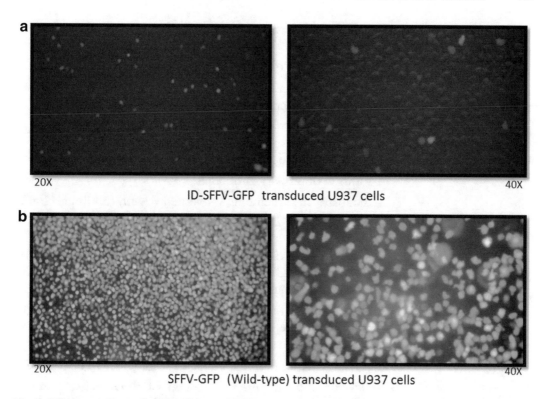

Fig. 4 GFP expression in ID-SFFV-GFP- and SFFV-GFP-transduced U937 cells on day 3 post-transduction (MOI 5). (**a**) <5 % of ID-SFFV-GFP-transduced U937 cells showed green fluorescence indicating GFP expression. (**b**) Virtually all SFFV-GFP-transduced U937 cells showed GFP expression. The cells were viewed at 20× and 40× magnifications

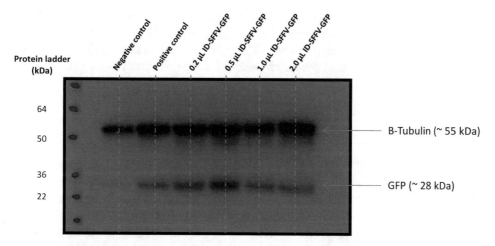

Fig. 5 Western blot analysis of ID SFFV-GFF-transduced U937 cells. Intracellular expression (~35 kDa) was determined 3 days post-transduction. GFP protein was detected in all samples at different virus volumes (0.2, 0.5, 1.0, and 2.0 μL). Cell lysate from untransduced 293T was used as negative controls. Whole-cell lysate from pTATκ-GFP-transfected 293T cells (with prior confirmation of the GFP expression) was used as a positive control (~28 kDa). Tubulin (~55 kDa) was used as loading control for each sample

3. Boil the mixture at 95 °C for 5–10 min before loading the samples onto 10 % SDS-polyacrylamide gel.

4. Run sample at 165 V for 35–45 min.

5. Transfer protein electrophoretically to Hybond ECL nitrocellulose membranes at 165 V for 2 h (*see* **Note 26**).

6. Block the membrane for 1 h in blocking buffer (Bb) (*see* **Note 27**).

7. Rinse the membrane three times in TBS-Tween 20 prior to addition of primary antibodies.

8. Incubate the membrane overnight with antibody buffer containing the primary antibody (1:1000 dilutions) at 4 °C (*see* **Note 28**).

9. The following day, rinse the membrane three times in TBS-Tween 20, and further expose to appropriate horseradish peroxidase-conjugated secondary antibodies at 4 °C for 1 h.

10. Rinse the membrane three times, and incubate with enhanced chemiluminescence reagent at room temperature for 5 min to detect immunoreactive bands.

11. Develop the film using a Photon Imaging system SRX-101A.

12. Develop the film in 30 s–1 min of developer/replenisher chemical, followed by 30 s–1 min of fixative/processing chemical, wash in dH$_2$O, and air-dry.

13. For future probing: Wrap the membrane in cling film, and store at –20 °C until needed (*see* **Note 29**). To re-probe the membrane with a different primary antibody, the previous antibody is first removed by stripping the membrane using 1× stripping buffer three times at 56 °C for 15 min. Rinse the membrane three times using TBS-Tween 20. Later, block the stripped membrane for 1 h in blocking buffer (*see* **Note 27**), and repeat **steps 8–11** for primary antibody probing as previously mentioned.

4 Notes

1. Add protease inhibitor cocktail in the last step. It contains enzymes to help protect the integrity of proteins during protein extraction and purification. If it is left too long at room temperature during the preparation of the LyB, it might degrade the enzyme function. It is also advisable to aliquot the LyB to preserve its function, and also can be kept for longer by minimizing the repeating freeze and thaw process.

2. The bovine albumin can also be used to substitute the skimmed milk powder as a part of blocking buffer components. Make sure that the fraction of this bovine albumin is fully dissolving in the buffer before using it.

3. Sodium azide is an inorganic compound that produces toxic gas. It is used as a preservative component in the antibody buffer to preserve the integrity, and function of the antibodies used in this case is for protein detection in western blot method.

4. The pH 6.96 of 2× HeBSS buffer is very crucial for the success of the plasmid transfection using the $CaPO_4$ chemical method. The efficiency of the transfection is affected by pH of the buffer. Therefore it is wise to optimize and adjust the pH as accurate as possible using the HCl.

5. In the case of in-house preparation of the SDS-PAGE gel, it is advisable to layer the top of the resolving gel buffer in the disposable cassette using absolute ethanol. This is to remove extra bubbles that form on the top and also to make sure that the edge top is even instead of crooked before layering with the stacking gel buffer.

6. Make sure to remove the ethanol by gently rinsing it a few times with water. Dry it with filter paper before adding the stacking gel buffer. Add the stacking gel buffer until it overloads the brim. This is to make sure that there are enough buffers when inserting and fixing the cassette comb.

7. The SDS-PAGE gel can be prepared in advance using the disposable cassette (or depends on the western blot system). This pre-cast gel can be kept in the 1× running buffer for at least 3 months.

8. Make sure that the ECL reagent is applied evenly on the membrane. Remove the excessive reagent by tapping the surface of the membrane with kimwipes or thin absorbent paper before applying the X-ray film. Make sure that it is done in the darkroom with safe lights to protect the X-ray film, and to prolong the ECL effect.

9. The standard molecular biology method with a slight modification is used to produce the vector expression plasmids encoding the gene marker (in this case is green fluorescent protein, GFP). This includes plasmid expansion and extraction using available commercial kits, PCR, enzymes digestion, etc..

10. It will take approximately 3 days to achieve at least 70–80% confluent of the 293T cells to grow in the 435 cm² triple-layer flasks. It is crucial for the $CaPO_4$ chemical transfection method, and to increase the virus titer. The reason is that some of the cells might die during the transfection process and thus it is wise to have the optimal number of the cells.

11. Important: Slowly, drop the mixture (one drop every second) to the 2× HeBSS. Do not do otherwise. This is to make sure that the plasmids precipitate evenly.

12. The incubation time for the coprecipitation of the plasmids is crucial as it will give enough time for the plasmid to form precipitation, and at the same time preserve the plasmid from degrading if it is left too long at room temperature. Thus, keep the incubation time within 20–30 min.

13. Mix well the DNA Ca-PO$_4$ coprecipitation mixture with the 80 mL complete media. Slowly and steadily pour the mixture down through the flask's bottle neck. This is to avoid the cell detached from the bottom of the flask as the 293T is considered fragile cells.

14. Let the mixture to evenly separate between the flask's compartments by 3–5-min vertical stand. This is to make sure that all bottom layer of the flask receive the equal volume of the mixture which will cover the whole surface.

15. When laying the flask horizontally, do it very quick but gently, so as not to detach the cells. If it is too slow, it might not cover the whole surface of the top compartment, as the mixture has slowly transferred to the lower bottom of the other compartment instead.

16. The fresh complete media must be replaced. The transfection media does decrease cell survival. Gently, replace the fresh media, to avoid cells from detaching.

17. Harvest the virus at 48 h, filter through 0.45 μM, and keep in the sterile contained at 4 °C (this procedure is repeated in the second harvest at 72 h). Replenish 80 mL of complete media.

18. Remove the remaining supernatant by putting the centrifuge container upside down for 5–10 min (do not exceed the time as it will dry the pellet).

19. Briefly, thaw the virus and discard the remaining lentiviral vector from the tube accordingly by following the hazardous protocol. Do not freeze the remaining lentiviral vector as it will degrade and will not be accurate for future transduction.

20. qRT-PCR method can be used to determine the lentiviral vector titer by quantitative detection of RNA genome copies of the envelope protein of the lentiviral vector. However, it does not reflect the lentiviral vector functionality. In some cases, it will be better to determine the titer by flow cytometry instead, especially for proteins that can be conjugated with fluorochrome antibodies, which is easy to measure.

21. We suggest starting at small volume: 0.2, 0.5, 1.0, and 2.0 μL (you may increase the volume accordingly). Four different lentiviral vector's volumes are sufficient to determine the titer. Always do the experiment in triplicate for statistical analysis.

22. Day 3 post-transduction is the optimal time to determine the lentiviral vector titer as it has been done for other lentiviral vectors.

Based on previous studies, the lentiviral vector enters target cells by day 3 post-transduction. However, in our previous experience, integrase-defective lentivirus will achieve the highest expression at day 3, and the expression will decrease over time (in our experiment almost zero expression by day 10 post-transduction) [21]. In wild-type SFFV-GFP-transduced cells, GFP expression is remained consistently at about 100%. Similar results were reported elsewhere, where the GFP expression dropped quickly within the first week after transduction [22–24]. Thus, the best time is at day 3 post-transduction for integrase-defective lentiviral vectors. It is advisable to plot graft for all data (triplicate). Choose the best lentiviral vector's volume that expresses 5–20% GFP, and calculate titer using the given formula.

23. It is important to know that different qPCR machines will have different settings. You might need to optimize accordingly using the protocol given by the manufacturer of the commercial kits used for the assay. Some commercial kits will advise different settings.

24. There are a few cationic polymers that can be used to enhance or increase the efficiency of transduction in certain cells. Polybrene acts by neutralizing the charge repulsion between virions and the cell surface. It can be toxic in some susceptible cells. Thus, it is recommended optimizing the concentration, so it will not kill the cells. Alternatively, DAEA-Dextran, which is less toxic and very effective for transient transfection, can be used as substitute.

25. Incubation must be carried out on ice, as the LyB contains protease cocktail inhibitors which need to be preserved at cold temperature. This will allow the protein's integrity from extracted cells to be well preserved.

26. Ideally, transfer the protein in cold room or keep the blot tank in container with ice. This is to avoid protein from degrading during the high voltage.

27. One hour is more than enough to block the unspecific protein on the membrane. However, it is also recommended to block the membrane overnight at 4 °C or cold room with continuous gentle shake.

28. In the case of detecting two or more different proteins with distance protein weight, both primary antibodies can be added together in the antibody buffer and incubate overnight at 4 °C. Alternatively, the second primary antibody can be detected by re-probing the membrane with special stripping buffer to remove the previous antibody and ECL reagent. Optimization of the concentration used to probe the protein is crucial to make sure that it binds the right protein, and to

eliminate high (or dark) background when developing the film later. It is also wise to use the monoclonal antibody instead of polyclonal to avoid the multiple bands due to truncated or unspecific proteins.

29. It is recommended to store at –20 °C for long-term analysis (can last up to 1 year) by wrapping using cling film. To re-probe, make sure that the frozen membrane is thawed at room temperature to avoid breakage before re-probe, or alternatively put the membrane in wash buffer to soften it. Membrane can also be kept in wash buffer if needed to re-probe within 1-month period.

Acknowledgments

This work was supported by the Ministry of Higher Education of Malaysia and Universiti Kebangsaan Malaysia. The work has been carried out at the King's College London, Department of Haematological Medicine, The Rayne Institute, London, UK. *Conflict of interest*: The authors declare no conflict of interest.

References

1. Meissner A, Wernig M, Jaenisch R (2007) Direct reprogramming of genetically unmodified fibroblasts into pluripotent stem cells. Nat Biotechnol 25:1177–1181

2. Park IH, Zhao R, West JA et al (2007) Reprogramming of human somatic cells to pluripotency with defined factors. Nature 451:141–146

3. Wernig M, Meissner A, Foreman R et al (2007) In vitro reprogramming of fibroblasts into a pluripotent ES-cell-like state. Nature 448:318–324

4. Zufferey R, Dull T, Mandel RJ et al (1998) Self-inactivating lentivirus vector for safe and efficient in vivo gene delivery. J Virol 72:9873–9880

5. Wanisch K, Yanez-Munoz RJ (2009) Integration-defective lentiviral vectors: a slow coming of age. Mol Ther 17:1316–1332

6. Yamashita M, Emerman M (2006) Retroviral infection of non- dividing cells: old and new perspectives. Virology 344:88–93

7. Nightingale SJ, Hollis RP, Pepper KA et al (2006) Transient gene expression by noninte-grating lentiviral vectors. Mol Ther 13:1121–1132

8. Aiuti A, Biasco L, Scaramuzza S et al (2013) Lentiviral hematopoietic stem cell gene therapy in patients with Wiskott-Aldrich syndrome. Science 341:1233151

9. Lewinski MK, Bisgrove D, Shinn P et al (2005) Genome-wide analysis of chromosomal features repressing human immunodeficiency virus transcription. J Virol 79:6610–6619

10. Hacein-Bey-Abina S, Von Kalle C, Schmidt M et al (2003) A serious adverse event after successful gene therapy for X-linked severe combined immunodeficiency. N Engl J Med 348:255–256

11. Okita K, Matsumura Y, Sato Y et al (2011) A more efficient method to generate integration-free human iPS cells. Nat Methods 8:409–412

12. Vargas J, Gusella GL, Najfeld V et al (2004) Novel integrase-defective lentiviral episomal vectors for gene transfer. Hum Gene Ther 15:361–372

13. Peluffo H, Foster E, Ahmed SG et al (2013) Efficient gene expression from integration-defective lentiviral vectors in the spinal cord. Gene Ther 20:645–657

14. Apolonia L, Waddington SN, Fernandes C et al (2007) Stable gene transfer to muscle using non-integrating lentiviral vectors. Mol Ther 15:1947–1954

15. Leavitt A, Robles G, Alesandro N et al (1996) Human immunodeficiency virus type 1 integrase

mutants retain in vitro integrase activity yet fail to integrate viral DNA efficiently during infection. J Virol 70:721–728

16. Engelman A (1999) In vivo analysis of retroviral integrase structure and function. Adv Virus Res 52:411–426

17. Shawand A, Cornetta K (2014) Design and potential of non-integrating lentiviral vectors. Biomedicines 2:14–35

18. Bayer M, Kantor B, Cockrell A et al (2008) A large U3 deletion causes increased in vivo expression from a nonintegrating lentiviral vector. Mol Ther 16:1968–1976

19. Lombardo A, Genovese P, Beausejour CM et al (2007) Gene editing in human stem cells using zinc finger nucleases and integrase-defective lentiviral vector delivery. Nat Biotechnol 25:1298–1306

20. Kingston RE, Chen CA, Rose JK (2003) Calcium phosphate transfection. Curr Protoc Mol Biol. Chapter 9, Unit 9.1

21. Nordin F, Abdul Karim N, Wahid SFA (2014) Transgene expression is transient in non-integrating lentiviral-based transduction system: an alternative approach. Regen Res 3:1–7

22. Philippe S, Sarkis C, Barkats M et al (2006) Lentiviral vectors with a defective integrase allow efficient and sustained transgene expression in vitro and in vivo. Proc Natl Acad Sci U S A 103:17684–17689

23. Cornu TI, Cathomen T (2007) Targeted genome modifications using integrase-defective lentiviral vectors. Mol Ther 15:2107–2113

24. Sloan R, Wainberg M (2011) The role of unintegrated DNA in HIV infection. Retrovirology 8:52

Chapter 13

Intrastriatal Delivery of Integration-Deficient Lentiviral Vectors in a Rat Model of Parkinson's Disease

Ngoc B. Lu-Nguyen, Martin Broadstock, and Rafael J. Yáñez-Muñoz

Abstract

Standard integration-proficient lentiviral vectors (IPLVs) are effective at much lower doses than other vector systems and have shown promise in several gene therapy approaches. Their main drawback is the potential risk of insertional mutagenesis. Novel biosafety-enhanced integration-deficient lentiviral vectors (IDLVs) offer a significant improvement and comparable transduction efficacy to their integrating counterparts in some central nervous system applications. We describe here methods for (1) production of IDLVs (and IPLVs), (2) IDLV/IPLV delivery into the striatum of a rat model of Parkinson's disease, and (3) *postmortem* brain processing.

Key words Integration-deficient lentiviral vectors, 6-OHDA, Intrastriatal injection, Parkinson's disease

1 Introduction

Gene therapy approaches have offered promise for many disorders, and lentiviral vectors (LVs) are one of the most attractive viral vector-based systems. LVs have many positive features derived from the biology of the corresponding natural viruses and their extensive vector development [1–3]. In particular, LVs can transduce a variety of cell types of the central nervous system (CNS), including dividing as well as nondividing cells, with stable long-term expression of the transgene [4, 5]. However, a potential obstacle for the routine clinical use of current integration-proficient LVs (IPLVs) is the risk of insertional mutagenesis caused by integration of the viral provirus into the host cell genome [6]. This risk could be addressed by using integration-deficient LVs (IDLVs), without a reduction in vector transduction efficiency if the target cell population does not divide significantly [7–9]. It may also be possible to use replicating IDLVs for stable expression from viral episomes in dividing cells [10].

Maurizio Federico (ed.), *Lentiviral Vectors and Exosomes as Gene and Protein Delivery Tools*, Methods in Molecular Biology, vol. 1448, DOI 10.1007/978-1-4939-3753-0_13, © Springer Science+Business Media New York 2016

IDLVs are commonly produced by targeted changes of individual amino acids within the catalytic active site of integrase (class I mutations), most frequently encoding a D64V change, which inhibit viral integration but leave other viral processes unaffected [11, 12]. This strategy has mediated nearly complete (99%) inhibition of viral integration without significantly affecting proviral synthesis or infectious titers [9, 11–13]. The failure to integrate into the host genome leads to increased levels of episomal viral DNA [8, 9, 14]. These viral episomes are mostly converted into circles that lack replication signals, and are stable in quiescent cells but progressively diluted in proliferating cells [9]. Hence, IDLVs are ideally suited for applications in the post-mitotic central nervous system (CNS) environment [9, 15, 16].

Very recently, we have assessed biosafety and transduction efficiency of IDLVs in an animal model of Parkinson's disease, the 6-hydroxydopamine (6-OHDA)-lesioned rat, with IPLVs used as a reference [17]. Examination of reporter gene (enhanced green fluorescent protein, *eGFP*) and therapeutic transgene (glial cell-derived neurotrophic factor, *GDNF*) expression has shown efficient, long-lived, and transcriptionally targeted expression from IDLVs in the striatum of injected rats. We have confirmed the lack of significant integration of IDLVs in injected rat brains by linear amplification-mediated PCR analysis followed by deep sequencing and insertion site analysis [17].

We regard these results as very encouraging for future IDLV-mediated gene therapy approaches. In this chapter, we provide a detailed description of protocols to produce IDLVs (and IPLVs). We also present methods for delivering LVs into the striatum of 6-OHDA-treated rats and for *postmortem* brain processing. We hope that the comprehensive descriptions in this chapter will promote a broader application and facilitate the study of IDLVs in the CNS.

2   Materials

2.1   Lentiviral Vector Production

1. HEK293T cells.

2. Culture medium: Dulbecco's modified Eagle's medium (DMEM) high glucose supplemented with 10% fetal bovine serum (FBS), 100 U/ml penicillin, 100 μg/ml streptomycin, stored at 4 °C.

3. 15 cm Tissue culture plates.

4. Tissue culture-grade water, stored at room temperature (RT).

5. 1× Endotoxin-free TE (Tris/EDTA) buffer, filter-sterilized through a 0.22 μm filter, stored at RT.

6. 2.5 M CaCl$_2$: Dissolved in water, filter-sterilized through a 0.22 μm filter, aliquoted, and stored at –20 or –80 °C.

7. 2× HBS: 100 mM HEPES, 281 mM NaCl, 1.5 mM Na$_2$HPO$_4$, dissolved in water, adjusted to pH 7.12 (pH is crucial), filtered through a 0.22 μm filter, aliquoted, and stored at –20 or –80 °C. Use freshly thawed reagent only.

8. 1 M MgCl$_2$: Dissolved in water, filter-sterilized through 0.22 μm filter, and stored at 4 °C.

9. DNase I: Stored at –20 °C.

10. Polyallomer ultracentrifuge tubes.

11. Ultracentrifuge compatible with SV32-Ti rotor (Beckman Coulter, UK).

2.2 Stereotactic Injection of LVs

1. Sprague-Dawley rats (250–300 g), maintained in a standard 12-h light/dark cycle with free access to food and water. Experiments are performed in accordance with the UK Animals (Scientific Procedures) Act, 1986.

2. Paxinos and Watson Rat Brain Atlas [18].

3. Stereotactic frame (World Precision Instruments, UK).

4. UltraMicroPump III (World Precision Instruments, UK).

5. Ideal Micro drill (Harvard Apparatus, UK).

6. Shaver.

7. Surgical tools (i.e., scalpels, scissors, tweezers, absorbable Vetsuture, Halsey needle holder).

8. 25 μl Injection syringe with compatible stainless steel 33 G needle (Hamilton, UK).

9. 5 ml Syringes.

10. 26 G Needles.

11. 5 % Emla cream (AstraZeneca, UK).

12. Aqupharm solution (0.18 % sodium chloride + 4 % glucose).

13. Isoflurane.

14. 100 % Oxygen.

15. 70 % Ethanol.

16. ddH$_2$O.

17. Heat pads.

18. Paper towels.

19. Clean cages with bedding, food, and water.

20. LVs, kept on ice during procedure.

2.3 6-OHDA
Lesioning

1. All materials listed in Subheading 2.2, except #20.

2. 6-Hydroxydopamine (6-OHDA): Dissolved in 0.9% sterile saline and 0.02% ascorbic acid (2.5 µg/µl). Store on ice, protect from light, and use within a day.

3. Pargyline (5 mg/ml) and desipramine (25 mg/ml): Dissolved in sterile water and stored at RT.

2.4 Postmortem
Brain Processing
and Immunohisto-
chemistry Staining

1. CO_2 chamber.

2. 1× Phosphate-buffered saline (PBS): 8 g NaCl, 0.2 g KCl, 1.44 g Na_2HPO_4, 0.24 g KH_2PO_4, dissolved in 1 L water, adjusted to pH 7.4, and stored at RT.

3. 4% Paraformaldehyde (PFA): Dissolved in 1× PBS, adjusted to pH 7.4, and preferably used within a day (or stored at −20 °C).

4. Vibrating microtome (Campden Instruments, UK).

5. Paintbrush.

6. Blocking buffer: 1% Bovine serum albumin (BSA) and 0.02% sodium azide, dissolved in 1× PBS-T (0.25% Triton X-100 in 1× PBS), and stored at 4 °C.

7. 1 M Tris buffer: Trizma base dissolved in water, adjusted to pH 7.8 with 1 M HCl, and stored at RT.

8. Sodium azide: 0.1% Stock dissolved in water and stored at RT.

9. Mowiol solution:

   • Stir 4.8 ml glycerol and 2.4 g Mowiol in 6 ml water for 2 h, RT.

   • Add 12 ml of 0.2 M Tris buffer pH 8.5, and 0.02% sodium azide.

   • Incubate solution in 50–60 °C water bath for 10 min, stirring frequently.

   • Centrifuge at 5000×g for 15 min.

   • Collect supernatant, aliquot, and store at −20 °C (*see* **Note 1**).

10. *p*-Phenylenediamine (PPD) solution: 0.1% PPD dissolved in water, protected from light, and stored at −20 °C.

11. Mounting solution: Mix one part of PPD solution with nine parts of Mowiol solution; maintain at RT, protect from light, and use within a day.

12. Antibodies (as required).

13. 4,6-Diamidino-2-phenylindole (DAPI): Dissolved in water, protected from light, and stored at −20 °C.

14. SuperFrost slides and cover slips.

3 Methods

All in vitro work in Subheading 3.1 is carried out under sterile cell culture conditions.

3.1 Production of LVs by Transient Calcium Phosphate Transfection [5, 9, 19]

1. Seed HEK293T cells in 15 cm plates (*see* **Note 2** for cell density) and culture until the cells are around 60% confluent ($\sim 2 \times 10^7$/plate/25 ml medium).

2. Two hours (minimum 30 min) prior to transfection of LV plasmids, replace the culture medium with 20 ml fresh medium per plate.

3. Prepare mixture of plasmid DNA in 15 or 50 ml Falcon tube. The amount below is for each 15 cm culture plate; scale up/down as required (*see* **Note 3**):

   • To produce second-generation LVs, use a three-plasmid system at molar ratio 1:1:2 of packaging:env:transfer plasmids:

     – Packaging plasmid (pCMVΔR8.74 for IPLVs or pCMVΔR8.74intD64V for IDLVs): 16.25 μg.

     – Envelope plasmid (pMD2.VSV-G): 7 μg.

     – Transfer plasmid (containing the transgene of interest within pHR' lentiviral backbone): 25 μg (if the size of promotor + transgene is ≤1500 bp) or 32 μg (if the size of promotor + transgene is ≤3000 bp).

   • To produce third-generation LVs, use a four-plasmid system at molar ratio 1:1:1:2 of packaging:rev:env:transfer plasmids:

     – Packaging plasmid (pMDLg/pRRE for IPLVs or pMDLg/pRREintD64V for IDLVs): 12.5 μg.

     – REV plasmid (pRSV-REV): 6.25 μg.

     – Envelope plasmid (pMD2.VSV-G): 7 μg.

     – Transfer plasmid (containing the transgene of interest within pRRL or pCCL lentiviral backbone): 25 μg (if the size of promotor + transgene is ≤1500 bp) or 32 μg (if the size of promotor + transgene is ≤3000 bp).

4. Make up the DNA mix to 112.5 μl with 1× TE buffer.

5. Top up with 1012.5 μl tissue culture-grade water.

6. Add 125 μl 2.5 M $CaCl_2$, vortex, and leave for 5 min, RT.

7. Add 1250 μl 2× HBS dropwise while vortexing DNA/$CaCl_2$ mix at full speed.

8. Immediately add the mix to HEK293T cells and gently mix with the culture medium.

9. Put cells back in incubator (maintained at 37 °C, 5% CO_2).

10. Sixteen hours post-transfection, remove the medium and replace with 18 ml fresh medium per plate.

11. Twenty-four hours after medium change, harvest cell supernatant, which contains viral vector particles (*see* **Note 4**).

12. Centrifuge at 2500 rpm ($540 \times g$) for 10 min, RT.

13. Filter supernatant through a 0.22 μm Nalgene filter (or a 0.45 μm Nalgene filter to minimize vector loss).

14. Transfer filtered medium to high-speed polyallomer centrifuge tubes (16 ml/tube).

15. Ultracentrifuge at 23,400 rpm ($50,000 \times g$) for 2 h, 4 °C.

16. Discard supernatant and keep tubes upside down on sterile paper towels for a few minutes to drain the remaining supernatant. Dry the last drops around the rim with paper towels.

17. Add 50 μl of DMEM without supplements (or 1× PBS if preferred) per tube.

18. Pipette up and down several times and transfer to 1.5 ml Eppendorf tube.

19. Centrifuge for 10 min at 4000 rpm ($864 \times g$), 4 °C, to remove any aggregates.

20. Transfer the supernatant to new Eppendorf tubes.

21. Adjust vector stock to 10 mM $MgCl_2$ with 1 M $MgCl_2$.

22. Add 5 U/ml DNase I and incubate for 30 min, 37 °C.

23. Aliquot and store at −80 °C.

24. Titrate vector stock to standardize the amount of vector injected (*see* **Note 5**).

3.2 Stereotactic Injection of LVs

1. Use Paxinos and Watson Rat Brain Atlas to determine injection site(s) (*see* **Note 6**).

2. Set up stereotactic frame with nose bar at −3.3 mm (below the horizontal).

3. Set up UltraMicroPump for automatic injection rate at 0.5 μl/min.

4. Autoclave all surgical tools prior to use.

5. Sterilize Hamilton syringe and needle with 70 % ethanol, then wash with ddH_2O, and prime with viral vectors to prevent adsorption of the vector during dosing.

6. Place rat into an anesthesia chamber and induce with 5 % isoflurane in 100 % O_2 until the animal goes into deep anesthesia (heart beats slowly and regularly).

7. Shave the head fur and place rat on a heat pad, within the stereotactic frame, with anesthesia maintained using approximately 2.5 % isoflurane in 100 % O_2.

8. Place rat into stereotaxic frame and hang incisors on incisor bar. The rat is ready for surgery following loss of pedal withdrawal reflex and eye-blink reflex. Monitor state of anesthesia throughout surgical procedure.

9. Cover two ear bars (of stereotactic frame) with Emla cream and set up the bars (*see* **Note 7**).

10. Make a longitudinal incision in the scalp starting from the midline between the eyes and extending for ~1 mm towards the tail.

11. Keep the scalp open with tweezers.

12. Gently wipe the skull with sterile paper towels.

13. Determine the position of bregma (*see* **Note 8**) and calculate the final values of AP and ML according to it.

14. Drill a burr hole into the skull at the identified position and pierce dura using a sterile needle.

15. Read the DV value, calculate the final value needed, and move the syringe down to the position corresponding to this value (*see* **Note 6**).

16. Inject LVs using UltraMicroPump at a rate of 0.5 μl/min (*see* **Note 6**).

17. During injection, rehydrate the rat with Aqupharm solution (10 ml/kg, *s.c.*).

18. After injection, leave the needle in place for ~3 min prior to retracting it.

19. Suture the scalp, place rat in a clean, warm cage, and wait until the animal regains consciousness.

20. Clean Hamilton needle and Vetsuture with 70% ethanol for the next injection.

21. After the last injection clean Hamilton syringe with 70% ethanol and then water before returning to its container.

3.3 6-OHDA Lesioning

1. Thirty minutes prior to surgery, inject rat with a combined solution of pargyline (5 mg/kg, i.p.) and desipramine (25 mg/kg, i.p.) (*see* **Note 9**).

2. Carry out all steps listed in Subheading 3.2. However,

   – In **step 5**: prime the syringe with 6-OHDA solution instead of LV stock.

   – In **step 15**: we inject 6-OHDA at the same locations as vector (*see* **Note 10**).

   – In **step 20**: discard remaining 6-OHDA.

3. Timing of 6-OHDA lesioning (*see* **Note 11**).

3.4 Postmortem Brain Processing

1. Sacrifice rats by CO_2 exposure and decapitate.

2. Open the skull with medium scissors or forceps, remove the whole brain, and transfer into 50 ml Falcon tubes filled with ice-cold 4% PFA (1 brain/tube, *see* **Note 12**).

3. Fix brains for 3–5 days at 4 °C.

4. Rinse brains with ice-cold 1× PBS.

5. Slice brains on a vibrating microtome at 50 μm thickness.

6. Collect brain sections using a paintbrush and keep in ice-cold 1× PBS during sectioning.

7. Wash in ice-cold 1× PBS (2×2 min) with gentle agitation.

8. Block in 1% BSA blocking buffer for 1 h, RT.

9. Incubate with primary antibody overnight, 4 °C (*see* **Note 13**).

10. Wash in 1× PBS (3×5 min) with gentle agitation.

11. Incubate with compatible secondary antibody for 1 h, RT (*see* **Note 13**). Protect samples from light after this step.

12. Wash in 1× PBS (3×5 min) with gentle agitation.

13. Incubate with DAPI (1 μg/ml) for 15 min, RT.

14. Wash in 1× PBS (3×5 min) with gentle agitation.

15. Use paintbrush to flatten brain sections onto SuperFrost slides (approximately three sections/slide).

16. Mount with mounting solution (50–100 μl/slide) and cover with cover slips.

17. Air-dry at RT and store at 4 °C.

---

4 Notes

1. Mowiol may not be dissolved completely but the pellet must be colorless. After centrifugation, collect and aliquot the supernatant and store at −20 °C until use. Do not disturb the pellet.

2. As growth rate of 293T cells is quite variable, adjust cells seeded accordingly.

3. Plasmid stocks and reagents are endotoxin free and of tissue culture grade. LV transfer plasmids are self-inactivating and contain a central polypurine tract/central termination sequence and Woodchuck hepatitis virus posttranscriptional regulatory element.

4. Replace culture medium again with 18 ml/plate of fresh medium for second harvest (after additional 24 h), if required. The first harvest usually provides the highest vector titers but the second harvest can have comparable yield.

5. We favor titration of the late reverse transcript by qPCR [20] in transduced cells harvested 24 h post-transduction, normalizing with the amount of endogenous β-actin gene, as described [9] and discussed [8]. It is important to harvest transduced cells at 24 h when titrating IDLVs (and matched IPLV stocks) by qPCR, to minimize loss of episomes due to cell proliferation-mediated dilution.

6. We obtained successful LV transduction with widespread *eGFP* expression within the striatum following two injections at (1) AP: +1.8 mm, ML: –2.5 mm relative to bregma and DV: –5.0 mm relative to dura, and (2) AP: 0.0 mm, ML: –3.5 mm relative to bregma and DV: –5.0 mm relative to dura. Vectors were injected at 5 μl/site, 10^9 viral qPCR transducing units/ml (*see* **Note 5**).

7. Two ear bars should be inserted at equivalent depth, usually around 7. If the bars are set at the right position, when you release incisors from the bar and use your index finger to gently press the head down or lift it up, the head will move rigidly and not drift downwards.

8. Be careful not to confuse bregma with lambda (just below bregma).

9. Pargyline and desipramine are used to increase the bioavailability and specificity of 6-OHDA for dopaminergic neurons.

10. We used 6-OHDA at 2.5 μg/μl and injected 2 μl/site at two sites into the striatum and observed 50 % death of dopaminergic neurons in the ipsilateral substantia nigra.

11. 6-OHDA lesioning can be administered before or after LV injection depending on the purpose of the study.

12. The volume of 4 % PFA should be 10–20 times that of the brain for complete fixation. We used 20 ml/brain.

13. Dilute antibodies in blocking buffer at concentrations according to manufacturers' recommendation or previous optimization.

Acknowledgements

This work received financial support from the EU FP7 program (project NEUGENE: grant agreement no. 222925), Royal Holloway, University of London, and University of Medicine and Pharmacy at Ho Chi Minh city, Vietnam. We thank Luigi Naldini for lentiviral plasmids.

References

1. Cannon JR, Sew T, Montero L et al (2011) Pseudotype-dependent lentiviral transduction of astrocytes or neurons in the rat substantia nigra. Exp Neurol 228:41–52

2. Dull T, Zufferey R, Kelly M et al (1998) A third-generation lentivirus vector with a conditional packaging system. J Virol 72: 8463–8471

3. Mátrai J, Chuah MK, VandenDriessche T (2010) Recent advances in lentiviral vector development and applications. Mol Ther 18:477–490

4. Jakobsson J, Ericson C, Jansson M et al (2003) Targeted transgene expression in rat brain using lentiviral vectors. J Neurosci Res 73: 876–885

5. Naldini L, Blömer U, Gallay P et al (1996) In vivo gene delivery and stable transduction of nondividing cells by a lentiviral vector. Science 272:263–267

6. Biasco L, Baricordi C, Aiuti A (2012) Retroviral integrations in gene therapy trials. Mol Ther 20:709–716

7. Banasik MB, McCray PB Jr (2010) Integrase-defective lentiviral vectors: progress and applications. Gene Ther 17:150–157

8. Wanisch K, Yáñez-Muñoz RJ (2009) Integration-deficient lentiviral vectors: a slow coming of age. Mol Ther 17:1316–1332

9. Yáñez-Muñoz RJ, Balaggan KS, MacNeil A et al (2006) Effective gene therapy with non-integrating lentiviral vectors. Nat Med 12: 348–353

10. Kymäläinen H, Appelt JU, Giordano FA et al (2014) Long-term episomal transgene expression from mitotically stable integration-deficient lentiviral vectors. Hum Gene Ther 25:428–442

11. Leavitt AD, Robles G, Alesandro N et al (1996) Human immunodeficiency virus type 1 integrase mutants retain in vitro integrase activity yet fail to integrate viral DNA efficiently during infection. J Virol 70:721–728

12. Engelman A (1999) In vivo analysis of retroviral integrase structure and function. Adv Virus Res 52:411–426

13. Apolonia L, Waddington SN, Fernandes C et al (2007) Stable gene transfer to muscle using non-integrating lentiviral vectors. Mol Ther 15:1947–1954

14. Nightingale SJ, Hollis RP, Pepper KA et al (2006) Transient gene expression by nonintegrating lentiviral vectors. Mol Ther 13: 1121–1132

15. Peluffo H, Foster E, Ahmed SG et al (2013) Efficient gene expression from integration-deficient lentiviral vectors in the spinal cord. Gene Ther 20:645–657

16. Philippe S, Sarkis C, Barkats M et al (2006) Lentiviral vectors with a defective integrase allow efficient and sustained transgene expression in vitro and in vivo. Proc Natl Acad Sci U S A 103:17684–17689

17. Lu-Nguyen NB, Broadstock M, Schliesser MG et al (2014) Transgenic expression of human glial cell line-derived neurotrophic factor from integration-deficient lentiviral vectors is neuroprotective in a rodent model of Parkinson's disease. Hum Gene Ther 25:631–641

18. Paxinos G, Watson C (2006) The rat brain in stereotaxic coordinates. Elsevier, San Diego

19. Naldini L, Blömer U, Gage FH et al (1996) Efficient transfer, integration, and sustained long-term expression of the transgene in adult rat brains injected with a lentiviral vector. Proc Natl Acad Sci U S A 93:11382–11388

20. Butler SL, Hansen MS, Bushman FD (2001) A quantitative assay for HIV DNA integration in vivo. Nat Med 7:631–634

Chapter 14

Development of Lentiviral Vectors for Targeted Integration and Protein Delivery

Diana Schenkwein and Seppo Ylä-Herttuala

Abstract

The method in this chapter describes the design of human immunodeficiency virus type 1 (HIV-1) integrase (IN)-fusion proteins which we have developed to transport different proteins into the nuclei of lentiviral vector (LV)-transduced cells. The IN-fusion protein cDNA is incorporated into the LV packaging plasmid, which leads to its incorporation into vector particles as part of a large Gag–Pol polyprotein. This specific feature of protein packaging enables also the incorporation of cytotoxic and proapoptotic proteins, such as frequently cutting endonucleases and P53. The vectors can hence be used for various protein transduction needs. An outline of the necessary methods is also given to study the functionality of a chosen IN-fusion protein in a cell culture assay.

Key words Integrase fusion protein, Targeted integration, Genomic safe harbor, Protein transduction, Vector production

1 Introduction

HIV-1 is a lentivirus belonging to the family of Retroviridae. All retroviruses integrate their genomes into the chromatin of the host cell as an obligatory step of the virus life cycle [1]. Before integration, the single-stranded RNA genome, of which there are two copies in each HIV-1 particle, is reverse transcribed into a cDNA molecule. This is transported to host cell nucleus through active transport and becomes subsequently permanently integrated into the chromatin of the target cell [2]. Integration is a semi-random process that relies on the activity of the viral IN. In the first step of integration, IN cleaves a dinucleotide from the 3′ ends of the viral long terminal repeats (LTRs) that were formed during the reverse transcription process. Next, IN produces a cut into the host chromatin. The last step, strand transfer, occurs when IN joins the cleaved 3′ ends of the viral LTR to the 5′ strands of the host DNA. Cellular DNA repair enzymes finalize the covalent attachment

Maurizio Federico (ed.), *Lentiviral Vectors and Exosomes as Gene and Protein Delivery Tools*, Methods in Molecular Biology, vol. 1448, DOI 10.1007/978-1-4939-3753-0_14, © Springer Science+Business Media New York 2016

of the two DNA molecules of different origins by cleaving off the unattached nucleotides and filling in the gaps of the ligation intermediates.

Integrated HIV-1 genomes are called proviruses. The sites of integration are not randomly distributed along the cellular chromatin, but they also occur without a strong preference for specific nucleotide sequences. Both the wild-type HIV-1 and vectors derived of it prefer genomic regions for integration that are gene rich and actively transcribed in the host cell [3–5]. Integration sites (IS) are most frequently found throughout the length of protein-encoding genes. This preference may be beneficial for HIV-1 in promoting high-level transcription of the provirus to ensure viral replication, but is problematic from the point of view of gene therapy, when the aim is to insert therapeutic genes safely into patient cells. To avoid interrupting cellular genes with integrated transgenes, or activating nearby genes through promoter insertion, therapeutic gene integration would be best targeted away from genes into so-called predetermined genomic safe harbor sites [6]. To date many different methods have been developed that aim to target integration into specific sites of the human genome. For example, for HIV-1 based vectors, it has been demonstrated that by modifying the DNA-binding capabilities of the IN cofactor protein LEDGF/p75, native LV integration preferences can be altered [7–9]. We have also shown that LV integration into a predetermined site can be increased significantly with the aid of IN-fusion proteins [10].

IN-fusion proteins were first described in the 1994, when it was found that sequence-specific DNA-binding proteins or domains were able to retarget integration into predetermined sites in vitro [11]. In the context of virions, IN-fusions were found to decrease the viability of viruses but integration was observed to be modestly targeted in in vitro experiments using extracted preintegration complexes that contained both the IN-fusion protein and a wild-type IN [12]. We took IN-fusion proteins into modern third-generation LVs and showed that they could be used for the delivery of desired proteins into transduced cell nuclei [13]. Moreover, such vectors were able to enrich vector integration in predetermined genomic safe harbor target sites when IN was fused to a meganuclease recognizing a sequence at these sites [10]. This chapter describes the original design of IN-fusion protein-encoding constructs which drive the packaging of the proteins into third-generation LV particles that can be used to study targeted integration or protein transduction. In addition, general outlines of the steps needed to test correct IN-fusion protein incorporation and functionality are provided.

2   Materials

2.1   Plasmids for the Production of Third-Generation LVs

For third-generation LV production, four plasmids are used [14]. One of these is a SIN vector construct carrying the transgene of interest under the control of a desired promoter located between the viral LTRs. An important safety feature of this construct is the deletion in the U3 part of the LTR which impedes the promoter activity from LTRs of the provirus [15]. The packaging plasmid contains genes for the structural proteins and enzymes to form the vector particles. A plasmid encoding the viral accessory protein Rev is needed to enhance the export of full-length and singly spliced mRNAs from the producer cell's nucleus [14]. Last, a plasmid containing the cDNA to produce a vector pseudotyping protein, such as the frequently used VSV-G, is needed.

As a control and for the *trans*-complementation of IN-fusion protein containing LV particles (IFLVs), a packaging plasmid carrying an inactive IN is needed. We used a pMDLg/pRRE plasmid where a point mutation was introduced to generate the inactivating D64V mutation [16] into IN. This plasmid was named pMDLg/pRRE-IN$_{D64V}$. When used in LV production alone, this plasmid leads to the production of integration-deficient LVs (IDLVs).

The IN-fusion protein to be packaged into the LV has to be cloned into the packaging plasmid pMLDg/pRRE (mainly for integration targeting studies where IN's activity is desired) or into the pMDLg/pRRE-IN$_{D64V}$ (preferred for protein transduction studies). This can be done by conventional molecular cloning methods (*see* **Note 1**) or by gene synthesis services, for which instructions are given in Subheading 3.1. LV production plasmids can be purchased from several commercial suppliers.

The different plasmids used to produce the different types of LVs in our work were as follows:

1. pLV-GFP: the plasmid encoding for the vector RNA genome with a PGK-EGFP transgene cassette.

2. pMDLg/pRRE: the unmodified packaging plasmid [14].

3. pMDLg/pRRE-IN$_{D64V}$: used to generate IDLVs and to *trans*-complement LVs for targeted integration.

4. pMDLg/pRRE carrying the IN-fusion protein: for IN-fusion protein-carrying LVs where IN's activity is desired, such as for targeted integration.

5. pMDLg/pRRE-IN$_{D64V}$ carrying the IN-fusion protein: for protein transduction purposes or when IN's activity is not desired.

6. pRSV-REV.

7. pMD2G.

2.2 Antibodies for Western Blot

1. A primary antibody specific for HIV-1 IN [e.g., antisera to HIV-1 IN peptide: aa 23–34 from NIH AIDS Research and Reference Reagent Program].

2. A secondary antibody recognizing the IN-specific primary antibody.

3. A primary antibody specific against the protein fused to IN.

4. A secondary antibody recognizing the fusion partner-specific primary antibody.

2.3 Cell Culture Testing of IN-Fusion Protein Vectors by a FACS-Based Analysis Method

1. A suitable cell line (e.g., MRC5 lung fibroblasts).

2. Cell culture vessels.

3. Complete cell culture media.

4. FACS tubes with and without cell strainer caps.

5. Phosphate buffered saline (PBS).

6. Trypsin or other cell dissociation medium.

7. PBS-BSA (1%).

8. Optional: fixation agent (e.g., 4% PBS-PFA).

9. Optional: transduction enhancers such as Polybrene.

10. Other basic BSL2 cell culture laboratory consumables and personal protection items.

11. Equipment: FACS, light microscope, fluorescence microscope, cell counter/hemocytometer, and tabletop centrifuge.

3 Methods

In order to generate LVs carrying desired IN-fusion proteins, first a proper packaging plasmid needs to be designed and cloned. Originally IN-fusion constructs were generated by molecular cloning, which is described in **Note 1**. This plasmid will be used in LV production. Once the LVs are produced and titered, correct incorporation of the fusion proteins is verified with Western blotting. Thereafter, the vectors can be used for functionality testing in cell culture assays as desired. For protein transduction purposes, the IN-fusion protein-carrying LV (IFLV) should contain an integration-deficient (e.g., D64V-mutated) IN fused to the protein of interest. The packaging plasmid used for vector production in this case is the pMDLg/pRRE-IN$_{D64V}$ carrying the fusion protein cDNA cloned to the 3′ end of IN$_{D64V}$. For targeted integration purposes, the IFLV is advised to contain the IN$_{D64V}$ in addition to the IN-fusion protein to maximize vector functionality. For these IFLVs, both the packaging plasmids pMDLg/pRRE with the fusion protein cDNA and the pMDLg/pRRE-IN$_{D64V}$ are used in LV production. In our hands, mixing equal amounts of the two plasmids has worked well.

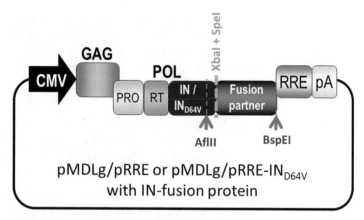

Fig. 1 A schematic representation of the packaging plasmid containing the IN-fusion protein and the relevant restriction enzyme sites in the construct. *CMV* cytomegalovirus immediate early promoter, *PRO* protease, *RT* reverse transcriptase, *IN* integrase, *RRE* Rev responsive element, *pA* polyadenylation signal, *GAG* group-specific antigen, *POL* polyprotein

3.1 Designing the IN-Fusion Protein-Encoding LV Packaging Plasmid

1. Start the design of the IN-fusion protein construct from the IN-sequence and the amino acid linker. The full sequence of the IN-cDNA used in the original protocol is given in **Note 2**. The unique restriction sites AflII and BspeI in pMDLg/pRRE are used to clone the IN-fusion cassette into the packaging plasmid (Fig. 1). Therefore the IN-fusion protein construct is to be synthetized starting from the AflII site of IN. Replace the stop codon of IN with a codon or codons encoding for a desired amino acid linker. If no other preferences exist, use the linker sequence described in **Note 2** that was generated during the original cloning procedure (*see* **Note 1**; XbaI site ligated to SpeI site).

2. Design the fusion partner cDNA. Check that the sequence of IN-fusion partner does not contain AflII and BspeI restriction enzyme sites to enable cloning of the construct into the packaging plasmid. If sites exist, introduce a silent mutation (not altering the amino acid sequence of the protein) into the cDNA to delete them. Replace the start codon of the fusion partner with a codon encoding for a desired amino acid of the linker. Insert the restriction site for BspEI (sequence: TCCGGA) after the stop codon of the fusion partner to enable cloning into the packaging plasmid.

3. Make sure that the designed IN-fusion construct sequence contains no unintended stop or start codons and that the restriction enzyme sites for AflII and BspEI, needed for cloning into the packaging plasmid, are unique and in place (Fig. 1).

4. Place an order for the synthesis of the IN-fusion construct preferably subcloned into a cloning plasmid from which it can be digested with AflII and BspEI for cloning purposes. Clone the fragment into the packaging plasmid pMDLg/pRRE (and/or pMDLg/pRRE-IN$_{D64V}$) opened with the same restriction enzymes.

5. Optional: order the cloning of the IN-fusion construct into the packaging plasmid pMDLg/pRRE using the restriction enzymes AflII and BspEI together with cDNA synthesis. Order a convenient amount of this plasmid for the laboratory stock.

6. Order or produce an endotoxin-free giga-prep of the packaging plasmid to be used for LV production.

3.2 Production and Titering of Lentiviral Vectors

1. Prepare third-generation LV preparations according to [17–19] or order vectors from a commercial supplier. For a valid functional assay, produce the following vector types:

   - An unmodified integration competent LV (ICLV).

   - The IN-fusion protein-carrying LV (IFLV). For protein transduction purposes: containing the integration-deficient (e.g., D64V-mutated) IN fused to the protein of interest (pMDLg/pRRE-IN$_{D64V}$ with the fusion protein cDNA as the packaging plasmid in vector production). For targeted integration: containing the IN-fusion protein and the integration-deficient IN protein packaged into the same vector particles (pMDLg/pRRE with the fusion protein cDNA and pMDLg/pRRE-IN$_{D64V}$ mixed in equal amounts in vector production).

   - Optional: An integration-deficient LV (IDLV) to serve as a control (using the packaging plasmid pMDLg/pRRE-IN$_{D64V}$ in vector production).

2. Titer the vectors with both a p24 particle assay (generally expressed as pg of p24/ml) to aid in quantifying viral particles and with a functional assay, to produce the biological titer, if possible. The particle titer is used to load and compare equal amounts of vectors in Western blots and functional assays and is a useful value because IN-fusion protein incorporation may decrease the biological titer of vectors.

3.3 Verification of Correct Fusion Protein Packaging with SDS–PAGE and Immunoblotting

1. Lyse LV preparations in Laemmli buffer and denature at 95 °C for 5 min before separation on 10–12% sodium dodecyl sulfate–polyacrylamide gel electrophoresis (SDS–PAGE) gels.

2. Perform SDS–PAGE using precast gels or with self-made gels. In our hands clear results confirming the packaging of IN-fusion proteins have been obtained by loading 500 ng of p24 per well. If using two different primary antibodies, load all vectors in duplicate (on separate gels if desired).

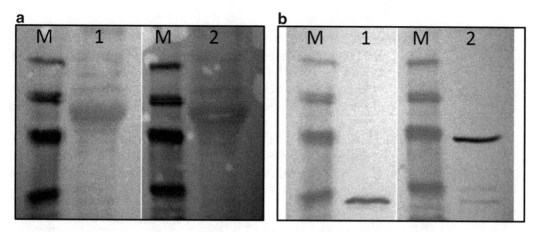

Fig. 2 Verification of the correct fusion partner packaging into LVs with Western blot. (**a**) Ponceau S-stained blots (**b**) HIV-1 IN antisera-probed blots. Samples on the blots: M, molecular weight marker, 1-ICLV, and 2-IFLV carrying the IN-I-Ppol fusion protein

3. Transfer the proteins resolved by SDS–PAGE to a nitrocellulose membrane (0.2 mm).

4. Detect all proteins on the membrane by staining the membranes with Ponceau S-dying solution to verify that equal amounts of vectors were loaded and transferred (Fig. 2a).

5. Probe the blot with antibodies. Use a primary antibody to HIV-1 IN and on a separate blot a specific antibody recognizing the other part of the fusion protein, if available. Detect proteins on the blots with the chosen method. We originally used the antisera to HIV-1 integrase (peptide, aa 23–34) at a 1:2000 dilution and the secondary antibody (Goat Anti-Rabbit IgG H+L–AP Conjugate) at an 1:3000 dilution and performed a colorimetric detection of the IN-fusion proteins using NBT/BCIP substrate solution (16 µl/ml of staining buffer). Typically this resulted in clearly visible specific bands corresponding to the size of the wt IN or the IN-fusion protein (Fig. 2b).

3.4 Cells Transductions

1. Select a suitable cell line for vector functionality testing. The selection of cell line depends on the specific vector/IN-fusion protein test. We have routinely used the MRC-5 lung fibroblasts, which have a finite dividing capacity of 42–46 population doublings before the onset of senescence, for various studies owing to their normal karyotype.

2. On the day before transduction, plate cells on at least triplicate wells of a six-well plate per each vector to be tested. Test at use least one concentration of the test vector. As controls, use a nonmodified control vector with the same MOI and at an equal p24-based particle amount, as well as one non-transduced control (altogether at least 12 wells). Plate cells such that on

the day of transduction they will be at 60–80% confluency (optimal plating amounts will depend on the cell type).

3. Calculate the amounts of vectors needed for the experiment. Multiplicity of infection (MOI) 1 based on the functional (i.e., biological, fluorescence-based) titer is a good starting point. Calculate how much of vector is being used per well in terms of ng of p24. Then calculate the amounts of control vector (unmodified ICLV) needed for the transduction of cells at MOI = 1 (TU/cell) and at the same p24 amount than the test vector. The volume of vector needed for the transduction of one well with a desired MOI is calculated as follows:

$$\text{Volume of LV required} \, (\mu l) = \frac{\text{M.O.I.} \times \text{Number of cells in well}}{\text{LV titer} \, (\text{TU} / \mu l)}$$

For example, to transduce 200,000 cells with the MOI of 2 using a vector which titer is 4.0×10^8 TU/ml, one would need

$$\times \, \mu l = \frac{2 \, \text{TU} / \text{cell} \times 2 \times 10^5 \, \text{cells}}{4.0 \times 10^5 \, \text{TU} / \mu l} = 1 \, \mu l.$$

4. On the day of transduction, thaw vectors on ice immediately prior to use and allow to warm to room temperature for 5 min before transduction.

5. Transduce cells. First make a suitable dilution of the vector in PBS or complete medium (solutions at room temperature) that can be directly pipetted onto the cells (freshly changed prewarmed medium in the well). Alternatively, dilute the vector immediately prior to use into prewarmed complete medium and exchange the old medium in correct wells immediately with the LV-containing medium.

6. Gently rock plates horizontally after the addition of the vector to ensure equal dispersion of the vector particles and return plates to an incubator (37 °C, 5% CO_2).

7. Exchange the medium in the wells with fresh complete medium on the next day after transduction.

3.5 FACS Analysis for Vector Functionality Testing

1. On day two post transduction, inspect the cells on a fluorescent microscope for EGFP expression and any signs of cytotoxicity (i.e., dead cells floating in the medium and decreased confluency). For optimal FACS results, cells should be equally confluent in each well. If this is not the case, adjust the volume of suspended cells used for FACS sample preparation and seeding onto new plates so that approximately equal amounts are used between different samples.

2. Prepare samples of each transduced well for FACS analysis. For choosing the time points for FACS analysis, *see* **Note 3**. Wash each well with prewarmed PBS and detach cells with trypsin.

Suspend cells into prewarmed medium well by gentle pipetting and take a suitable volume (e.g., 2/3) of the cell suspension into a labeled FACS tube and close lid. Depending on the cell line and the well confluency, remove a suitable volume of the remaining suspension in the original plate onto new six-well plates (e.g., 1/5–1/10 of the original volume of suspension) containing 2 ml of prewarmed fresh medium, rotate, and return to the incubator. Pellet cells in the FACS tubes and wash the cell pellet with PBS. Suspend the cell pellet into PBS containing 1% BSA (or FBS). The volume of the buffer will depend on the number of cells. Filter suspension immediately prior to running the samples (e.g., using FACS tubes with a cell strainer cap).

3. Run samples in a FACS device with appropriate settings.

4. Compare the percentage of fluorescent cells between the different vectors and time points of cell harvesting. To determine the so-called integration efficiency of a vector, normalize the value of the last time point (e.g., day 10) to the percentage of fluorescing cells on the day of maximal expression (e.g., day 2) post transduction. From this comparison one can estimate what percentage of the initially transduced cells remains fluorescent, i.e., what percentage of vectors that promoted GFP expression were integrated into the cellular genome.

5. Harvest and freeze transduced cells in aliquots at or after day 10 post transduction for future analysis of vector IS (examples of possible methods for IS extraction are given in **Note 4**). Optionally the fluorescing cells can be separated from the non-transduced ones by fluorescence-assisted cell sorting prior to long-term storage at −70 or −80 °C.

6. To detect successful protein transduction with IFLVs that carry other fusion proteins than fluorescent proteins, *see* **Note 5**.

4   Notes

1. Regarding the cloning strategy for the IN-fusion constructs, the unique restriction sites AflII and BspEI in pMDLg/pRRE were used originally to clone the IN-fusion cassette into the packaging plasmid. AflII cleaves IN at the latter half of the gene, and BspEI cuts the packaging plasmid after the stop codon of IN in *pol* and before the RRE element (Fig. 1). The IN-fusion protein becomes transcribed and translated as a part of the large Gag–Pol polyprotein and therefore the start codon of the fusion partner cDNA needs to be deleted. In the original protocol, the start codon of the fusion partner was replaced with a SpeI cleavage site (sequence: ACTAGT) that was used

for IN-fusion cloning. The IN-fusion protein cDNAs were first constructed and subcloned into the cloning plasmid pBluescript II. The cDNAs for IN and the fusion partner were amplified by PCR with primers introducing the correct restriction enzyme cleavage sites and codon modifications as described in Subheading 3.1. PCR fragments were purified with a cleanup kit and individually blunt end ligated into the EcoRV site of pBluescript II. The plasmid carrying IN-cDNA in the correct orientation was digested with XbaI and gel extracted. SpeI was used to digest the fusion partner cDNA which was subsequently gel extracted and ligated to the plasmid carrying the IN-cDNA. Ligation of the fusion partner cDNA to the 3' end of IN in the correct orientation was verified with different restriction enzymes. The enzymes AflII and BspEI were used to digest the IN-fusion cDNA (lacking part of the 5' sequence of IN) and the gel-extracted fragment was ligated into pMDLg/pRRE digested with AflII and BspEI and gel extracted (lacking the 3' end of IN; see Fig. 1).

2. Due to the original cloning steps, the IN-cDNA in the final pMDLg/pRRE differs from that of the parental packaging plasmid by three nucleotides. These three nucleotides correspond to the differences between the IN-sequence of pMDLg/pRRE and that of the plasmid pLJS10 which harbors the HIV-1 HXB2 IN gene. Below the nucleotide sequence of the all of the IN-cDNA is described as it is in all of the packaging plasmids created by use that encode for IN-fusion proteins. The first part of the IN-sequence is derived from the packaging plasmid pMDLg/pRRE (shown as bold letters below), and the latter part (after the unique TTAAG AflII site) is derived from the IN-sequence from the HIV clone HXB2 (GenBank: K03455.1), contained in the plasmid pLJS10 (highlighted with italics below). The three nucleotide mismatches between these sequences after the relevant AflII site of IN cause two amino acid changes to the IN-sequence (Table 1). In addition to the short linker formed by the ligation of a cleaved XbaI site

Table 1
Codon differences between the HIV-HXB2 IN-sequence and the pMDLg/pRRE IN-sequence downstream of the AflII site and the amino acids they encode for

Codon sequence in pMDLg/pRRE	Codon sequence in pLJS10 (HIV-HXB2)	Affected amino acid in pMDLg/pRRE	Final amino acid in fusion construct (and amino acid in HIV-HXB2)
GAT	AAT	D233	N233
GTT	CTT	V235	L235
ATC	ATT	I269	I269

to a SpeI site (underlined below), some IN-fusion proteins contained a nuclear localization signal between the two protein cDNAs. It should be noted that not all proteins likely function as (IN)-fusion proteins, and in some cases, optimizing the linker between the two proteins may be necessary.

The Nucleotide Sequence of the IN-cDNA in Our IN-Fusion Constructs:

**CTATTTTTAGATGGAATAGATAAGGCCCAAG
AAGAACATGAGAAATATCACAGTAATT
GGAGAGCAATGGCTAGTGATTTTAACCTACCA
CCTGTAGTAGCAAAAGAAATAGTAGCCA-
GCTGTGATAAATGTCAGCTAAAAGGGGAAGCC
ATGCATGGACAAGTAGACTGTAGCCCAGGAAT
ATGGCAGCTAGATTGTACACATTTAGAAGGAA-
AAGTTATCTTGGTAGCAGTTCATGTAGCCAGT
GGATATATAGAAGCAGAAGTAATTCCAG
CAGAGACAGGGCAAGAAACAGCATACTT
CCTCTTAAAATTAGCAGGAAGATGGCCAG
TAAAAACAGTACATACAGACAATGGC
AGCAATTTCACCAGTACTACAGTTAA-
GGCCGCCTGTTGGTGGGCGGGGATCAAG-
CAGGAATTTGGCATTCCCTACAATCCCCAAA
GTCAAGGAGTAATAGAATCTATGAATAAAG-
AATTAAAGAAAATTATAGGACAGGTAAGA
GATCAGGCTGAACATC** *TTAAGACAGCAGTACA-
AATGGCAGTATTCATCCACAATTTTAAAAGAAA-
AGGGGGGATTGGGGGGTACAGTGCAGG-
GGAAAGAATAGTAGACATAATAGCAACAG-
ACATACAAACTAAAGAATTACAAAAACAAA
TTACAAAAATTCAAAATTTTCGGGTTTAT
TACAGGGACAGCAGA* aat *CCA* ctt *TGG
AAAGGACCAGCAAAGCTCCTCTGGAAAGG-
TGAAGGGGCAGTAGTAATACAAGATAAT
AGTGACATAAAAGTAGTGCCAAGAAGAAA
AGCAAAGATCATTAGGGATTATGGAAAACA-
GATGGCAGGTGATGATTGTGTGGCAAGTAGAC-
AGGATGAGGAT*<u>*TCTAGT.*</u>

3. In order to study the integration capability of the LVs, the percentage of fluorescing cells is measured over a time window that is long enough to allow transient expression from nonintegrated vector genomes to seize. Good starting points for FACS sample preparation are, for example, days 2, 4, 7, and 10 post transduction. The first one or two analyzed time points should represent the day of maximal transgene expression after transduction. There are differences between cell lines in how quickly maximal expression is achieved and the optimal FACS analysis time points should be experimentally tested. By the

last FACS sampling time point (day 10 or later), the expression from nonintegrated vectors has generally decreased to a level that is close to cell line-specific background fluorescence. In the example, Subheading 3.4, the cell samples are not fixed and FACS analysis is performed immediately after sample preparation.

4. Many different methods have been developed to extract the unknown genomic sequence surrounding a known integrated vector or virus sequence. Some methods rely on cleaving the genomic DNA surrounding the provirus sequence with restriction enzymes, after which a linker cassette is ligated into the genomic DNA that serves as the binding site for known primer sequences. Together with provirus-specific primers, they are used to amplify the IS sequence surrounding the known vector DNA. The most frequently used of such methods are the linear amplification-mediated PCR (LAM-PCR) [20] and ligation-mediated PCR (LM-PCR) [21]. Methods that rely on the use of restriction enzymes to fragment genomic DNA are prone to so-called restriction bias that may result in unequal retrieval of IS from different parts of the genome [22, 23]. Alternative Re-free methods include, for example, the nonrestrictive linear amplification-mediated PCR (nrLAM-PCR) [24], a MuA transposase-based PCR method [25], and the flanking-sequence exponential anchored–PCR (FLEA–PCR) [26]. Instead of restriction enzymes, the genomic DNA can also be first sheared with sonication after which the process can continue similar to LM- or LAM-PCRs or their variants [27, 28]. Such methods can generally yield a better coverage of all possible genomic integration sites and be used more reliably for the estimation of clonal contributions of differently modified cells in a polyclonal population. All the above mentioned methods are described in detail in the corresponding references. The selection of the IS extraction method depends on the amount of starting material, the availability of necessary equipment, and, for example, on the need to reliably analyze the sizes of provirus-modified cell clones. IS sequence-containing amplicons that are generally bar-coded at least at one end by specific sequence identificators are sequenced with next-generation sequencing methods and the results analyzed bioinformatically.

5. The testing of successful protein transduction by LVs depends on the IN-fusion protein in question. With fluorescent fusion proteins, such as the IN-mCherry generated by us, microscopy techniques can be used. To detect the functionality of pro-apoptotic and cytotoxic fusion proteins, there are several commercial assays and kits available. IN-fusion proteins that are designed for the targeted integration of vectors generally

require the use of IS extraction methods (*see* **Note 4**), large-scale sequencing, and bioinformatic data analysis.

Acknowledgments

This work was supported by grants from Finnish Academy, ERC, the Sigrid Juselius Foundation, the Eemil Aaltonen Foundation, the Instrumentarium Science Foundation, and the Ella and Georg Ehrnrooth Foundation.

References

1. Goff SP (2007) Retroviridae: the retroviruses and their replication. In: Knipe DM, Howley PM (eds) Fields virology, 5th edn. Lippincott Williams & Wilkins, Philadelphia, pp 1999–2069

2. Freed EO, Martin MA (2007) HIVs and their replication. In: Knipe DM, Howley PM (eds) Fields virology, 5th edn. Lippincott Williams & Wilkins, Philadelphia, pp 2107–2186

3. Schröder ARW, Shinn P, Chen H et al (2002) HIV-1 integration in the human genome favors active genes and local hotspots. Cell 110:521–529

4. Wang GP, Ciuffi A, Leipzig J et al (2007) HIV integration site selection: analysis by massively parallel pyrosequencing reveals association with epigenetic modifications. Genome Res 17:1186–1194. doi:10.1101/gr.6286907

5. Berry C, Hannenhalli S, Leipzig J, Bushman FD (2006) Selection of target sites for mobile DNA integration in the human genome. PLoS Comput Biol 2:e157. doi:10.1371/journal.pcbi.0020157

6. Sadelain M, Papapetrou EP, Bushman FD (2011) Safe harbours for the integration of new DNA in the human genome. Nat Rev Cancer 12:51–58. doi:10.1038/nrc3179

7. Gijsbers R, Ronen K, Vets S et al (2010) LEDGF hybrids efficiently retarget lentiviral integration into heterochromatin. Mol Ther 18:552–560. doi:10.1038/mt.2010.36

8. Ferris AL, Wu X, Hughes CM et al (2010) Lens epithelium-derived growth factor fusion proteins redirect HIV-1 DNA integration. Proc Natl Acad Sci U S A 107:3135–3140. doi:10.1073/pnas.0914142107

9. Silvers RM, Smith JA, Schowalter M et al (2010) Modification of integration site preferences of an HIV-1-based vector by expression of a novel synthetic protein. Hum Gene Ther 21:337–349. doi:10.1089/hum.2009.134

10. Schenkwein D, Turkki V, Ahlroth MK et al (2013) rDNA-directed integration by an HIV-1 integrase-I-PpoI fusion protein. Nucleic Acids Res 41:e61. doi:10.1093/nar/gks1438

11. Bushman FD (1994) Tethering human immunodeficiency virus 1 integrase to a DNA site directs integration to nearby sequences. Proc Natl Acad Sci U S A 91:9233–9237

12. Bushman FD, Miller M (1997) Tethering human immunodeficiency virus type 1 preintegration complexes to target DNA promotes integration at nearby sites. J Virol 71:458–464

13. Schenkwein D, Turkki V, Kärkkäinen H-R et al (2010) Production of HIV-1 integrase fusion protein-carrying lentiviral vectors for gene therapy and protein transduction. Hum Gene Ther 21:589–602

14. Dull T, Zufferey R, Kelly M et al (1998) A third-generation lentivirus vector with a conditional packaging system. J Virol 72:8463–8471

15. Zufferey R, Dull T, Mandel RJ et al (1998) Self-inactivating lentivirus vector for safe and efficient in vivo gene delivery. J Virol 72:9873–9880

16. Kulkosky J, Jones KS, Katz RA et al (1992) Residues critical for retroviral integrative recombination in a region that is highly conserved among retroviral/retrotransposon integrases and bacterial insertion sequence transposases. Mol Cell Biol 12:2331–2338

17. Follenzi A, Naldini L (2002) Generation of HIV-1 derived lentiviral vectors. Methods Enzymol 346:454–465

18. Follenzi A, Naldini L (2002) HIV-based vectors. Preparation and use. Methods Mol Med 69:259–274

19. Tiscornia G, Singer O, Verma IM (2006) Production and purification of lentiviral vec-

tors. Nat Protoc 1:241–245. doi:10.1038/nprot.2006.37

20. Schmidt M, Schwarzwaelder K, Bartholomae C et al (2007) High-resolution insertion-site analysis by linear amplification-mediated PCR (LAM-PCR). Nat Methods 4:1051–1057. doi:10.1038/nmeth1103

21. Kustikova OS, Baum C, Fehse B (2008) Retroviral integration site analysis in hematopoietic stem cells. Methods Mol Biol 430:255–267. doi:10.1007/978-1-59745-182-6_18

22. Harkey MA, Kaul R, Jacobs MA et al (2007) Multiarm high-throughput integration site detection: limitations of LAM-PCR technology and optimization for clonal analysis. Stem Cells Dev 16:381–392. doi:10.1089/scd.2007.0015

23. Gabriel R, Eckenberg R, Paruzynski A et al (2009) Comprehensive genomic access to vector integration in clinical gene therapy. Nat Med 15:1431–1436. doi:10.1038/nm.2057

24. Paruzynski A, Arens A, Gabriel R et al (2010) Genome-wide high-throughput integrome analyses by nrLAM-PCR and next-generation sequencing. Nat Protoc 5:1379–1395. doi:10.1038/nprot.2010.87

25. Brady T, Roth SL, Malani N et al (2011) A method to sequence and quantify DNA integration for monitoring outcome in gene therapy. Nucleic Acids Res 39:e72. doi:10.1093/nar/gkr140

26. Pule MA, Rousseau A, Vera J et al (2008) Flanking-sequence exponential anchored-polymerase chain reaction amplification: a sensitive and highly specific method for detecting retroviral integrant-host-junction sequences. Cytotherapy 10:526–539. doi:10.1080/14653240802192636

27. Gillet NA, Malani N, Melamed A et al (2011) The host genomic environment of the provirus determines the abundance of HTLV-1-infected T-cell clones. Blood 117:3113–3122. doi:10.1182/blood-2010-10-312926

28. Firouzi S, López Y, Suzuki Y et al (2014) Development and validation of a new high-throughput method to investigate the clonality of HTLV-1-infected cells based on provirus integration sites. Genome Med 6:46. doi:10.1186/gm568

Part IV

Production, Detection, and Engineering of Exosomes

Chapter 15

Biogenesis and Functions of Exosomes and Extracellular Vesicles

Florian Dreyer and Andreas Baur

Abstract

Research on extracellular vesicles (EVs) is a new and emerging field that is rapidly growing. Many features of these structures still need to be described and discovered. This concerns their biogenesis, their release and cellular entrance mechanisms, as well as their functions, particularly in vivo. Hence our knowledge on EV is constantly evolving and sometimes changing. In our review we summarize the most important facts of our current knowledge about extracellular vesicles and described some of the assumed functions in the context of cancer and HIV infection.

   Key words Exosomes, Extracellular vesicles, Biomarker, HIV, ESCRT

1   Introduction

In recent years the function of extracellular vesicles (EVs) attracted increasing interest, particularly in cancer and viral research. Described to harbor and deliver a diverse repertoire of functional molecules to recipient cells, including genetic information, EVs seemingly constitute a new layer of complexity in multicellular organisms, which has been recognized only a few years ago. Based on the latest research, EVs have been described, for example, to support tumor growth, formation of metastasis, and immune evasion and stimulate HIV viral replication. Seminal work was published in 2008 when Skog et al. reported that glioblastoma cells secrete EVs containing mRNA transcripts harboring tumor-specific mutations [1]. Importantly, circulating EVs derived from glioblastoma patients also contained mutated mRNA transcripts encoding the EGFRvIII which were not detectable in healthy individuals [1]. In 2009 Muratori et al. published that HIV-infected cells shed large amounts of EV for reasons that were not clear at that time [2]. Meanwhile, EVs are associated with many more diseases and conditions and even parasites seem to release EV. Based on these findings, it is anticipated that circulating EVs

Maurizio Federico (ed.), *Lentiviral Vectors and Exosomes as Gene and Protein Delivery Tools*, Methods in Molecular Biology, vol. 1448, DOI 10.1007/978-1-4939-3753-0_15, © Springer Science+Business Media New York 2016

have a far greater importance in living organisms than previously thought and EV research is expected to increase significantly. In this chapter, we will concentrate on the current knowledge of EVs in general and reflect on some aspects of these novel factors in cancer and HIV infection.

2   Extracellular Vesicles

Intercellular communication represents an event of vital importance for multicellular organisms. It has been believed for decades that this process is solely mediated by the secretion of single soluble factors secreted into the extracellular space. However, the discovery that EVs contain a multitude of factors including signaling molecules, enzymes, and miRNA added a new layer of complexity to our understanding of intercellular communication. EVs are small and defined spherical structures limited by a lipid bilayer which are secreted into extracellular space [3]. Latest research identified EVs as autocrine stimulators as well as short- and long-distance messengers, which are taken up and processed by recipient cells to elicit various cellular responses. In addition, different types of EVs have been described, which differ with respect to their subcellular origin, their biophysical and/or biochemical properties, their receptor composition, and possibly their content (Table 1).

In addition to the EV types described in Table 1, Muratori and coworkers described a new type of EVs that are shed in clusters, or microvesicle clusters (MC), and do not originate, like typical exosomes, from multivesicular bodies (MVBs) or the plasma membrane, as, for example, microvesicles [2] (see below). These clusters were found to be released not only by HIV-infected T cells in vitro and in vivo but also after classical stimulation of T cells, for example, by PHA/PMA.

Current research focuses mainly on the investigation of two types of EVs, exosomes, and microvesicles. The term exosomes was coined by Trams et al. who described the release of EVs with 5′-nucleotidase activity from various normal and neoplastic cell lines [4]. These EVs had an average diameter of 500–1000 nm and were accompanied by a second vesicle population with a diameter of ~40 nm [4]. Subsequently it had been reported that reticulocytes actively secrete microvesicles of ~50–100 nm in diameter, mediated by fusion events of multivesicular endosomes with the cellular plasma membrane [5, 6]. These microvesicles were referred to as exosomes. In recent years exosomes have been extensively investigated and many biological functions were unraveled and have been attributed to these vesicles [7–11]. However, since exosomes are difficult to discriminate and/or purify from EV of other origin, many EV-induced biological functions reported in the

Table 1
Types and characteristics of EVs

Feature	Exosomes	Microvesicles	Ectosomes	Membrane particles	Exosome-like vesicles	Apoptotic vesicles
Size	50–100 nm	100–1000 nm	50–200 nm	50–80 nm	20–50 nm	50–500 nm
Density in sucrose	1.13–1.19 g/ml	ND	ND	1.04–1.07 g/ml	1.1 g/ml	1.16–1.28 g/ml
Appearance by electron microscopy	Cup shape	Irregular shape and electron-dense	Bilamellar round structures	Round	Irregular shape	Heterogeneous
Sedimentation	$100,000 \times g$	$10,000 \times g$	$160,000–200,000 \times g$	$100,000–200,000 \times g$	$175,000 \times g$	$1200 \times g$, $10,000 \times g$ or $100,000 \times g$
Lipid composition	Enriched in cholesterol, sphingomyelin, and ceramide, contain lipid rafts, expose phosphatidylserine	Expose phosphatidylserine	Enriched in cholesterol and diacylglycerol, expose phosphatidylserine	ND	Do not contain lipid rafts	ND
Main protein markers	Tetraspanins (CD63, CD9), Alix, and TSG101	Integrins, selectins, and CD40 ligand	CR1 and proteolytic enzymes, no CD63	CD133; no CD63	TNFRI	Histones
Intracellular origin	Internal compartments (endosomes)	Plasma membrane	Plasma membrane	Plasma membrane	Internal compartments?	ND

Reprinted by permission from Macmillan Publishers Ltd: Nature Reviews Immunology, Thery et al. [53], copyright 2009

literature are not necessarily induced by exosomes alone. Nevertheless, EVs that originate from MVB and are released after fusion of the MVB with the plasma membrane are considered as exosomes.

3 Biogenesis of EVs

Various types of EVs have been identified and the same cell can produce multiple species of secreted vesicles. These different types of vesicles are generated at distinct subcellular locations and exhibit common as well as distinct key features (Fig. 1 and Table 1). With respect to their biogenesis, mainly three types of EVs have been investigated, namely, exosomes, microvesicles (Fig. 1), and microvesicle clusters (MC). Hallmarks of exosome biogenesis are first an endocytic event at the plasma membrane [5, 6], and, after the maturation of early endosomes to the late endosomes [12], the

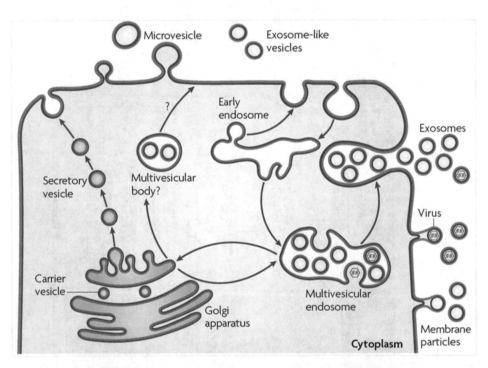

Fig. 1 Overview of multiple EV species and their subcellular origin. Vesicle trafficking between various subcellular compartments represents a fundamental cellular mechanism mediated through carrier vesicles which remain intracellular. On the other hand, cells generate vesicles destined for secretion. Various types of secreted vesicles exist, and they may differ in respect of their subcellular origin, their biogenesis pathway, their cargo uploading mechanisms, and their molecular composition. In addition they can differ in size and various other biophysical and biochemical characteristics. In general, one and the same cell can generate and secrete multiple EV species like vesicles, exosomes, membrane particles, or exosome-like vesicles. [Reprinted by permission from Macmillan Publishers Ltd: Nature Reviews Immunology, Thery et al. [53], copyright 2009]

formation of intraluminal vesicles (ILVs) by inward budding of the endosomal membrane, which gives rise to multivesicular bodies (MVBs) [13] (Fig. 2a). The process of MVB biogenesis is mediated by at least two distinct pathways and involves the sorting of various molecules into ILVs. The first pathway leading to MVB formation requires the *endosomal sorting complex required for transport* (ESCRT). This multimolecular machinery is consistent of ESCRT0, ESCRTI, ESCRTII, and ESCRTIII and is recruited to the endosomal membrane where the individual steps of ILV biogenesis are orchestrated [14]. This involves the recognition of ubiquitinated cargo proteins by ESCRT0, ESCRTI, and ESCRTII and the invagination of the late endosomal membrane mediated by ESCRTI and ESCRTII, a process facilitated through curvature-inducing factors [14, 15] (Fig. 2a). Recruitment of ESCRTIII to the site of membrane invagination occurs through binding to ESCRTII and leads to the deubiquitination of cargo proteins, the promotion of vesicle abscission, and thereby to the generation of ILVs [15, 16]. The second pathway of MVB formation is independent of the ESCRT machinery and is based on the specific lipid composition of the endosomal membrane. Raft-based microdomains are present on the limiting plasma membrane of endosomal compartments and contain high amounts of sphingolipids which represent substrates for the neutral sphingomylinase2 (nSMase2) [17–20]. At the endosomal membrane, nSMase2 is able to convert sphingolipids to ceramide which in turn induces coalescence of microdomains into larger structures thereby promoting domain-induced budding and formation of ILVs [18]. Following the formation of MVBs, they are either destined for the degradative or the secretory pathways, which are both governed by Rab GTPases [17]. While Rab7 can mediate the degradation through the fusion of MVBs with lysosomal compartments [17], several other Rab proteins like Rab5b, Rab9a, RAB27a, RAB27b, and Rab35 were reported to be crucial for intracellular MVB trafficking and secretion events [21, 22]. The final release of ILVs occurs upon MVB fusion with the cellular plasma membrane, a process which is yet not well investigated but probably mediated, at least in part, by *soluble N-ethylmaleimide-sensitive factor attachment protein receptors* (SNAREs), like the vesicle-associated membrane protein (VAMP) TI-VAMP/VAMP7 [23]. Once the ILVs are secreted, they are termed exosomes. Until today they represent the only known type of EVs of endosomal origin (Fig. 2a). The capacity to secrete exosomes differs from cell type to cell type and can occur on a constitutive or inducible basis. For example, dendritic cells (DCs) [24] and macrophages [25] secrete EVs on a constitutive bases, while mast cells [26] or T cells [27] have to be activated. In addition, the release of exosomes has been described for DCs [28, 29] and for B cells [30] upon interactions with T cells. In tumor

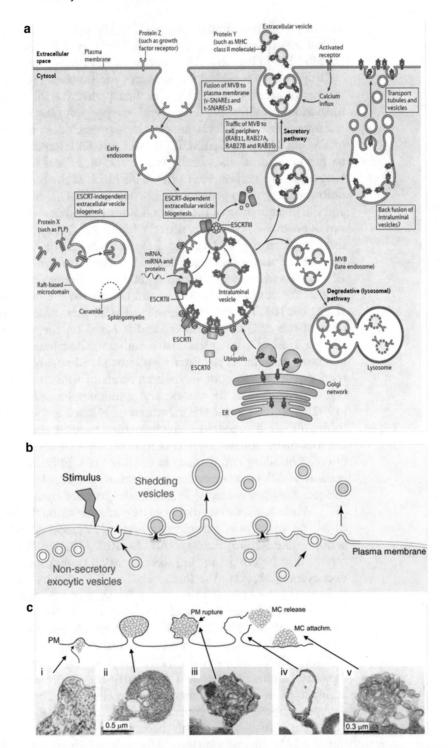

Fig. 2 Biogenesis and secretion of exosomes, microvesicles, and microvesicle clusters. (**a**) Exosomes, 40–100 nm in diameter, are generated by formation of intraluminal vesicles (ILVs) in an ESCRT- or sphingomyelinase-dependent manner into an endosomal compartment or MVB. These structures can enter either the degradative or the secretory route. MVBs destined for exosome generation follow the secretory

cells genotoxic stress leads to an increased activation of p53 transcription factors and, among other changes, to an enhanced p53 and tumor suppressor-activated pathway 6 (TSAP6) expression, which mediates augmented exosome secretion [31, 32].

The biogenesis of microvesicles differs considerably from that of exosomes; however, much less is known about the cellular processes leading to their generation. The formation of microvesicles occurs at the cellular plasma membrane [33]. Prior to their shedding, cytoplasmic protrusions are generated by the cell, which undergoes fission events, and finally microvesicles pinch off the cellular membrane [34]. The mechanisms underlying these shedding events are not well elucidated yet; however, microdomain-induced budding processes seem to be involved in these secretion events [35]. Despite the fact that microvesicles can be generated by resting cells, stimulation events leading, e.g., to increased intracellular calcium levels result in cellular membrane remodeling and an enhanced microvesicle secretion [34, 36]. Furthermore it has been reported that microvesicle secretion can be stimulated using phorbol esters [37] (Fig. 2b).

Microvesicle clusters (MC) have been described first by Muratori et al. in 2009. In this study, it was reported that stimulation of an HIV Nef-inducible Jurkat cell line, or stimulation of Jurkat cells with PHA or PMA, leads to the formation and secretion of MC. In contrast to exosomes or microvesicles, MC were composed of a large number of individual microvesicles (60–80 nm) and had a size of ~5–800 nm. The secretion process of MC, however, differed considerably from the aforementioned mechanisms. The budding event seemed to be initiated by the recruitment of small vesicles from the cytoplasm to the cellular membrane, which

Fig. 2 (continued) pathway, translocate to the cellular periphery where they fuse with the plasma membrane, and release their ILVs into the extracellular space. Once secreted, ILVs are termed exosomes. MVBs that enter the degradative pathway fuse with lysosomes where their cargo is degraded, a process of critical importance for the attenuation of signaling events. [Reprinted by permission from Macmillan Publishers Ltd: Nature Reviews Immunology, Robbins and Morelli [17], copyright 2014.] (**b**) Microvesicles, 100–1000 nm in diameter, are generated at the plasma membrane in a constitutive manner or upon stimuli. Nonsecretory exocytic vesicles (*blue*) seem to release their vesicular content at the sites of microvesicle generation thereby contributing to the microvesicle biogenesis. In addition, membrane-remodeling events take place leading to the generation of a plasma membrane composition distinct from surrounding areas, but similar to those of exocytosed vesicles (*red*). In the final stage, these areas bud off from the plasma membrane giving rise to secreted microvesicles. The mechanisms underlying the proposed membrane-remodeling or membrane-sorting events remain to be elucidated. (**c**) Microvesicle clusters are 5–800 nm in diameter consisting of smaller vesicle and tubules of about 60–80 nm in diameter. Prior to their secretion, microvesicles accumulate beneath the cell membrane where they bulge the plasma membrane until it ruptures releasing the microvesicle clusters. They remain coherent and attach as vesicle aggregate to the cell surface of bystander cells. *PM* plasma membrane, *MC attachm.* microvesicle cluster attachment

subsequently bulged into a ball-like structure and finally ruptured to release MC into the extracellular space [2]. After their secretion, these clusters remained stable and attached as whole complexes to the surface of bystander cells [2]. Furthermore it was reported that despite the unconventional release mechanism, the identified microvesicles share a number of biophysical and biochemical characteristics with exosomes. For example, they flotated in a sucrose gradient at a density of 1.13–1.19 g/ml and contained high amounts of CD63. Further evidence was provided that the described secretion process may be ERK1/2 dependent; however, the underlying molecular mechanisms leading to the biogenesis and secretion of microvesicle clusters remained unclear [2] (Fig. 2c).

4   Molecular Composition of EVs

During their biogenesis and prior to their secretion, various molecules are uploaded into the lumen of EVs. These molecules include various types of proteins like major histocompatibility complex (MHC) class I and II molecules, costimulatory molecules, tetraspanins, proteases, cytokines, growth factors, and death ligands. In addition, EVs can also contain genetic information like mRNA and miRNA molecules and also active enzymes. Even the presence of retrotransposon elements has been reported [38]. Despite this diverse repertoire, the molecular profile of EVs can be generally divided into two groups. The first group includes proteins relevant for the individual EV biogenesis pathways and for EV secretion [39]. These factors are found in EVs across various cell types and include, e.g., TSG101, Alix, or Rab proteins. The second group involves molecules that are specifically uploaded into vesicles by certain cell types thereby assigning EVs a characteristic cell-type fingerprint [39]. These factors involve, e.g., cytokines; surface receptors, like B cell or T cell; or signaling molecules and enzymes.

Apart from this classification, the selective sorting of molecules into EVs is commonly observed. For example, an accumulation of specific factors was observed, while others were barely detectable despite being present in parental cells [40–44]. Little is known about these selective shuttling mechanisms. However, ubiquitylation may represent a sorting signal, targeting proteins to late endosomes, where they are captured and transported into ILVs through the ESCRT machinery [17] (Fig. 2). In addition, it has been reported that plasma membrane anchor tags such as myristoylation, prenylation, and palmitoylation WHICH can target proteins to the site of vesicle budding and into EVs [45]. Hence, in addition to ubiquitylation, posttranslational lipid modifications seem to play a role in shuttling of proteins into EVs. Furthermore, CD43, a transmembrane sialoglycoprotein, has been implicated in mediating the selective protein upload into EVs [45, 46]. For example, in breast cancer cells, CD43 interacts with DICER which is uploaded into EVs [46]. Upon CD43 silencing, however, DICER levels significantly decreased in breast cancer EVs, while they increased in the nucleus and in the cytoplasm [46].

MicroRNAs on the other hand seem to be specifically uploaded into EVs, at least in part through shuttling sequences. It has been reported that sumoylated heterogeneous nuclear ribonucleoprotein (hnRNP) A2B1 specifically binds to miRNAs containing these shuttling motifs, leading to their uploading into ILVs [47]. In addition, posttranscriptional modifications of miRNAs through nontemplate nucleotide additions mediate their uploading into EVs [48]. Accordingly, it has been reported that 3′-end uridylated miRNAs appear to be enriched in EVs, while 3′-end adenylated miRNAs seem to be enriched in their parental cells [48]. Furthermore, the cellular expression level of individual miRNAs and their cognate target mRNA transcripts seem to influence the miRNA shuttling into EVs. In general, individual miRNAs are enriched in EVs in case of a high cellular miRNA/target mRNA expression ratio (i.e. high cellular expression of individual miRNAs and low cellular expression of their cognate target mRNA transcripts) [49]. Conversely, a low cellular miRNA/target mRNA expression ratio led to a decreased shuttling of miRNAs into EVs [49]. The detailed molecular mechanisms, however, remain to be elucidated.

Apart from these studies investigating specific EV uploading mechanisms, it has been suggested recently that the molecular cargo of EVs is not only functional in recipient cells but also in the vesicles itself. Hence, not only mature miRNAs but also pre-miRNA transcripts are present in EVs of breast cancer cells along with key components of the miRNA biogenesis machinery, i.e. DICER, TRBP, and AGO2 [46]. Remarkably, especially DICER and TRBP were functional in EVs, and the coordinated interaction of all factors mediated the cell-independent miRNA maturation with gene-silencing activity in recipient cells [46]. Importantly, these processes were observed in vivo using circulating EVs from breast cancer patients [46].

5   EVs in Physiological and Pathophysiological Conditions

In physiological and pathophysiological conditions, EVs act as multimolecular messengers by an autocrine and paracrine manner and proximal or distal from their site of origin. Long-distance EV transfer is very likely as EVs have been detected in various bodily fluids including peripheral blood, cerebrospinal fluid, urine, and saliva [50]. They are able to extravasate from the blood stream into various tissues like lungs or bones [51]. In addition, they seem to be able to pass the blood-brain barrier and to enter the brain, mediating gene silencing in neurons, microglia, and oligodendrocytes [52]. Basically, the interaction of EVs with recipient cells is mediated by:

1. A direct binding of EV lipids and/or transmembrane proteins with cellular surface proteins and/or receptors.

2. Membrane fusion events and integration of EV membrane-bound factors and lipids into the cellular membrane.

3. A cellular uptake of EVs by macropinocytosis and a subsequent fusion with other endosomal structures.

4. A cellular uptake and release of their molecular cargo into the cellular interior [53].

These uptake mechanisms are not mutually exclusive but reflect complementary processes allowing the transfer of proteins, mRNAs, and miRNAs to specific locations in recipient cells [54–56]. Hence, EVs can exert pleiotropic functions on multiple biological processes. For example, under physiological conditions EVs may contribute to blood coagulation [57], wound healing [58], or the regulation of immune responses against the fetus during pregnancy [59].

However, EVs also play major roles under pathophysiological conditions like in autoimmune [60] and inflammatory diseases [61], infectious diseases [62], or cancer [62]. Especially in cancer various and partly contradicting roles have been attributed to EVs. In general, cancer cells are able to stimulate themselves and/or modulate their microenvironment to favor tumor growth and progression and to suppress immune reactions [63]. Recently, various studies point at the relevance of EVs in mediating these effects. For example, it has been reported by Al-Nedawi et al. that glioma cells harboring the EGFRvIII mutation upload this mutated protein into EVs and transfer it to cancer cells lacking the EGFRvIII receptor. As a consequence, transforming signaling pathways like MAPK and Akt pathways have been activated in recipient cells and an altered EGFRvIII regulated gene expression was detectable, which finally led to morphological transformations and to an increased anchorage-independent growth capacity [55]. Peinado et al. demonstrated that melanoma exosomes are able to promote the metastatic phenotype of primary tumors through the education of bone marrow progenitor cells. This process is mediated by the exosomal transfer of the receptor tyrosine kinase MET to bone marrow progenitor cells. Furthermore, melanoma exosomes induced vascular leakiness at pre-metastatic sites and altered bone marrow progenitor cells toward a provasculogenic phenotype [51]. In addition to their crucial contribution to cancer growth and progression tumor, EVs are also involved in suppressing immune reactions. Accordingly, malignant melanoma, for example, exploits a mechanism referred to as tumor counterattack. Andreola et al. reported that melanoma cells are able to express and shuttle membrane-bound FasL into MVBs, while this death ligand was not detectable on the melanoma cell surface [64]. Upon secretion these EVs could induce Fas-mediated T cell apoptosis in a paracrine manner [64], while the secreting melanoma cells could escape an autocrine FasL-vesicle-induced cell death [65, 66].

On the other hand, EVs secreted by immune cells also play a role in pathophysiological conditions. Similar to EVs from cancer cells, multiple features have been attributed to immune cell EVs. This involves their role as mediators of the immune responses. In this context most studies focused on the analysis of DC EVs [56, 67–69]. Initially it was shown by Raposo et al. that EVs derived from B cells carry MHC class II molecules that can induce antigen-specific CD4+ T cell responses in vitro, although the efficiency of antigen presentation was estimated to be inferior as compared to B cells [70]. Zitvogel et al. then demonstrated that DCs also secrete EVs which harbor functional MHC class I, MHC class II, and T cell costimulatory molecules. In this study it was also reported that EVs derived from mouse DCs pulsed with tumor peptides caused tumor growth arrest and tumor eradication in 40–60% when injected in murine tumor models. These effects were described to be mediated by T cells [24]. In a subsequent study, Wolfers et al. extended these findings to tumor cell-derived EVs and demonstrated that they harbor tumor antigens. Upon injection of tumor EVs in a murine tumor model, significant antitumor effects were reported. However, tumor EVs could not directly induce CD8+ T cell activation in vitro despite the presence of MHC class I. Instead, CD8+ T cell activation was only observed when tumor EVs were first loaded onto DCs. The injection of tumor EV loaded DCs into murine tumor models and then led to a significant tumor growth delay and a curing rate of 33% [8].

Based on these and other findings, phase I clinical trials were carried out which recently have been completed [71, 72]. In one of these studies, DC EVs have been loaded with melanoma-associated antigen (MAGE) A3 peptides and were used for the vaccination of patients bearing MAGE-A3+ advanced melanomas [72]. The vaccination of 15 melanoma patients finally revealed one individual with an objective response, one with a minor response, and two patients with disease stabilizations. These observations were partly associated with tumor regressions. On the cellular level however, no MAGE-A3-specific CD4+ and CD8+ T cell responses could be determined, but, instead, an enhanced natural killer (NK) cell effector function was reported for eight patients. These surprising results were then further investigated and it has been shown by Viaud et al. that DC EVs can promote the proliferation and activation of NK cells in a natural killer group 2 member D (NKG2D) and interleukin-15 receptor α (IL-15Rα)-dependent manner. This suggested a mechanistic explanation on how DC EVs can induce tumor regression in vivo [73]. In addition it was recently reported that mouse DC EVs, independently of antigen presentation events, can directly induce apoptosis in various tumor cell lines in a caspase-dependent manner. This process was described to be mediated by tumor necrosis factor (TNF), FasL, and/or tumor necrosis factor-related apoptosis-inducing ligand (TRAIL) expressed in the correct orientation on the DC EV surface [74].

While numerous studies have concentrated on the role of EV in cancer, rather little is known about the role of EV in HIV infection. Similar as in the cancer field, there are no confirmed data on the relative concentration of HIV-specific EV in circulation nor where they originate. The first report came in 2009, when Muratori and colleagues reported that HIV-infected PBMC in vivo and in vitro secrete large amounts of MC in a Nef-dependent manner. At that time, the results were hampered by the fact that there was no obvious function of these vesicles, as there was little known about vesicle functions in general. In 2013 the same group published the molecular mechanism by which Nef induces the release of vesicles [75]. Nef seemed to target and associate with proteins of an integrin-associated signaling complex that included ADAM10 and ADAM17 proteases. The Nef-induced vesicles uploaded these ADAM proteases and could stimulate the release of TNF in target cells. Supporting these findings, vesicles purified from the plasma of HIV-infected individuals, but not of healthy controls, contained both ADAM proteases and Nef. As TNF is the most important activator of HIV replication in vivo, these results provide a first logical explanation of why these vesicles are relevant in HIV infection and pathogenesis. Supporting this conclusion, the group of M. Federico has shown that HIV-/Nef-induced vesicles can stimulate resting T cells to replicate HIV in an ADAM17-dependent manner [76, 77]. This suggested that HIV-/Nef-induced vesicles are potentially critical to enable HIV replication in the predominantly resting T cell compartment.

6   EVs as Novel Biomarkers

Based on their molecular cargo, which appears to be altered in pathophysiological conditions, EVs have been suggested as biomarkers for diagnostic purposes. Accordingly, it has been reported that a protein signature present in circulating exosomes of melanoma patients was identified which could be linked to distinct clinical tumor stages. Skog et al. demonstrated that circulating EVs derived from glioblastoma patients contained mRNA transcripts reflecting mutations typically found in these tumors. Hence, the authors reported that EGFRvIII transcripts were detectable in 28% of the glioblastoma patients analyzed. Furthermore they determined the presence of mutated mRNA transcripts in two patients in which the mutation was not detectable in the primary tumor sample thereby confirming the general genetic heterogeneity of tumor cell populations. In addition, protein signatures, mutated mRNA transcripts, and aberrant miRNA expression patterns have been used to characterize various tumor types. Taylor et al. demonstrated that miRNAs are readily detectable in circulating EVs derived from ovarian cancer patients using the miRNA microarray technology. The authors identified a set of eight miRNAs which was found to be significantly enriched in ovarian cancer patients compared to individuals with benign disease, while this miRNA signature was not detectable in circulating EVs derived from healthy individuals [78]. Furthermore, Ogata-Kawata et al. reported the identification of a signature consisting of seven miRNAs derived from circulating EVs of colorectal cancer patients. Compared to healthy individuals, this signature was significantly enriched in primary colorectal cancer patients. Upon surgical resection, however, these miRNAs were again significantly downregulated [79].

Taken together, these studies demonstrate the enormous potential of circulating EVs as easy accessible novel biomarkers for cancer and possibly other diseases. It is likely that they can also be used for the monitoring of disease progression or for the evaluation of therapy responses. In addition it is conceivable that circulating EVs from sensitive physiologic sensing systems like the immune system, but not from the limited number of residual cancer cells, may reflect another promising surrogate biomarker source for the detection of residual cancer cells and for the clinical classification, surveillance, and therapy once the molecular determinants have been identified.

References

1. Skog J et al (2008) Glioblastoma microvesicles transport RNA and proteins that promote tumour growth and provide diagnostic biomarkers. Nat Cell Biol 10:1470–1476

2. Muratori C et al (2009) Massive secretion by T cells is caused by HIV Nef in infected cells and by Nef transfer to bystander cells. Cell Host Microbe 6:218–230

3. Bollati V et al (2014) Susceptibility to particle health effects, miRNA and exosomes: rationale and study protocol of the SPHERE study. BMC Public Health 14:1137

4. Trams EG et al (1981) Exfoliation of membrane ecto-enzymes in the form of microvesicles. Biochim Biophys Acta 645:63–70

5. Harding C, Heuser J, Stahl P (1983) Receptor-mediated endocytosis of transferrin and recycling of the transferrin receptor in rat reticulocytes. J Cell Biol 97:329–339

6. Pan BT et al (1985) Electron microscopic evidence for externalization of the transferrin receptor in vesicular form in sheep reticulocytes. J Cell Biol 101:942–948

7. Skokos D et al (2001) Mast cell-dependent B and T lymphocyte activation is mediated by the secretion of immunologically active exosomes. J Immunol 166:868–876

8. Wolfers J et al (2001) Tumor-derived exosomes are a source of shared tumor rejection antigens for CTL cross-priming. Nat Med 7:297–303

9. Kadiu I et al (2012) Biochemical and biologic characterization of exosomes and microvesicles as facilitators of HIV-1 infection in macrophages. J Immunol 189:744–754

10. Li J et al (2013) Exosomes mediate the cell-to-cell transmission of IFN-alpha-induced antiviral activity. Nat Immunol 14:793–803

11. Chatila TA, Williams CB (2014) Regulatory T cells: exosomes deliver tolerance. Immunity 41:3–5

12. Poteryaev D et al (2010) Identification of the switch in early-to-late endosome transition. Cell 141:497–508

13. Thery C, Zitvogel L, Amigorena S (2002) Exosomes: composition, biogenesis and function. Nat Rev Immunol 2:569–579

14. Williams RL, Urbe S (2007) The emerging shape of the ESCRT machinery. Nat Rev Mol Cell Biol 8:355–368

15. Rusten TE, Vaccari T, Stenmark H (2012) Shaping development with ESCRTs. Nat Cell Biol 14:38–45

16. Hurley JH, Hanson PI (2010) Membrane budding and scission by the ESCRT machinery: it's all in the neck. Nat Rev Mol Cell Biol 11:556–566

17. Robbins PD, Morelli AE (2014) Regulation of immune responses by extracellular vesicles. Nat Rev Immunol 14:195–208

18. Trajkovic K et al (2008) Ceramide triggers budding of exosome vesicles into multivesicular endosomes. Science 319:1244–1247

19. Wu BX, Clarke CJ, Hannun YA (2010) Mammalian neutral sphingomyelinases: regulation and roles in cell signaling responses. Neuromolecular Med 12:320–330

20. Kharaziha P et al (2012) Tumor cell-derived exosomes: a message in a bottle. Biochim Biophys Acta 1826:103–111

21. Ostrowski M et al (2010) Rab27a and Rab27b control different steps of the exosome secretion pathway. Nat Cell Biol 12:19–30; sup pp 11–13

22. Hsu C et al (2010) Regulation of exosome secretion by Rab35 and its GTPase-activating proteins TBC1D10A-C. J Cell Biol 189:223–232

23. Fader CM et al (2009) TI-VAMP/VAMP7 and VAMP3/cellubrevin: two v-SNARE proteins involved in specific steps of the autophagy/multivesicular body pathways. Biochim Biophys Acta 1793:1901–1916

24. Zitvogel L et al (1998) Eradication of established murine tumors using a novel cell-free vaccine: dendritic cell-derived exosomes. Nat Med 4:594–600

25. Bhatnagar S et al (2007) Exosomes released from macrophages infected with intracellular pathogens stimulate a proinflammatory response in vitro and in vivo. Blood 110:3234–3244

26. Raposo G et al (1997) Accumulation of major histocompatibility complex class II molecules in mast cell secretory granules and their release upon degranulation. Mol Biol Cell 8:2631–2645

27. Blanchard N et al (2002) TCR activation of human T cells induces the production of exosomes bearing the TCR/CD3/zeta complex. J Immunol 168:3235–3241

28. Buschow SI et al (2009) MHC II in dendritic cells is targeted to lysosomes or T cell-induced exosomes via distinct multivesicular body pathways. Traffic 10:1528–1542

29. Nolte-'t Hoen EN et al (2009) Activated T cells recruit exosomes secreted by dendritic cells via LFA-1. Blood 113:1977–1981

30. Muntasell A et al (2007) T cell-induced secretion of MHC class II-peptide complexes on B cell exosomes. EMBO J 26:4263–4272

31. Lespagnol A et al (2008) Exosome secretion, including the DNA damage-induced p53-dependent secretory pathway, is severely compromised in TSAP6/Steap3-null mice. Cell Death Differ 15:1723–1733

32. Yu X, Harris SL, Levine AJ (2006) The regulation of exosome secretion: a novel function of the p53 protein. Cancer Res 66:4795–4801

33. Deolindo P, Evans-Osses I, Ramirez MI (2013) Microvesicles and exosomes as vehicles between protozoan and host cell communication. Biochem Soc Trans 41:252–257

34. Cocucci E, Racchetti G, Meldolesi J (2009) Shedding microvesicles: artefacts no more. Trends Cell Biol 19:43–51

35. Conde D et al (2005) Tissue-factor-bearing microvesicles arise from lipid rafts and fuse with activated platelets to initiate coagulation. Blood 106:1604–1611

36. Quesenberry PJ, Aliotta JM (2010) Cellular phenotype switching and microvesicles. Adv Drug Deliv Rev 62:1141–1148

37. Cocucci E et al (2007) Enlargeosome traffic: exocytosis triggered by various signals is followed by endocytosis, membrane shedding or both. Traffic 8:742–757

38. Balaj L et al (2011) Tumour microvesicles contain retrotransposon elements and amplified oncogene sequences. Nat Commun 2:180

39. Gutierrez-Vazquez C et al (2013) Transfer of extracellular vesicles during immune cell-cell interactions. Immunol Rev 251:125–142

40. Thery C et al (1999) Molecular characterization of dendritic cell-derived exosomes. Selective accumulation of the heat shock protein hsc73. J Cell Biol 147:599–610

41. Mittelbrunn M et al (2011) Unidirectional transfer of microRNA-loaded exosomes from T cells to antigen-presenting cells. Nat Commun 2:282

42. Hessvik NP et al (2012) Profiling of microR-NAs in exosomes released from PC-3 prostate cancer cells. Biochim Biophys Acta 1819: 1154–1163

43. Li CC et al (2013) Glioma microvesicles carry selectively packaged coding and non-coding RNAs which alter gene expression in recipient cells. RNA Biol 10:1333–1344

44. Gezer U et al (2014) Long non-coding RNAs with low expression levels in cells are enriched in secreted exosomes. Cell Biol Int 38: 1076–1079

45. Shen B et al (2011) Protein targeting to exosomes/microvesicles by plasma membrane anchors. J Biol Chem 286:14383–14395

46. Melo SA et al (2014) Cancer exosomes perform cell-independent microRNA biogenesis and promote tumorigenesis. Cancer Cell 26:707–721

47. Villarroya-Beltri C et al (2013) Sumoylated hnRNPA2B1 controls the sorting of miRNAs into exosomes through binding to specific motifs. Nat Commun 4:2980

48. Koppers-Lalic D et al (2014) Nontemplated nucleotide additions distinguish the small RNA composition in cells from exosomes. Cell Rep 8:1649–1658

49. Squadrito ML et al (2014) Endogenous RNAs modulate microRNA sorting to exosomes and transfer to acceptor cells. Cell Rep 8:1432–1446

50. Yuana Y et al (2013) Extracellular vesicles in physiological and pathological conditions. Blood Rev 27:31–39

51. Peinado H et al (2012) Melanoma exosomes educate bone marrow progenitor cells toward a pro-metastatic phenotype through MET. Nat Med 18:883–891

52. Alvarez-Erviti L et al (2011) Delivery of siRNA to the mouse brain by systemic injection of targeted exosomes. Nat Biotechnol 29:341–345

53. Thery C, Ostrowski M, Segura E (2009) Membrane vesicles as conveyors of immune responses. Nat Rev Immunol 9:581–593

54. Valadi H et al (2007) Exosome-mediated transfer of mRNAs and microRNAs is a novel mechanism of genetic exchange between cells. Nat Cell Biol 9:654–659

55. Al-Nedawi K et al (2008) Intercellular transfer of the oncogenic receptor EGFRvIII by microvesicles derived from tumour cells. Nat Cell Biol 10:619–624

56. Montecalvo A et al (2012) Mechanism of transfer of functional microRNAs between mouse dendritic cells via exosomes. Blood 119:756–766

57. Biro E et al (2003) Human cell-derived microparticles promote thrombus formation in vivo in a tissue factor-dependent manner. J Thromb Haemost 1:2561–2568

58. Zhang B et al (2015) HucMSC-exosome mediated-Wnt4 signaling is required for cutaneous wound healing. Stem Cells 33(7): 2158–2168

59. Taylor DD, Akyol S, Gercel-Taylor C (2006) Pregnancy-associated exosomes and their modulation of T cell signaling. J Immunol 176:1534–1542

60. Saenz-Cuesta M, Osorio-Querejeta I, Otaegui D (2014) Extracellular vesicles in multiple sclerosis: what are they telling us? Front Cell Neurosci 8:100

61. Buzas EI et al (2014) Emerging role of extracellular vesicles in inflammatory diseases. Nat Rev Rheumatol 10:356–364

62. Silverman JM, Reiner NE (2011) Exosomes and other microvesicles in infection biology: organelles with unanticipated phenotypes. Cell Microbiol 13:1–9

63. Hanahan D, Weinberg RA (2011) Hallmarks of cancer: the next generation. Cell 144: 646–674

64. Andreola G et al (2002) Induction of lymphocyte apoptosis by tumor cell secretion of FasL-bearing microvesicles. J Exp Med 195: 1303–1316

65. Raisova M et al (2000) Resistance to CD95/Fas-induced and ceramide-mediated apoptosis of human melanoma cells is caused by a defective mitochondrial cytochrome c release. FEBS Lett 473:27–32

66. Irmler M et al (1997) Inhibition of death receptor signals by cellular FLIP. Nature 388:190–195

67. Delcayre A, Shu H, Le Pecq JB (2005) Dendritic cell-derived exosomes in cancer immunotherapy: exploiting nature's antigen delivery pathway. Expert Rev Anticancer Ther 5:537–547

68. Naslund TI et al (2013) Dendritic cell-derived exosomes need to activate both T and B cells to induce antitumor immunity. J Immunol 190:2712–2719

69. Sobo-Vujanovic A et al (2014) Dendritic-cell exosomes cross-present Toll-like receptor-ligands and activate bystander dendritic cells. Cell Immunol 289:119–127

70. Raposo G et al (1996) B lymphocytes secrete antigen-presenting vesicles. J Exp Med 183:1161–1172

71. Morse MA et al (2005) A phase I study of dexosome immunotherapy in patients with advanced non-small cell lung cancer. J Transl Med 3:9

72. Escudier B et al (2005) Vaccination of metastatic melanoma patients with autologous dendritic cell (DC) derived-exosomes: results of the first phase I clinical trial. J Transl Med 3:10

73. Viaud S et al (2009) Dendritic cell-derived exosomes promote natural killer cell activation and proliferation: a role for NKG2D ligands and IL-15Ralpha. PLoS One 4:e4942

74. Munich S et al (2012) Dendritic cell exosomes directly kill tumor cells and activate natural killer cells via TNF superfamily ligands. Oncoimmunology 1:1074–1083

75. Lee JH et al (2013) HIV Nef, paxillin, and Pak1/2 regulate activation and secretion of TACE/ADAM10 proteases. Mol Cell 49: 668–679

76. Arenaccio C et al (2014) Exosomes from human immunodeficiency virus type 1 (HIV-1)-infected cells license quiescent CD4+ T lymphocytes to replicate HIV-1 through a Nef- and ADAM17-dependent mechanism. J Virol 88:11529–11539

77. Arenaccio C et al (2014) Cell activation and HIV-1 replication in unstimulated CD4+ T lymphocytes ingesting exosomes from cells expressing defective HIV-1. Retrovirology 11:46

78. Taylor DD, Gercel-Taylor C (2008) MicroRNA signatures of tumor-derived exosomes as diagnostic biomarkers of ovarian cancer. Gynecol Oncol 110:13–21

79. Ogata-Kawata H et al (2014) Circulating exosomal microRNAs as biomarkers of colon cancer. PLoS One 9:e92921

80. Schorey JS, Bhatnagar S (2008) Exosome function: from tumor immunology to pathogen biology. Traffic 9:871–881

81. Azmi AS, Bao B, Sarkar FH (2013) Exosomes in cancer development, metastasis, and drug resistance: a comprehensive review. Cancer Metastasis Rev 32:623–642

Chapter 16

Generation, Quantification, and Tracing of Metabolically Labeled Fluorescent Exosomes

Carolina Coscia, Isabella Parolini, Massimo Sanchez, Mauro Biffoni, Zaira Boussadia, Cristiana Zanetti, Maria Luisa Fiani, and Massimo Sargiacomo

Abstract

Over the last 10 years, the constant progression in exosome (Exo)-related studies highlighted the importance of these cell-derived nano-sized vesicles in cell biology and pathophysiology. Functional studies on Exo uptake and intracellular trafficking require accurate quantification to assess sufficient and/or necessary Exo particles quantum able to elicit measurable effects on target cells. We used commercially available BODIPY® fatty acid analogues to label a primary melanoma cell line (Me501) that highly and spontaneously secrete nanovesicles. Upon addition to cell culture, BODIPY fatty acids are rapidly incorporated into major phospholipid classes ultimately producing fluorescent Exo as direct result of biogenesis. Our metabolic labeling protocol produced bright fluorescent Exo that can be examined and quantified with conventional non-customized flow cytometry (FC) instruments by exploiting their fluorescent emission rather than light-scattering detection. Furthermore, our methodology permits the measurement of single Exo-associated fluorescence transfer to cells making quantitative the correlation between Exo uptake and activation of cellular processes. Thus the protocol presented here appears as an appropriate tool to who wants to investigate mechanisms of Exo functions in that it allows for direct and rapid characterization and quantification of fluorescent Exo number, intensity, size, and eventually evaluation of their kinetic of uptake/secretion in target cells.

Key words Exosomes, Metabolic labeling, BODIPY fatty acids, Differential centrifugation, Lipid analysis, Flow cytometry, Exosome uptake

1 Introduction

Since their discovery, microvesicles and exosomes (Exo) stimulated a surge of interest in the study of their biogenesis, cell targeting, and cellular effects. Exo are 50–100 nm-sized vesicles released by almost all cell types, which have been especially highlighted for their role in intercellular communication, in both physiological and pathological conditions including cancer [1, 2]. Exo biogenesis starts with the inward budding of membrane portions of late

Maurizio Federico (ed.), *Lentiviral Vectors and Exosomes as Gene and Protein Delivery Tools*, Methods in Molecular Biology, vol. 1448, DOI 10.1007/978-1-4939-3753-0_16, © Springer Science+Business Media New York 2016

endosomes to form intraluminal vesicles (ILVs) that mature into multivesicular bodies (MVBs). Upon fusion with the plasma membrane, MVBs release an Exo swarm in the extracellular space that, by entering biological fluids, reaches their cell targets ultimately delivering their cargo of specific signals [3]. Despite the recent expansion of studies in the Exo field, there is a paucity of effectual methods for the reliable quantification and characterization of these vesicles. Nowadays quantification of Exo is often based on the level of total amount of proteins in vesicle preparations, but bulk protein contamination of ultracentrifuged vesicles makes quantification poorly reproducible among different preparations. A now rather diffused technology, nanoparticle tracking analysis (NTA), although promising, harbors several limitations because it has the tendency to overestimate the number of vesicles and seems less accurate for analysis of heterogeneous-sized preparations [4]. Flow cytometry, on the other hand, is a powerful technique allowing for single-particle detection and high-throughput, multiparameter analysis, but the fact that Exo vesicles have sizes below 200 nm constitutes a major challenge for the detection of small particles on the basis of their light-scattering signal, as performed in conventional FC. In recent years in the attempt to overcome such a bias, a successful new methodological approach consisting of fluorescent-labeled cell-derived vesicles coupled with high-resolution flow cytometry (hFC) analysis has been developed [4–6]. Although extremely valuable to directly analyze quantitatively and qualitatively individual cell-derived vesicles, this approach requires an optimized custom configuration of the commercially available Becton Dickinson (BD) Influx™ high-end flow cytometer that hampers its diffusion as a widely used method. Furthermore, fluorescent probes commonly used to obtain bright fluorescent vesicles preparations such as lipophilic dyes (e.g., PKH67, Di-dyes) [4] require additional washing steps to remove free unbound dye, while others, like CFSE [7], or lipid- (FM) specific dyes [8] are nonspecifically incorporated making extracellular vesicles quantification less precise. From our previous experience in labeling EVs [9], we developed a novel approach to obtain brightly fluorescent exosomes that can be examined and quantified with conventional non-customized FC instruments, i.e., Gallios (Beckman Coulter) or Canto (BD) and can be quantitatively traced in acceptor cells. Our methodology is based on cell treatment with BODIPY®-labeled fatty acid analogues that upon uptake enter the cellular lipid metabolism ultimately producing fluorescent Exo as a direct result of biogenesis. The great advantage of using fluorescent fatty acid analogues is that they enter the cellular lipid metabolic pathway without affecting the natural lipid metabolism or perturb the lipid homeostasis inside the cell. Nascent Exo, once released in the cell medium, can be routinely isolated by well-established differential centrifugation protocols (Fig. 1a) that can be coupled with density gradient floatation (Fig. 1b). Purified fluorescent Exo

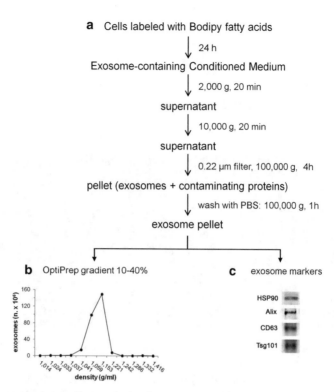

a Cells labeled with Bodipy fatty acids

↓ 24 h

Exosome-containing Conditioned Medium

↓ 2,000 g, 20 min

supernatant

↓ 10,000 g, 20 min

supernatant

↓ 0.22 µm filter, 100,000 g, 4h

pellet (exosomes + contaminating proteins)

↓ wash with PBS: 100,000 g, 1h

exosome pellet

b OptiPrep gradient 10-40%

c exosome markers

HSP90
Alix
CD63
Tsg101

Fig. 1 Exosome purification. (**a**) The experimental workflow used for fluorescent Exo isolation based on differential ultracentrifugation. Exo-containing conditioned medium from BODIPY fatty acid-labeled cells is processed by differential centrifugation to remove intact cells and cell debris. Resuspended Exo plus contaminating proteins pellet is filtered using a 0.22 µm membrane filter before last centrifugation step. The speed and length of each centrifugation are indicated. The final Exo pellet is resuspended in PBS and can be either directly FC counted or (**b**) further purified by running overnight on an 10–40 % OptiPrep density gradient. The fluorescent peak displays a density ranging from 1.06 to 1.15 g/mL typical of Exo [10, 11]. (**c**) Western blot analysis of purified exosomes (5×10^7) probed with antibodies against Exo markers HSP90, Alix, CD63, and Tsg101

display a density ranging from 1.06 to 1.15 g/mL typical of Exo [10, 11] and are positive for Exo markers (Alix, Tsg101, CD63, HSP90) (Fig. 1c). We used both green fluorescent hexadecanoic acid (BODIPY FL C_{16}) (C16) and red fluorescent dodecanoic acid (BODIPY 558/568 C_{12}) (C12) that are reported to incorporate well into cells [12, 13] but as far as we know never to label MVBs. The characteristics that highlight BODIPY-conjugated lipids as close to natural membrane molecules cannot be extended to synthetic lipophilic fluorescent probes so far largely introduced for Exo research, especially when they are used to trace membrane trafficking of Exo following cell uptake. Metabolic labeling of Exo is thus an effective tool that may consent precise quantification of the natural extent and timing of Exo production related to cell cycle, type, and culture conditions. Furthermore our methodology

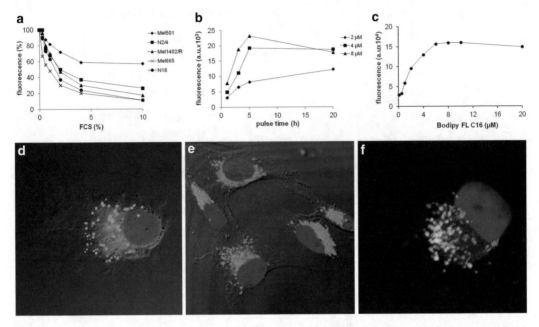

Fig. 2 Metabolic labeling of Me501 cells with BODIPY fatty acids. (**a**) FCS dependence of C16 incorporation in different cell lines. Cell-associated fluorescence is analyzed by FC. In all cell lines tested 0.3% FCS ensures optimal C16 cell incorporation. (**b**) Time dependence of C16 incorporation into Me501 cells. Cell-associated fluorescence is maximal after 5 h incubation with all C16 concentrations tested. (**c**) C16 concentration dependence of Me501 cell incorporation. After 5 h incorporation, a plateau is reached at 7 μM probe concentration. (**d**, **e**) Confocal microscopy cross sections of Me501 cells metabolically labeled for 5 h with (**d**) C16 or (**e**) C12 showing fluorescence localization in the ER/late endosomal/MVB compartments. (**f**) Colocalization of C16 with anti-bis(monoacylglycero)phosphate (BMP) antibody, an Exo-specific lipid [14]. As expected, BMP is completely absent on plasma membrane and consequently from microvesicles budding from the plasma membrane (ectosomes)

enables the measuring of single Exo-associated fluorescence transfer to cells, thus making quantitative the correlation between Exo uptake and activation of cellular processes (Fig. 2).

In conclusion we can infer that metabolically labeled vesicles positive for Exo markers (HSP90/Alix/CD63/Tsg101) are likely to represent a real Exo population that can be characterized and measured as a single particle by means of affordable FC instruments available to a wider scientific community.

2   Materials

2.1   Cell Culture

1. Human melanoma Me501 cells.

2. Cell culture medium: RPMI 1640, complete with required nutrients and antibiotics (e.g., L-glutamine, penicillin/streptomycin) and supplemented with 10% (v/v) fetal calf serum (FCS) heat inactivated and filtered through a 0.22 μm filter.

3. Tissue culture flasks.

2.2 Cell Labeling with BODIPY Fatty Acid Analogues

1. Green fluorescent fatty acid: BODIPY FL C_{16} (4,4-difluoro-5,7-dimethyl-4-bora-3a,4a-diaza-s-indacene-3-hexadecanoic acid) (C16). Resuspend powder in methanol at 1 mM final concentration. Make 100 μL aliquots in Eppendorf tubes and store at –20 °C (up to 12 months) (*see* **Note 1**).

2. Red fluorescent fatty acid: BODIPY 558/568 C_{12} (4,4-difluoro-5-(2-thienyl)-4-bora-3a,4a-diaza-s-indacene-3-dodecanoic acid) (C12). Resuspend powder in methanol at 1 mM final concentration. Make 100 μL aliquots in Eppendorf tubes and store at –20 °C (up to 12 months).

3. Cell-labeling medium: cell culture medium, 0.3% FCS (*see* **Note 2**).

4. 2 mL round bottom tube (Eppendorf) (*see* **Note 3**).

5. Bovine serum albumin (BSA) essentially fatty acid-free 2% in PBS (*see* **Note 4**).

6. KOH 20 mM.

7. Phosphate-buffered saline (PBS).

8. Microfuge.

9. ThermoMixer (Eppendorf).

2.3 Exo Isolation

1. Exo production medium: RPMI 1640 supplemented with all the nutrients and antibiotics and 10% exosome-depleted FBS (Exo-FBS) (*see* **Notes 5** and **6**).

2. 50 mL conical tubes (Falcon).

3. Beckman ultracentrifuge.

4. SW41 Ti Rotor, Swinging Bucket (Beckman Coulter).

5. SW60 Ti Rotor, Swinging Bucket (Beckman Coulter).

6. Polyallomer konical™ tubes appropriate for the ultracentrifuge SW41 Ti Rotor and SW60 Ti Rotor (Beckman Coulter) (*see* **Note 7**).

7. Sterile PBS.

8. Stock OptiPrep™ solution: 60% (w/v) aqueous iodixanol.

2.4 Analysis of Fluorescent Lipids

1. *Lipid extraction*: extraction solvent: chloroform/methanol 2:1 (v/v) [15].

2. Double-distilled water (ddH$_2$O).

3. 15 mL polypropylene centrifuge tubes or glass tubes.

4. Vortex.

5. Centrifuge.

6. N$_2$ tank.

7. *TLC analysis*: silica gel plates with fluorescence indicator.

8. Solvent mixture for separation of neutral lipids (*see* **Notes 8** **and 9**): hexane/diethyl ether/acetic acid (70:30:1, v/v).

9. Solvent mixture for separation of phospholipids (*see* **Note 9**): chloroform/methanol/32% ammonia (65:35:5, v/v) [16].

10. Lipid stain mixture: 3% copper acetate and 8% ortofosforic acid. Make 100 mL in a glass container.

11. Neutral lipid standards: triglyceride, cholesterol, and cholesterol ester. Make a pool in chloroform/methanol 2:1 (v/v) containing 20 μg of triglycerides and 5/10 μg each of cholesterol, cholesterol ester in 20 μL.

12. Phospholipid standards: phosphatidylcholine (PC), phosphatidylethanolamine (PE), phosphatidylserine (PS), phosphatidylinositol (PI), sphingomyelin (SM), cardiolipin (CL), and bis(monoacylglycerol)phosphate (BMP). Make a pool in chloroform/methanol 2:1 (v/v) containing 20 μg of each standard in 20 μL.

13. Filter paper.

14. Glass syringe (Hamilton).

15. TLC glass tank.

16. Glass tray of suitable size to accommodate TLC plate.

17. Oven.

18. Typhoon Phosphorimager for fluorescence detection (GE Healthcare).

19. Scanner.

2.5 Protein Quantitation (Bradford Assay)

1. BSA standard stock (2 mg/mL).

2. Protein Assay Dye Reagent Concentrate (Bio-Rad).

3. Test tubes.

4. PBS.

5. Cell lysis buffer: 10 mM Tris–HCl pH 7.4, 150 mM NaCl, 60 mM octylglucosyde, 5 mM EDTA, 1% Triton, Protease Inhibitor Cocktail Tablet, 1 in 10 mL (Sigma) (*see* **Note 10**).

6. Plastic or quartz cuvettes.

7. Spectrophotometer.

2.6 Western Blot Analysis

1. Blotting System (Bio-Rad) and transfer membranes (Hybond C Extra, GE Healthcare Life Sciences).

2. TBST: 10 mM Tris–HCl pH 8, 150 mM NaCl, 0.1% (w/v) Tween 20.

3. Blotto: 5% (w/v) skim milk powder in TBST.

4. Transfer buffer: 20 mM Tris–HCl, pH 7.4, 150 mM glycine, 20% methanol.

5. Running buffer: 25 mM Tris–HCl, pH 7.4, 192 mM glycine, 0.1% SDS.

6. Ponceau S staining solution: 0.5% (w/v) Ponceau S, 1% acetic acid.

7. Mouse anti-TSG101mAb (Santa Cruz): 1:200 in Blotto.

8. Rabbit polyclonal anti-CD63 Ab (System Bioscience): 1:1000 in Blotto.

9. Mouse anti-Hsp90 mAb (Santa Cruz):1:200 in Blotto.

10. Mouse anti-Alix mAb (Abcam):1:1000 in Blotto.

11. HRP conjugated secondary antibody 1:3000 in TBST.

12. ECL SuperSignal West Pico Chemiluminescent Substrate (PIERCE).

13. FluorChem™ Q System (Protein Simple).

2.7 Flow Cytometry (FC)

1. Size and number calibration beads: green fluorescent (505/515) Flow Cytometry Submicron Particle Size Reference Kit (Life Technologies).

2. Exo counting beads: Flow-Count Fluorospheres (Beckman Coulter).

3. PBS filtered through 0.22 μm membrane filter.

4. 5 mL polypropylene round bottom tubes (Beckman Coulter).

5. Gallios Flow Cytometer and Kaluza Software (Beckman Coulter) or similar.

2.8 Fluo-Exo Cell Transfer Assay

1. HBSS (Hank's Balanced Salt Solution), 20 mM HEPES.

2. ToPro-3 (viability dye): make 1 mM stock in DMSO (*see* **Note 11**).

3. 96 well plates.

4. Orbital shaker.

5. 5 mL polypropylene round bottom tubes (Beckman Coulter).

6. Fluorescence intensity calibration beads: Quantum™ FITC-5 MESF (Molecules of Equivalent Soluble Fluorophores) (Bangs Laboratories, Inc.).

3 Methods

3.1 BODIPY Fatty Acid Preparation

1. Thaw an aliquot of C16 or C12 (*see* **Note 12**).

2. Place the tube with lid open under a fume hood and evaporate off the solvent under a stream of N2 at room temperature (RT).

3. Add 30 μL KOH, 20 mM (*see* **Note 13**).

4. Vortex until complete solubilization.

5. Spin 20 s at 12,100 × g with microfuge.

6. Put tube in ThermoMixer at 60 °C for 10 min (*see* **Note 14**).

7. Add 70 μL BSA 2 % in PBS (v/w) and mix by pipetting (*see* **Note 15**).

3.2 Cell Labeling with BODIPY Fatty Acids

1. Adherent cells (Me501) are cultured to 50 % confluency in cell culture medium in 75 cm² flasks at 37 °C with 5 % CO_2 (*see* **Note 16**).

2. Remove medium and wash with 5 mL PBS.

3. Add 4 mL of cell-labeling medium containing 7 μM BODIPY fatty acids (*see* **Note 17**).

4. Incubate 5 h in at 37 °C with 5 % CO_2 (*see* **Note 17**).

5. Remove medium, wash cells twice with PBS to eliminate probe in excess, add 36 mL/flask of Exo production medium, and return cells to the incubator for 24 h (*see* **Note 18**).

6. Collect cell culture supernatant (exosome-containing conditioned medium, ECM) and proceed with Exo isolation or keep at 4 °C (*see* **Note 19**).

3.3 Fluorescent Exo Isolation

1. Transfer ECM to a 50 mL centrifuge tube.

2. Centrifuge 20 min at 2000 × g, 4 °C and discard pellet.

3. Transfer supernatant to 12 mL ultracentrifuge tubes (for SW41 Ti Rotor) (*see* **Note 20**).

4. Centrifuge 20 min at 10,000 × g, 4 °C and discard pellet.

5. Filter supernatant with 0.22 μm membrane filter and place in a fresh 12 mL polyallomer tube (SW41 Ti).

6. Centrifuge 4 h at 100,000 × g (*see* **Note 21**).

7. Discard supernatant and add PBS to fill the tube (*see* **Note 22**).

8. Centrifuge 1 h at 100,000 × g.

9. Discard supernatant and resuspend Exo pellet with 100 μL of PBS (*see* **Notes 23** and **24**).

10. For a further step of purification, perform an OptiPrep™ (iodixanol) gradient separation as follows: add Exo (260 μL in PBS) to 1 mL of 60 % OptiPrep™.

11. Prepare a discontinuous gradient: 60 % (w/v), 40 % (w/v), 30 % (w/v), and 10 % (w/v) solutions of OptiPrep™ by diluting 60 % stock with PBS.

12. In a 4.5 mL tube suitable for *SW60* Ti Rotor, place at the bottom Exo diluted in OptiPrep™ and then gently lay 0.5 mL 40 % OptiPrep™, 0.5 mL 30 % OptiPrep™, and 1.8 mL 10 % OptiPrep™.

13. Centrifuge 18 h at 192,000 × g.

14. Collect 12×330 µL fractions and FC count as described in Subheading 3.7 (*see* **Note 25**).

15. To determine the density of a fraction, run in parallel a control OptiPrep™ gradient. Collect fractions as described above and measure the refractive index on 5 µL of each fraction with a refractometer (*see* **Note 26**).

3.4 Analysis of Fluorescent Lipids

1. *Lipid extraction*: transfer Exo or cells in PBS to a 15 mL tube and add ddH$_2$O to reach 1.5 mL final volume.

2. Add 6 mL chloroform/methanol 2:1 (v/v) (*see* **Note 27**).

3. Vortex and centrifuge 20 min at $2,240 \times g$ at RT.

4. Remove aqueous upper phase (containing non-lipid cellular material) and interface.

5. Evaporate the lower chloroform phase under a gentle nitrogen stream at 50 °C. It takes about 20 min.

6. Add to each tube a suitable volume of chloroform/methanol 2:1 (v/v) in order to have the equivalent of 5–10×10^7 Exo or 5×10^5 cells in 20 µL (*see* **Notes 28** and **29**).

7. *TLC analysis*: mark lanes needed for samples and standards with a fine point pencil and a ruler, making the loading mark at least 1 cm from the bottom of the plate (*see* **Note 30**).

8. Using a glass syringe, spot or streak 20 µL of the lipid sample and pooled standards. Allow sample to dry.

9. For neutral lipid separation (Fig. 3a/d): line the TLC tank with filter paper and pour 30 mL of solvent mixture. Put the lid on the tank and let the solvent equilibrate for at least 30 min (*see* **Note 31**). When ready to run samples, pour 10 mL of fresh solvent mixture in a glass tray that can accommodate the TLC plate and place at the bottom of the TLC tank.

10. For phospholipid separation (Fig. 3e/f): pour 100 mL of fresh solvent mixture in the TLC tank.

11. Lower the loaded TLC plate into the chromatography tank making sure the samples are above the surface of the developing solvent (*see* **Notes 32** and **33**).

12. Place the lid on the tank and allow the solvent to ascend to about 1 cm from the top of the TLC plate (*see* **Note 34**).

13. Remove plate from the tank and air-dry in a fume hood (*see* **Note 35**).

14. Scan plates with a Typhoon Phosphorimager system.

15. Quantify the fluorescence intensity of the lipid bands using available software (ImageQuant).

16. After quantification of fluorescent bands, nonfluorescent lipid standards can be visualized by immersing the TLC plate for 10 min in a glass tray containing 100 mL of staining solution.

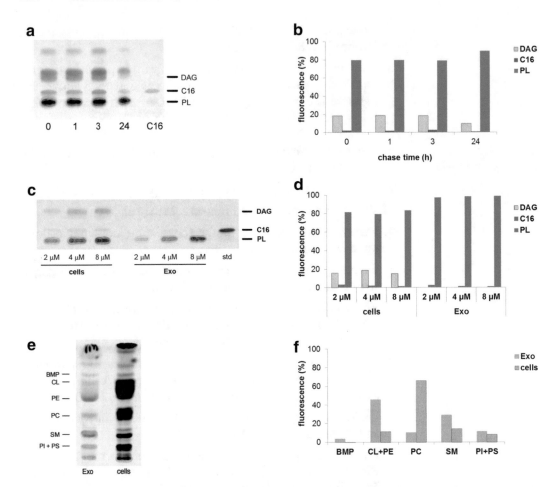

Fig. 3 Lipid analysis of C16-labeled cells and Exo. (**a**) Cells were treated for 5 h with 7 μM C16 and chased in complete media. At different time points, lipids were extracted and subjected to TLC analysis for neutral lipids. (**b**) Quantification of relative density of lipid spots shows that at the end of the incubation time, most fluorescent probe is incorporated into phospholipids/DAG and only very little is still present as free probe as determined by comparing cells and Exo. (**c**) Cells were treated with different concentrations of C16 and after 24 h cells and Exo were collected and analyzed by TLC for neutral lipids. (**d**) Quantification of relative density of lipid spots shows that in contrast to cells, Exo contain mostly phospholipids and virtually no free C16. (**e**) Cells and Exo lipid extracts are analyzed by TLC for phospholipids showing that C16 is metabolized in all the major phospholipid classes including Exo-specific BMP whose relative ratio is much higher in Exo if compared to cells. (**f**) Quantification of relative ratio of lipid spots shows that differences in relative amounts of phospholipids between Exo and cells are representative of their unlabelled counterpart [14] with the exception of BMP which is greatly enriched in Exo. Abbreviations used: *SM* sphingomyelin, *CL* cardiolipin, *PS* phosphatidylserine, *PI* phosphatidylinositol, *PE* phosphatidylethanolamine, *PC* phosphatidylcholine, *BMP* bis(monoacylglycero) phosphate

17. Remove the plate, air-dry (*see* **Note 36**), and bake in preheated oven for 10 min at 120 °C.

18. Scan image and analyze with Alphaview or other software.

3.5 Protein Quantitation (Bradford Assay)

1. Prepare a duplicate set of BSA dilutions, starting with 40 µg/mL and performing twofold dilutions in dH_2O (six dilutions). 800 µL for each dilution will be needed.

2. Prepare a blank reference standard not containing protein (800 µL of dH_2O).

3. Add cell lysate (*see* **Note 37**), Exo, or OptiPrep™ fractions (*see* **Note 38**), to 800 µL of dH_2O (final volume) (*see* **Note 39**).

4. Add 200 µL of Protein Assay Dye Reagent Concentrate.

5. Vortex and transfer samples and standards into cuvettes.

6. Read OD at 590 nm within 10 min.

3.6 Western Blot Analysis

1. For each lane, prepare a tube with 5×10^7 exosomes (counted as described in Subheading 3.7) or ~20 µg cell lysate (~5×10^4 cells) (*see* **Note 37**).

2. Add SDS sample buffer to each tube and heat for 5 min at 95 °C (*see* **Note 40**).

3. Load samples on a 10 % or 12 % gel.

4. Perform electrophoresis at constant 160 V for 1 h 30 min.

5. Following electrophoresis, electro-transfer proteins onto nitro-cellulose membranes using the Blotting System.

6. At the end of the run, check the quality of the protein transfer by incubating the nitrocellulose membrane for 1–2 min in Ponceau S solution (*see* **Note 41**).

7. Move the membrane to a clean tray and wash with dH_2O until red protein bands become visible.

8. Acquire the image of Ponceau stained membrane by a densitometer or scanner.

9. Block membranes with Blotto for 1 h at RT. Care should be taken not to touch and disrupt the membrane.

10. Probe the membranes with primary antibodies (i.e., anti-HSP90, anti-Alix, anti-TSG101, anti-CD63) O/N in Blotto at 4 °C (*see* **Notes 42** and **43**). Wash membrane three times in TTBS for 10 min.

11. Incubate membrane with HRP-labeled secondary antibody for 1 h at RT. Wash membrane three times in TTBS for 10 min.

12. Prepare the ECL working solution of the SuperSignal West Pico Chemiluminescent Substrate (*see* **Note 44**) by mixing Reagent 1 and Reagent 2 at 1:1 ratio (v/v) (*see* **Note 45**). Incubate the membrane in the ECL working solution for 60 s.

13. Visualize the protein bands using FluorChem™ Q System (Protein Simple).

**3.7 FC Analysis
of Fluo-Exo**

Although it is well known that FC based on light-scattering detection of vesicles and particles smaller than 300 nm is severely hampered by noise derived from buffers, optics, and electronics, we present here a protocol apt to discriminate fluorescently labeled vesicles from nonfluorescent noise by applying fluorescence threshold triggering. With this setup and by using control 100–500 nm fluorescent beads, we can distinguish Exo from noise events on the basis of fluorescence. One hundred nanometer beads of known number are also used as internal reference standard in each FC acquisition. Numerous repeated acquisitions of different dilutions of beads show linearity and reproducibility of measurements demonstrating that quantification of fluorescent Exo is accurate (Fig. 4):

1. Set FL1 discriminator to 1 on histogram and FL1/LogSS dot plot in order to fix the threshold on fluorescence intensity just above the PBS background noise (*see* **Note 46**).

2. Acquire PBS samples and increase FL1 voltage until PBS background noise is barely visualized.

3. Add 20 μL to Flow-Count Fluorospheres (*see* **Note 47**) to 200 μL of PBS. Set instrument at flux high; fix the stopping gate on 2000 Flow-Count Fluorospheres on correctly drawn region in a FL channel different from FL1, e.g., FL5 (Fig. 4c) (*see* **Note 48**). Modify FL1 voltage (*see* **Note 49**) in order to count no more than 150 events of background noise in respect to 2000 Flow-Count Fluorospheres (*see* **Note 50**).

4. Add 100,000 of each 0.1, 0.2, 0.5, and 1.0 μm sizes and number calibration beads to 200 μL of PBS in separated tubes.

5. Acquire at least 5000 diluted beads to set the mean fluorescence of the different-sized beads (Figs. 4a and b). Analyze the samples by plotting fluorescence at 525/40 nm (FL1) versus log scale side scatter (LogSS). The level of fluorescence threshold will exclude the PBS background noise only (Fig. 4a, histogram and dot plot) but will allow a clear identification of the smaller beads of 0.1 and 0.2 μm sizes (Fig. 4a, histogram and dot plot) (*see* **Note 51**).

6. *FC exosome count*: prepare sample by mixing 5 μL of Exo resuspended in PBS with 20 μL of Flow-Count Fluorospheres (*see* **Notes 47** and **52**) in 200 μL PBS final volume and a blank tube containing PBS as control of background noise.

7. Set instrument at flux high, fix the stopping gate on 2000 Flow-Count Fluorospheres on previously drawn (Subheading 3.7, **step 3**) region in a FL channel different from FL1, e.g., FL5 (Fig. 4c) (*see* **Note 48**), and register the events in the exosome region correctly drawn in FL1 (Fig. 4d) (*see* **Note 53**).

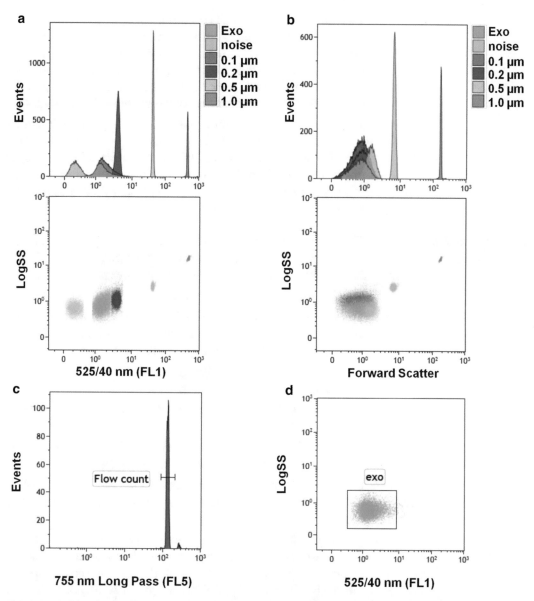

Fig. 4 Flow cytometry analysis of C16-Exo. C16-Exo, fluorescent beads ranging in size from 0.1 to 1.0 μm and background noise (noise) were analyzed for fluorescence (**a**, 525/40 nm FL1) and size (**b**, forward scatter). For more clarity, in these histograms and dot plots, the noise signal is shown although in the analyses it should not appear as described in Subheading 3.7. The pair color/sample of the legend matches with sample colors reported in the histograms (*upper side*) and dot plots (*lower side*) of (**a**) and (**b**). Two thousand Flow-Count Fluorospheres were used to determine Exo number. Exo sample was resuspended in PBS with Flow-Count Fluorospheres. The instrument was set to fix the stopping gate on 2000 Flow-Count Fluorospheres on correctly designed linear region in FL5 channel (**c**), while the number of Exo was registered in the rectangular Exo region previously drawn in FL1 (**d**)

8. To determine if there is a correspondence between the number as indicated on the package of 0.1 μm size standard fluorescent beads and the bead number counted by FC acquisition, prepare a tube with 10^7 beads of 0.1 μm size standard fluorescent with 20 μL of Flow-Count beads (*see* **Note 47**) in 200 μL PBS and follow the instructions reported in step 4 (*see* **Note 54**).

9. Total Exo and size standard fluorescent beads number can be established according to the formula: $x = ((y \times a/b)/c) \times d$ where y = events counted at 2000 counting beads; a = number of counting beads in the sample; b = number of counting beads registered (2000); c = volume of sample analyzed; and d = total volume of exosome preparation.

3.8   Fluo-Exo Cell Transfer Assay

1. The day before the experiment, seed 5×10^4 cells per well in a 96 well plate in duplicate for each Exo concentration (0–500 Exo per cell) plus one well for cell counting (*see* **Note 55**).

2. Gently remove media from cells and wash once with PBS.

3. To each well add 100 μL HBBS, 20 mM HEPES containing different amounts of Exo. To a well add 100 μL HBBS, 20 mM HEPES without Exo to test for autofluorescence.

4. Incubate 4 h at 37 °C with gentle shaking in an incubator equipped with an orbital shaker.

5. Remove medium, wash once with PBS, and add about 100 μL PBS.

6. Detach cells by gently pipetting and transfer to a fresh tube. Add PBS to reach 200 μL final volume (*see* **Note 56**).

7. Dead cells are excluded from analysis by adding ToPro-3 to ~20 nM final concentration just prior to FC analysis (*see* **Note 57**).

8. *Quantification of Exo and cells associated fluorescence* (Fig. 5): to quantify both Exo and cell-associated Exo, prepare a Quantum™ FITC-5 MESF standard curve by setting up five tubes with 50 μL PBS and three drops (~120 μL) of each bead with different amounts of fluorescein plus a blank tube with only PBS. Prepare a tube with Exo in PBS.

9. Acquire Exo, cell samples, and Quantum™ FITC-5 MESF beads with FC and determine arithmetic means for each sample.

10. To determine MESF per Exo and cells, transform fluorescence data (arithmetic mean) of Exo using the QuickCal analysis template provided with each Quantum™ MESF lot.

11. Transform MESF associated to cells in number of Exo transferred by using the formula: transferred Exo number = [cell fluorescence (MESF) – autofluorescence (MESF)]/MESF associated to a single Exo.

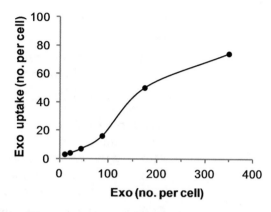

Fig. 5 Analysis of Exo transfer to cells. Me501 cells were incubated for 4 h with the indicated concentrations of fluorescent Exo. Single Exo-associated fluorescence is determined as described in Subheading 3.8, **step 8**. Flow cytometry analysis shows dose-dependent uptake of exosomes

4   Notes

1. When handling fluorescent probes, perform all the operations in the dark.

2. The amount of BODIPY fatty acid cell incorporation is dependent on FCS concentration in culture media and varies with cell type (Fig. 2a). The FCS concentration that gives the best uptake of the fluorescent probe should be determined prior to labeling a new cell type.

3. With this type of tube, we had better recovery of probe from tube walls.

4. BODIPY fatty acids are complexed to BSA to avoid lipotoxicity induced by free fatty acids. BSA must be fatty acid-free for optimal binding with BODIPY fatty acids [17].

5. In our hands Exo-FBS has proven to give the best recovery of fluorescent Exos in terms of Exo number.

6. Some batches of Exo-FBS may present turbidity; in this case centrifuge 5 min at $560 \times g$ and filter through 0.45 μm membrane filter.

7. If sterility is required, use sterile centrifuge and ultracentrifuge tubes and perform all steps in a tissue culture hood.

8. For separation of neutral lipids, TLC tank must be pre-saturated with the solvent mixture prior to immerse TLC plates as described in Subheading 3.4, **step 9**.

9. Prepare 100 mL solution and keep in an airtight container until ready to use. It can be reutilized in future experiments.

10. The same lysis buffer is used for Western blot analysis of cells.

11. Store at 4 °C. Prior to use make a 1:1000 dilution in PBS (50× stock).

12. It has to be noted that for Exo quantification experiments, we have only used C16 since the FC laser excitation required for C12 (ranging from 558 to 568 nm) has been difficult to achieve with common instruments equipped with 488 nm argon-ion laser resulting in poor and unreproducible Exo quantification. On the other hand, metabolic labeling of Exo with C12 can be successfully applied in experiments where Exo are tracked by other means, i.e., confocal microscopy, in vivo imaging, or FC equipped with optional lasers.

13. KOH is necessary to avoid micelle formation and to solubilize fatty acids in aqueous solutions.

14. If BODIPY fatty acid is not completely solubilized, after 5 min in ThermoMixer, vortex vigorously and extend incubation at 60 °C for additional 5 min.

15. It can be prepared in advance and stored at –20 °C. It can be frozen and thawed multiple times.

16. Cells must be in exponential growth rate when labeled with BODIPY fatty acids to allow for maximal probe incorporation.

17. Add 28 μL of 1 mM stock BODIPY fatty acid to 4 mL of medium. In Me501, a primary melanoma cell line, we obtained optimal fluorescence cell incorporation after 5 h incubation with C16 (Fig. 2b) at a probe concentration of 7 μM (Fig. 2c). C16 concentration and time of incubation may vary with different cell types. It has also to be noted that when a new cell type is used, several control experiments should be performed to ensure that fluorescent fatty acid analogues are metabolized as would be expected for native fatty acids. In particular they should include proof of esterification into phospholipids and neutral lipids by TLC and absence of unesterified C16 (Subheading 2.4) (Fig. 3a/f). Fluorescence intensity of Exo should also be checked to make sure they still can be FC counted (Subheading 3.7).

18. The volume of medium during the step of Exo secretion is critical for an abundant Exo recovery. 24–36 mL is optimal for a 75 cm² flask.

19. Can be stored at 4 °C up to a week.

20. It is only necessary to use sterile equipment if the final use of exosomes is going to require sterility. Otherwise very clean, but not necessarily sterile, tubes are required.

21. Best recovery of fluorescent Exo can be obtained by ultracentrifugation for 4 h.

22. This step is required to remove proteins in excess that could disturb Exo FC counting and western blot analysis.

23. Exo in PBS can be stored up to 2 days at 4 °C before FC counting.

24. Store Exo at –20 °C. Avoid repeated freezing and thawing and check again Exo number after thawing.

25. Iodixanol up to 60% (5 μL in 200 μL PBS) does not interfere with FC counting and protein determination by the Bradford method.

26. As an alternative measure the absorbance (optical density) of the fractions as described [18].

27. Up to 10^6 cells and 1×10^{10} Exo can be extracted with this volume of solvent.

28. This is the minimal amount of lipids to load in each lane to obtain a good resolution.

29. Tightly closed samples can be stored at 4 °C until needed.

30. Lanes must be 1 cm wide and distant 1 cm from each other.

31. Presaturation of the tank is an essential step to obtain a good separation of neutral lipid species.

32. Sample spots should remain above the surface of the developing solvent; otherwise samples could leach in the solvent.

33. For neutral lipid separation, the bottom edge of the TLC plate must be put in the glass tray.

34. Separation usually takes 10–15 min for neutral lipids and 30–40 min for phospholipid separation.

35. Plates can also be quickly dried with a hair dryer.

36. After baking fluorescent bands are not visible anymore on TLC plates.

37. Prepare cell lysates as follows: to $1–2 \times 10^6$ cell pellet, add 300 μL of lysis buffer and incubate 30 min at 4 °C on ice, centrifuge 5 min at $2000 \times g$, and discard pellet. Use 2 μL of lysate for protein determination. Prepare lysis buffer as described in Subheading 2.5, **step 5**.

38. Forty times of dilutions of 60% iodixanol (5 μL in 200 μL PBS) do not interfere with protein determination by the Bradford method.

39. The color changes immediately. If the color of some samples is obviously out of line with the BSA standard curve, prepare new tubes immediately with more or less sample.

40. Some antibodies against Exo markers, e.g., CD63 and CD81, give better resolution if sample buffer does not contain 2-mercaptoethanol or dithiothreitol (DTT).

41. Ponceau S allows reversible staining of total proteins blotted on nitrocellulose membranes.

42. All antibody incubations are carried out using gentle orbital shaking.

43. For a complete list of Exo marker antibodies, check 10.

44. If no protein band is visible, use ECL SuperSignal West Dura (PIERCE) for higher sensitivity.

45. Two milliliters per membrane is sufficient.

46. PBS must be filtered through a 0.22 μm filter which is used to dissolve the EV samples. Be careful to resuspend exosome population with a 0.22 μm-filtered PBS to remove eventual precipitates that could be mistakenly registered as events. Before running samples check instrument performance following the procedures suggested by the manufacturer.

47. Corresponding to 19,020 beads, but it depends on the batch.

48. On the Gallios instrument used to set up this protocol, it corresponds to 520 V.

49. Corresponding to about 2–3 events per second, in the presence of more events per seconds, follow the cleaning procedures suggested by the manufacturer; otherwise if the cleaning procedures fail, the PBS preparation must be verified.

50. This step is necessary to bypass the lack of exosome visualization by using a threshold set on size-based forward scatter. In fact the FS of background noise, 0.1 and 0.2 μm, are indistinguishable (Fig. 4b, histogram and dot plot).

51. To establish the right amount of Exo to be counted for each cell type/culture condition, make multiple dilutions of Exo in PBS to verify linearity and choose the right dilution for further measurements.

52. Each Fluorosphere contains a dye which has a fluorescent emission range from 525 to 700 nm when excited at 488 nm.

53. Verify that Exo population (Figs. 4a and b, green histograms and dots) lies below the 0.2 μm size in terms of fluorescence intensity (Figs. 4a and b, blue histograms and dots) but above the excluded background noise (Figs. 4a and b, turquoise histograms and dots).

54. To check for precision of instrument and reproducibility of measurements, it is necessary to determine if 0.1 μm beads counted at different dilutions display linearity.

55. Just prior to the transfer assay, count cells in a well to determine cell number per well.

56. Strongly adherent cells may require a trypsin/EDTA and centrifugation step before being resuspended in PBS.

57. Use 4 μL of 50× stock in 200 μL.

Acknowledgment

This work was supported by the Italian Ministry of Health (grant RF-2011-02347300). We thank Mario Falchi for his expert assistance with confocal imaging.

References

1. Cocucci E, Meldolesi J (2015) Ectosomes and exosomes: shedding the confusion between extracellular vesicles. Trends Cell Biol 25(6):364–372. doi:10.1016/j.tcb.2015.01.004

2. Felicetti F, Parolini I, Bottero L et al (2009) Caveolin-1 tumor-promoting role in human melanoma. Int J Cancer 125(7):1514–1522. doi:10.1002/ijc.24451

3. Thery C, Ostrowski M, Segura E (2009) Membrane vesicles as conveyors of immune responses. Nat Rev Immunol 9(8):581–593. doi:10.1038/nri2567

4. Maas SLN, de Vrij J, van der Vlist EJ et al (2015) Possibilities and limitations of current technologies for quantification of biological extracellular vesicles and synthetic mimics. J Control Release 200:87–96. doi:10.1016/j.jconrel.2014.12.041

5. Nolte-'t Hoen EN, van der Vlist EJ, Aalberts M et al (2012) Quantitative and qualitative flow cytometric analysis of nanosized cell-derived membrane vesicles. Nanomedicine 8(5):712–720. doi:10.1016/j.nano.2011.09.006

6. van der Vlist EJ, Nolte-'t Hoen EN, Stoorvogel W et al (2012) Fluorescent labeling of nanosized vesicles released by cells and subsequent quantitative and qualitative analysis by high-resolution flow cytometry. Nat Protoc 7(7):1311–1326. doi:10.1038/nprot.2012.065

7. Kormelink TG, Arkesteijn GJ, Nauwelaers FA et al (2015) Prerequisites for the analysis and sorting of extracellular vesicle subpopulations by high-resolution flow cytometry. Cytometry A 89:135–147. doi:10.1002/cyto.a.22644

8. Pospichalova V, Svoboda J, Dave Z et al (2015) Simplified protocol for flow cytometry analysis of fluorescently labeled exosomes and microvesicles using dedicated flow cytometer. J Extracell Vesicles 4:25530. doi:10.3402/jev.v4.25530

9. Parolini I, Federici C, Raggi C et al (2009) Microenvironmental pH is a key factor for exosome traffic in tumor cells. J Biol Chem 284(49):34211–34222. doi:10.1074/jbc.M109.041152

10. Thery C, Amigorena S, Raposo G et al (2006) Isolation and characterization of exosomes from cell culture supernatants and biological fluids. Curr Protoc Cell Biol 30:3.22.21–3.22.29. doi:10.1002/0471143030.cb0322s30

11. Tauro BJ, Greening DW, Mathias RA et al (2012) Comparison of ultracentrifugation, density gradient separation, and immunoaffinity capture methods for isolating human colon cancer cell line LIM1863-derived exosomes. Methods 56(2):293–304. doi:10.1016/j.ymeth.2012.01.002

12. Thumser AE, Storch J (2007) Characterization of a BODIPY-labeled fluorescent fatty acid analogue. Binding to fatty acid-binding proteins, intracellular localization, and metabolism. Mol Cell Biochem 299(1–2):67–73. doi:10.1007/s11010-005-9041-2

13. Wang H, Wei E, Quiroga AD et al (2010) Altered lipid droplet dynamics in hepatocytes lacking triacylglycerol hydrolase expression. Mol Biol Cell 21(12):1991–2000. doi:10.1091/mbc.E09-05-0364

14. Record M, Carayon K, Poirot M et al (2014) Exosomes as new vesicular lipid transporters involved in cell-cell communication and various pathophysiologies. Biochim Biophys Acta 1841(1):108–120. doi:10.1016/j.bbalip.2013.10.004

15. Folch J, Lees M, Sloane Stanley GH (1957) A simple method for the isolation and purification of total lipides from animal tissues. J Biol Chem 226(1):497–509

16. Kobayashi T, Stang E, Fang KS et al (1998) A lipid associated with the antiphospholipid syndrome regulates endosome structure and function. Nature 392(6672):193–197. doi:10.1038/32440

17. Bhattacharya AA, Grüne T, Curry S (2000) Crystallographic analysis reveals common modes of binding of medium and long-chain fatty acids to human serum albumin1. J Mol Biol 303(5):721–732. doi:10.1006/jmbi.2000.4158

18. Schröder M, Schäfer R, Friedl P (1997) Spectrophotometric determination of iodixanol in subcellular fractions of mammalian cells. Anal Biochem 244(1):174–176. doi:10.1006/abio.1996.9861

Chapter 17

Cardiac Myocyte Exosome Isolation

Zulfiqar A. Malik, Tingting T. Liu, and Anne A. Knowlton

Abstract

Exosomes are cell-derived small extracellular membrane vesicles (50–100 nm in diameter) actively secreted by a number of healthy and diseased cell types. Exosomes can mediate cellular, tissue, and organ level micro communication under normal and pathological conditions by shuttling proteins, mRNA, and microRNAs. Prior to vesicle molecular profiling, these exosomes can be isolated from conditioned cell media or bodily fluids such as urine and plasma in order to explore the contents and functional relevance. Exosome purification and analyses are a fast-growing research field. Regardless of several advances in exosome purification and analyses methods, research still faces several challenges. Despite tremendous interest in the role of extracellular vesicles, there is no general agreement on dependable isolation protocols. Therefore, there is an urgent need to establish reliable protocol of exosome purification and analysis. Here, we report a simple cost-effective isolation and analysis of cardiac myocyte exosomes from conditioned media.

Key words Exosomes, Cardiac myocytes, Cell signaling, Heart, Acetyl choline esterase, Protocol

1 Introduction

Exosomes form in the multivesicular body (MVB, Fig. 1a) and were originally described as a means to remove unwanted proteins and organelles from the cell [1, 2]. However it is now evident that exosomes, which are small lipid vesicles, have a broad range of functions including protein removal and intercellular signaling. Exosomes, which are secreted by most cell types, are 50–100 nM in diameter (Fig. 1b) and contain proteins, mRNA, microRNA, and DNA, all of which vary depending on the inducing agent and cell source. Electron microscopy of negative staining of fixed exosomes isolated from cardiac myocytes is shown in Fig. 1c. The trigger(s) for the creation of exosomes, which form through invagination of the membrane of the MVB, which is itself formed from invagination of the cell membrane, remain to be defined. As a result of these serial invaginations, the outer surface of the exosome is derived from the outer surface of the cell. The MVB can

Maurizio Federico (ed.), *Lentiviral Vectors and Exosomes as Gene and Protein Delivery Tools*, Methods in Molecular Biology, vol. 1448, DOI 10.1007/978-1-4939-3753-0_17, © Springer Science+Business Media New York 2016

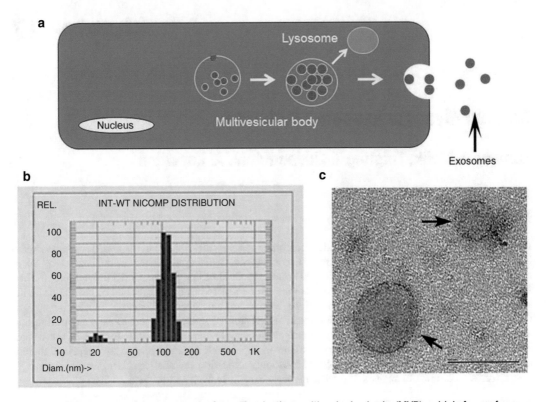

Fig. 1 (**a**) Cartoon summarizes exosome formation in the multivesicular body (MVB), which forms from an invagination of the plasma membrane. The exosomes then form via invagination of the MVB membrane. The MVB can either fuse with a lysosome, leading to degradation of contents, or fuse with the plasma membrane, releasing the exosomes into the extracellular space. (**b**) Nanotrac particle sizing profile. Exosomes peak at 100 nm. (**c**) EM of exosomes from plasma sample. Bar is 100 nm

either fuse with a lysosome, leading to destruction, or empty its contents extracellularly through fusion with the cell membrane. The control of this switch point remains unknown.

It is now recognized that exosomes bear proteins, lipids, and RNAs, mediating intercellular communication between different cell types in the body and thus affecting normal and pathological conditions. In the last few years, the role of exosomes in signaling and cancer and their potential as diagnostic and therapeutic agents have been widely recognized. Exosome research has burgeoned into an exciting field with over 350 articles on exosomes published in the last 3 years alone. Exosomes are found in all biological fluids, including urine, plasma, and ascites. Several protein families are commonly present in exosomes, including integrins, metabolic enzymes, cytoskeletal proteins, and heat shock proteins, particularly HSP90a and HSP70 [3, 4].

Due to the great potential of exosomes as a diagnostic and therapeutic tool, there is a need to understand their structure and function [5–10]. It is imperative to develop efficient reagents, tools, and protocols for exosome isolation, characterization, and analysis of their RNA and protein contents. Commonly used methods for exosome purification involve differential centrifugation, ultrafiltration, size-exclusion chromatography, and high-speed ultracentrifugation [11, 12]. The most frequently used methods of exosome purification involve differential ultracentrifugation (56%) followed by density gradient or cushion-based ultracentrifugation (27%) and ExoQuick precipitation [13]. Beside these traditional isolation techniques, commercially available easy-to-use precipitation solutions, such as ExoQuick™ and Total Exosome Isolation™ (TEI), have also been used in the last few years. Unfortunately, many studies fail to assess the quality and purity of isolated exosome populations before performing functional assays. One important challenge is the lack of standard methods to obtain highly pure and well-characterized exosome populations. In this paper, we detail our approach to isolation of exosomes produced by isolated adult rat cardiac myocytes. Furthermore, we enumerate the quality control methods we use for all our preparations to ensure that exosomes were isolated. Finally, we detail our approach to evaluate the reliability and impact of single-step purification of cardiac myocyte exosomes from conditioned media on purity, size, morphology, and proteome content.

2   Materials

Prepare all solutions using ultrapure water and analytical grade reagents to attain sensitivity at 25 °C. Diligently follow all waste disposal regulations when disposing waste materials. It is necessary to wash and autoclave all tools and bottles to be used in isolation. Wash only with Alconox, which is safe for washing equipment used in cell work.

2.1 Rat Cardiac Myocyte Isolation Components

For exosome isolation, adult cardiac myocytes are isolated from 3-month-old male Sprague-Dawley rats, as previously detailed [14]. For the isolation of myocytes, we need the following components:

1. Nalgene beakers (500 ml).
2. Nalgene bottles (500 ml, 1 L).
3. Nalgene bottle—bottom half.
4. Nalgene bottles—top half with mesh filter inserts.
5. Large pair of scissors.
6. Small pair of scissors.
7. Forceps (large and small).
8. Bulldog clamp.

9. Suture long enough to tie aorta to cannula.

10. Rubber cell scraper.

11. Sterilizer.

12. Tyrode's buffer (135 mM NaCl, 5.4 mM KCl, 1 mM $MgCl_2$, 0.33 mM NaH_2PO_4, 10 mM HEPES, 10 mM glucose).

13. Collagenase enzyme (Worthington).

14. Laminin (10 mg/ml in DMEM).

15. P35 (35 mm) and P100 (100 mm) plates.

16. Ketamine and Xylazine for anesthesia.

17. Heparin.

18. Perfusion pump.

19. Water bath.

20. Human serum albumin, as low endotoxin vs. FBS.

21. $CaCl_2$.

22. Butanedione monoxime—only in selected settings where isolation will be difficult, such as for myocytes from aged hearts.

23. 70% Ethanol.

2.2 Sample Collection Components

Cells are grown in media 199 supplemented with penicillin, streptomycin, insulin, and human serum albumin.

2.3 Exosome-Free Human Serum Albumin Purification Components

1. Beckman ultracentrifuge with SWTi-30 rotor.
2. Ultracentrifuge tubes.

2.4 Exosome Purification

1. Ethanol (100% tissue culture grade).
2. RNase-/DNase-free microtubes and pipette tips.
3. Falcon 50 ml conical centrifuge tubes.
4. Benchtop centrifuge (Thermo Scientific Sorvall).
5. ExoQuick precipitation reagent-EXOTC10A-1 (System Biosciences, Mountain View, CA).
6. Amicon Ultra filter (Millipore, Billerica, MA).

2.5 Exosome Quality Analysis Equipment and Solutions

1. DPBS (phosphate-buffered saline) pH 7.4.
2. Particle sizer (NICOMP 380 zls, PSS, Port Richey, FL).
3. NanoDrop spectrophotometer.
4. Plate reader (SpectraMax M Series Multi-Mode).
5. BCA assay (Pierce, Rockford, IL).
6. BSA 2 mg/ml standards (Pierce).

2.6 Exosome Protein Analysis by SDS-PAGE and Western Immunoblotting

1. Separating buffer (4× solution): 1.5 M Tris (hydroxymethyl) aminomethane (Tris–HCl), pH 8.7, 0.4 % SDS.

2. Stacking buffer (4× solution): 0.5 M Tris–HCl, pH 6.8, 0.4 % SDS.

3. 30 % Acrylamide/bis solution (37.5:1 with 2.6 % C) and N,N,N,N-tetramethylethylenediamine.

4. Ammonium persulfate: 10 % solution in water prepared immediately prior to use.

5. Running buffer (10× solution): 250 mM Tris–HCl, 1920 mM glycine, 1 % (w/v) SDS, pH 8.3.

6. SDS lysis buffer (5×): 0.3 M Tris–HCl (pH 6.8), 10 % SDS, 25 % B-mercaptoethanol, 0.1 % bromophenol blue, 45 % glycerol. Leave one aliquot at 4 °C for current use and store remaining aliquots at –20 °C.

7. Bromophenol blue solution: Dissolve 0.1 g in 100 ml water.

8. Page Ruler Prestained Protein Ladder (Thermo Scientific Pierce).

9. Transfer buffer (Tris-glycine): 25 mM Tris, 190 mM glycine, plus 0.05 % (w/v) SDS.

10. Nitrocellulose membrane (0.45 μm, Bio-Rad Laboratories) and thick filter paper (Bio-Rad Laboratories).

11. Tris-buffered saline, as a 10× solution (Bio-Rad Laboratories) with 0.5 % Tween-20 (TBS-T).

12. Blocking buffer: 5 % (w/v) nonfat dried milk (Bio-Rad Laboratories).

13. Mini PROTEAN 3 system glass plates (Bio-Rad Laboratories).

14. Medium binder clips ($1^1/_4$ in.).

15. Plastic container.

16. Primary antibody: Mouse anti-HSP60 (Enzo Life Sciences, Farmingdale, NY).

17. Secondary antibody: Anti-mouse IgG conjugated to horseradish peroxidase (GE Health Care Life Sciences/Amersham).

18. Chemiluminescent substrates for horseradish peroxidase (Pierce).

19. Autoradiography film, two sided. (Thermo Scientific Pierce).

3 Methods

To isolate exosomes, adult cardiac myocytes are prepared from the hearts of 3-month-old male rats, as previously described [14]. Adult cardiac myocytes are cultured in media containing human serum albumin. As serum samples contain exosomes, the human serum albumin is first centrifuged at $164,000 \times g$ for 2 h to remove all exosomes, as previously described [15].

3.1 Myocyte Isolation

1. Isolate adult rat cardiac myocytes with the Langendorff method, where the heart is perfused retrograde with type II collagenase through the aortic cuff. It is important to not advance the cannula into the ventricle, as the coronaries will then not be perfused. Sterile, cell culture grade water is needed for the isolation (*see* **Note 1**).

2. Make sure that water bath and pump are working so that solutions are maintained at 37 °C. PH of the solution needs to be 7.4 at all times for optimal digestion of the heart and good cell quality.

3. Give heparin as an IP injection 30 min before removing the heart for myocyte isolation (*see* **Note 2**). As the heart is perfused through the aortic cuff, the height of the column of fluid determines the pressure. For optimal isolation, pressure should be in physiologic range.

4. Place a bubble trap in place at the top of the system, as a bubble in the perfusion system acts like an embolus in the coronary artery, preventing perfusion and leading to poor digestion and thus poor-quality cardiac myocytes.

5. Rinse the heart in ice cold media before hanging it. At this point excess tissue can be trimmed off.

6. Rapidly hang the heart on the perfusion apparatus to minimize the time the heart is not perfused with oxygen (*see* **Note 3**). All tubing used in the procedure needs to be clinical grade so as to not leach chemicals into the perfusate.

7. Maintain the cleanliness of the system without using harsh/toxic chemicals. It is essential to having good cell isolations. If kept clean, tubing needs only to be changed every 6 months or longer, depending on frequency of use (*see* **Note 4**). This procedure yields 80 % rod-shaped cardiac myocytes and 8–10 million cells with quality isolation. Figure 2 shows a rat heart failure heart perfused on the isolation apparatus and the cardiac myocytes obtained from this heart. Yield of cells from a diseased heart is somewhat less than from a healthy heart.

3.2 Exosome Isolation by ExoQuick Precipitation

1. For the isolation of exosomes by precipitation, culture cardiac myocytes in media 199 supplemented with penicillin, streptomycin, insulin, and exosomes free human serum albumin media in ten P100 plates for 2 h. The diagram in Fig. 3 summarizes initial steps for exosome isolation.

2. Replace the supplemented media 199 with media 199 which contains all the above components, except albumin. This step is necessary because large amounts of protein, which is sticky, will make it difficult to purify exosomes. Myocytes and many other cells can be cultured without albumin for several hours without deleterious effects.

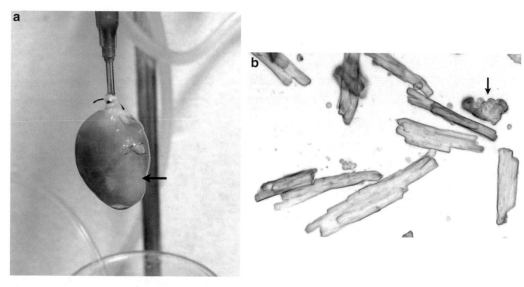

Fig. 2 (**a**) Isolated rat heart perfusion in preparation for isolation of cardiac myocytes. This heart has heart failure secondary to large infarct (*arrow*). (**b**) Ischemic heart failure cells isolated from the heart in (**a**). Most of cells are rods. *Arrow points* to dying cell that has folded up into a rounded shape. We are able to maintain these cells in culture for up to 24 h vs. the 48 h duration of culture with cardiac myocytes from a normal rat heart

3. We have found that both hypoxia/reoxygenation and ethanol, at levels found with intoxication, induce exosome production by cardiac myocytes. Treat cardiac myocytes with 65.1 mM cell culture grade ethanol (*see* **Note 5**) and incubate them for 2 h at 37 °C or with 2 h of hypoxia in an anaerobic chamber (Forma) and 1 h of reoxygenation, as previously described [16]. Both of these are mild injuries and do not cause significant cell damage. Ethanol treatment leads to the production of ROS, which stimulates exosome production, as previously reported [16].

4. At conclusion of the treatment times outlined above, collect the media and centrifuge at $300 \times g$ for 10 min at 4 °C to remove any nonadherent cells.

5. Centrifuge the media a second time at $4700 \times g$ for 30 min at 4 °C to remove cellular debris and extracellular DNA.

6. Collect the resulting supernatant, which contains the exosomes, and concentrate it at 4 °C from 50 ml to 140 μl with 100,000 molecular weight cutoff concentrating filters (Amicon Ultra Centrifugal filters), as per directions of the manufacturer.

7. Add ExoQuick to the concentrated media to complete isolation of the exosomes. ExoQuick, which essentially precipitates the exosomes (*see* **Note 6**), is added at a 1:1 ratio in a screw capped tube, mixed gently with a pipette, and incubated overnight (at least 12–15 h) at 4 °C.

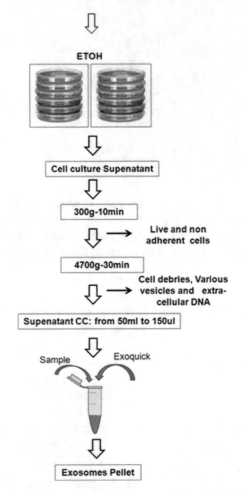

Fig. 3 Schematic provides overview of steps from cell culture plate to purified exosomes

8. The next day centrifuge the mixture at $1800 \times g$ for 30 min at 4 °C.

9. Aspire the supernatant and centrifuge the pellet at $1800 \times g$ for 5 min at 4 °C to remove all the residual solution.

10. Aspire the supernatant and dissolve the exosome pellet in DPBS pH 7.4 for exosome quality analysis and study.

3.3 Exosome Quality Analysis

1. Determine the quantity of protein by the BCA microassay method using BSA as a standard. Measure total protein as an index of the amount of exosomes present.

2. Exosomes are too small to readily visualize. The quality of exosome preparations is confirmed by measuring the hydrodynamic radius and the particle size distribution in terms of intensity, number, and volume by dynamic light scattering (DLS) on a Nicomp 380 DLS submicron particle sizer. Particle sizing by DLS is the most versatile and useful set of techniques for measuring sizes, size distributions, and (in some cases) shapes of nanoparticles in liquid (*see* **Note 7**).

3. Acetylcholinesterase activity, which reflects the amount of cell membrane present, is used to indirectly assess the quantity of exosomes isolated along with the measurement of total protein by BCA assay (Pierce, Rockford, IL), as previously described [13, 14]. Acetylcholine esterase activity is measured by adding 5-5′-dithiobis-(2-nitrobenzoic acid) (DTNB), acetylcholine iodide (ATC) in a 1:1 ratio with 10 μg of exosomes (total protein) in a cuvette and measuring absorbance at 412 nm [17]. Acetylcholinesterase (AchE) is an enzyme present in many tissues including nervous tissue, muscle, and red blood cells, which catalyzes the hydrolysis of acetylcholine and acetic acid. AChE has a very high catalytic activity, with each molecule of AChE degrading about 25,000 molecules of acetylcholine (ACh) per second. DTNB allows quantification of the thiocholine produced from the hydrolysis of acetylthiocholine by AChE in solutions. The absorption intensity of the DTNB adduct is used to measure the amount of thiocholine formed, which is proportional to the AChE activity. AChE activity is one way of confirming that one has highly consistent preparations of exosomes [15, 16] (*see* **Note 8**).

4. Perform SDS-PAGE by the method of Laemmli [18]. Proteins from each exosome isolate are standardized to the original sample volume and equal volumes are applied per lane of 12% SDS-PAGE gel.

5. Perform Western immunoblotting to analyze the presence of proteins of interest [16].

6. Transfer the SDS-PAGE gel to a nitrocellulose membrane and block for 1 h at room temperature with nonfat dried milk (*see* **Note 9**).

7. After blocking, probe the membrane for $1^{1}/_{2}$ h at 4 °C with primary antibody, wash, and then develop with secondary antibody linked to HRP (horseradish peroxidase).

8. Visualize the bound immune complexes using chemiluminescence (ECL, *see* **Note 10**) which leads to the development of bands on radiographic film. The resulting bands are qualified by digitizing the X-ray film image.

4 Notes

1. The water used for the cardiac myocytes isolation is very important. Small amounts of calcium or endotoxin in the water can damage the cardiac myocytes. Water must be sterile and cell culture grade. The water source cannot be casually changed without careful thought and testing. For example, a malfunctioning deionizing/water purification in one lab led to poor isolations, until someone made the connection between the sudden change in water quality secondary to equipment malfunction coinciding with problems with cardiac myocyte isolations. We find it best to purchase cell culture grade water for preparation of isolated cells.

2. Use 400–450 IU heparin for a 250–300 g rat given as an IP injection 30 min before the heart is to be removed. This gives heparin time to circulate and inhibit clotting. Adjust heparin dose for body weight.

3. Check the condition of the cells at every step by examining a drop under the microscope. If right after mincing there aren't mostly living cells (rods), then the problem is with the solutions or the perfusion. It is also very important to hang the heart as quickly as possible and run fluid rapidly while hanging to avoid air emboli. Alternatively one can cannulate the aorta with the heart immersed in media.

4. New tubing that is not cell culture or medical grade can lead to the leaching of chemicals into the perfusate, even with a small section of tubing. This can be lethal for the cardiac myocytes. We use Tygon tubing for our work. Tubing can last 6 months or more depending on frequency of isolations and care of equipment. A decline in cell yield or quality can be tip-off that it is time to change the tubing. After an isolation we flush the system with 200 ml of 70 % ethanol (mixed from a 100 % pure ethanol stock), drain the system to remove all ethanol, and then flush with 200 ml sterile cell culture grade water. We drain system to remove all fluid.

5. Untreated adult cardiac myocytes in culture produce a very minimal amount of exosomes. Exosome production by cardiac myocytes is increased by ethanol treatment. Treatment with cell culture grade ethanol, at concentrations found in humans

consuming alcoholic beverages, is done for 2 h and greatly increases exosome production. The ethanol concentration corresponds to legally intoxicated levels and levels found with the consumption of multiple alcoholic drinks [18].

6. We prefer to prepare exosomes by the ExoQuick method approach that meets our daily needs of experiments and also involves less labor than the serial centrifugation we have used previously [13].

7. DLS measurements are conducted at 25 °C by adding 200 μl of 0.5–1.0 mg/ml of total protein (based on BCA assay measurement of total protein in an aliquot of exosomes) in a glass tube (Fig. 2b). There are 1024 correlation channels equipped with a 15 mW He-Ne laser diode at 632.8 nm and a photodiode detector set at a 90° angle. Light scattering is recorded for 900 s with two replicate measurements and each exosome preparation is representative of five technical replicates. This step is important as it is the only confirmation that one has isolated vesicles of appropriate size.

8. The total reaction volume per cuvette is 1 ml, consisting of 10 μl (1 μg/μl) isolated exosomes, 450 μl of ATC (2.8 mM) and DTNB (0.3 mM), and 90 μl DPBS pH 7.4. The enzyme is preincubated at room temperature for a few minutes. The absorbency is measured continuously every 5 min for 30–60 min at 412 nm at room temperature using a NanoDrop 2000C spectrophotometer. The values are plotted using Graph Pad Prism5 and different exosome preparations compared. We have found that AChE activity correlates with exosome counts.

9. We have found that the powdered nonfat dried milk marketed by Bio-Rad gives much cleaner blots than the cheaper powdered milk products available in the grocery store.

10. Chemiluminescent substrates available in the market are not exactly fit for the detection and reflection of all the protein band density to measure equally, either they are very strong or weak ECLs. To get precise amount of band intensity in Western blots that should reflect the amount of protein loaded on SDS-PAGE, we mixed right proportion of two different chemiluminescent substrates (Pico and Femto-ECL) for the detection of horseradish peroxidase (HRP) activity from antibodies and other Western blot probes.

Acknowledgments

Supported by HL077281 and HL07907 both to AAK

References

1. Johnstone RM, Adam M, Hammond JR et al (1987) Vesicle formation during reticulocyte maturation: association of plasma membrane activities with released vesicles (exosomes). J Biol Chem 262:9412–9420

2. Johnstone RM, Mathew A, Mason AB et al (1991) Exosome formation during maturation of mammalian and avian reticulocytes: evidence that exosome release is a major route for externalization of obsolete membrane proteins. J Cell Physiol 147:27–36

3. Thery C, Zitvogel L, Amigorena S (2002) Exosomes: composition, biogenesis and function. Nat Rev Immunol 2:569–579

4. Simons M, Raposo G (2009) Exosomes: vesicular carriers for intercellular communication. Curr Opin Cell Biol 21:575–581

5. Schorey JS, Bhatnagar S (2008) Exosome function: from tumor immunology to pathogen biology. Traffic 9:871–881

6. Mittelbrunn M, Sánchez-Madrid F (2012) Intercellular communication: diverse structures for exchange of genetic information. Nat Rev Mol Cell Biol 13:328–335

7. Van Niel G, Porto-Carreiro I, Simoes S et al (2006) Exosomes: a common pathway for a specialized function. J Biochem 140:13–21

8. Lakkaraju A, Rodriguez-Boulan E (2008) Itinerant exosomes: emerging roles in cell and tissue polarity. Trends Cell Biol 18:199–209

9. Xu D, Tahara H (2013) The role of exosomes and microRNAs in senescence and aging. Adv Drug Deliv Rev 65:368–375

10. Vlassov AV, Magdaleno S, Setterquist R et al (2012) Exosomes: current knowledge of their composition, biological functions, and diagnostic and therapeutic potentials. Biochim Biophys Acta 1820:940–948

11. Szczepanski MJ, Szajnik M, Welsh A et al (2011) Blast-derived microvesicles in sera from patients with acute myeloid leukemia suppress natural killer cell function via membrane-associated transforming growth factor-β1. Haematologica 96:1302–1309

12. Hong CS, Muller L, Whiteside TL et al (2014) Plasma exosomes as markers of therapeutic response in patients with acute myeloid leukemia. Front Immunol 5:160

13. Van Deun J, Mestdagh P, Sormunen R et al (2014) The impact of disparate isolation methods for extracellular vesicles on downstream RNA profiling. J Extracell Vesicles 3:10

14. Sun L, Chang J, Kirchhoff SR, Knowlton AA (2000) Activation of HSF and selective increase in heat shock proteins by acute dexamethasone treatment. Am J Physiol 278:H1091–H1096

15. Gupta S, Knowlton AA (2007) HSP60 trafficking in adult cardiac myocytes: role of the exosomal pathway. Am J Physiol Heart Circ Physiol 292:H3052–H3056

16. Malik ZA, Kott KS, Poe AJ et al (2013) Cardiac myocyte exosomes: stability, HSP60, and proteomics. Am J Physiol Heart Circ Physiol 304:H954–H965

17. Ellman GL, Courtney KD, Andres V et al (1961) A new and rapid colorimetric determination of acetylcholinesterase activity. Biochem Pharmacol 7:88–95

18. Laemmli UK (1970) Cleavage of structural proteins during the assembly of the head of bacteriophage T4. Nature 227:680–685

Chapter 18

Incorporation of Heterologous Proteins in Engineered Exosomes

Francesco Manfredi, Paola Di Bonito, Claudia Arenaccio, Simona Anticoli, and Maurizio Federico

Abstract

Engineering exosomes to upload heterologous proteins represents the last frontier in terms of nanoparticle-based technology. A limited number of methods suitable to associate proteins to exosome membrane has been described so far, and very little is known regarding the possibility to upload proteins inside exosomes. We optimized a method of protein incorporation in exosomes by exploiting the unique properties of a nonfunctional mutant of the HIV-1 Nef protein referred to as Nef^{mut}. It incorporates at high extents in exosomes meanwhile acting as carrier of protein antigens fused at its C-terminus. Manipulating Nef^{mut} allows the incorporation into exosomes of high amounts of heterologous proteins which thus remain protected from external neutralization/degradation factors. These features, together with flexibility in terms of incorporation of foreign antigens and ease of production, make Nef^{mut}-based exosomes a convenient vehicle for different applications (e.g., protein transduction, immunization) whose performances are comparable with those of alternative, more complex nanoparticle-based delivery systems.

Key words Exosomes, Nef, Protein delivery, Fusion proteins, Insect cells

1 Introduction

Exosomes are vesicles of 50–100 nm which form intracellularly upon inward invagination of endosome membranes [1] leading to formation of intraluminal vesicles (ILVs) which then become part of multivesicular bodies (MVBs). They are intracellular organelles originating from endosomes and consisting of a limiting membrane enclosing ILVs. MVBs traffic either to lysosomes for degradation or to plasma membrane, thereby releasing their vesicular contents in the extracellular milieu. Vesicles released by this mechanism are defined exosomes.

Before budding, HIV and related lenti- and retroviruses interact with cell factors also involved in exosome biogenesis, i.e., Alix, Tsg101, and other components of the endosomal sorting complex required for transport (ESCRT) [2]. HIV budding occurs at lipid

Maurizio Federico (ed.), *Lentiviral Vectors and Exosomes as Gene and Protein Delivery Tools*, Methods in Molecular Biology, vol. 1448, DOI 10.1007/978-1-4939-3753-0_18, © Springer Science+Business Media New York 2016

rafts, i.e., cell membrane microdomains enriched in cholesterol, phospholipids with saturated side chains, and sphingolipids. Also exosomal membranes contain lipid raft microdomains [3]. The convergence of exosome and HIV biogenesis implies the possibility that viral products incorporate in exosomes. This was indeed demonstrated in the case of both Gag [4] and Nef [5, 6] HIV-1 proteins. Nef is thought to associate with exosomes as consequence of anchoring of its N-terminal myristoylation to lipid raft microdomains at the limiting membrane of MVBs.

HIV-1 Nef is a 27 kilodalton (kDa) protein lacking enzymatic activities [7]. It is the first HIV product synthesized in infected cells, thereby being expressed at levels comparable with those of HIV structural proteins. After synthesis at free ribosomes, Nef reaches both intracellular and plasma membranes to which it tightly interacts through both its N-terminal myristoylation and a stretch of basic amino acids located in alpha helix loop 1. Nef acts as a scaffold/adaptor element in triggering activation of signal transducing molecules like p21 PAK-2, NF-κB, STATs, ERK1-2, and Vav and Src family kinases. In most cases, it occurs upon Nef association with lipid raft microdomains. They are used as platform in cell trafficking and signaling, as well as for budding of diverse virus species including HIV [8], whose lipid composition in fact tightly resembles that of lipid raft microdomains [3]. The fact that exosome membranes also are enriched in lipid raft microdomains [9] explains why Nef can be found in both exosomes and HIV viral particles.

We identified a $^{V}153^{L}$ $^{E}177^{G}$ Nef mutant incorporating at quite high levels in HIV-1 particles, HIV-1-based virus-like particles (VLPs) [10], and exosomes [11]. The incorporation efficiency still increases when this mutant is engineered with an N-terminal palmitoylation through $^{G}3^{C}$ mutation [12], expectedly a consequence of an improved association with lipid rafts. This Nef mutant (referred to as Nef^{mut}) is defective for almost all Nef functions, and its efficiency of incorporation in nanovesicles does not change significantly when it is fused with foreign proteins.

Two alternative methods to upload exosomes with foreign products have been described: the first one exploits the binding of C1C2 domains of lactadherin to exosome lipids resulting in the association of foreign antigen with the external side of exosome membranes [13, 14]. The other one relies on coating exosomes with *Staphylococcus aureus* enterotoxin A tailed with a highly hydrophobic *trans*-membrane domain [15]. Both techniques result in a modification of the external contents of exosomes. Differently, manipulating Nef^{mut} allows the incorporation of high amounts of proteins into exosomes which thus remain protected from external neutralization/degradation factors. These features, together with ease of production and the demonstrated flexibility in terms of incorporation of foreign antigens, make Nef^{mut}-based exosomes a convenient candidate for both protein transduction and immunogen delivery whose performances are expected to be comparable with those of alternative, already characterized nanoparticle delivery systems.

Spodoptera frugiperda (Sf9) cells have long been used for the production of recombinant proteins expressed by either baculovirus *Autographa californica* nuclear polyhedrosis virus (AcNPV) genetic systems or stable transformation with specific plasmids [16]. Large-scale technologies for Sf9 cell culture for recombinant proteins production have also been well established [17]. Several pharmaceutical products obtained from Sf9 cells have been proven to be safe in humans and are currently on the market. The discovery that the intercellular communication among prokaryotes and eukaryotes relies also on the production of micro- and nanovesicles has opened the possibility to manipulate and use such vesicles as carriers of therapeutics. Little is known about the production of nanovesicles from Sf9 insect cells. Interestingly, our recent unpublished observations indicate that Sf9 cells produce high quantities of exosome-like nanovesicles which can be engineered upon intracellular expression of Nef^{mut}.

2 Materials

2.1 Vector Preparation

1. Immediate-early CMV promoter-regulated eukaryotic vector where the sequences of the Nef^{mut}-based fusion protein can be accommodated (*see* **Note 1**).

2. Eukaryotic vector expressing the G protein from vesicular stomatitis virus (VSV-G) or an alternative envelope protein allowing pH-dependent fusion (e.g., from Ebola virus).

3. Insect vector regulated by AcNPV-derived hr5 enhancer and ie-1 immediate-early promoter to express Nef^{mut} in Sf9 insect cells (*see* **Note 2**).

2.2 Exosome-Producing Cell Systems

1. Dulbecco's Modified Eagle's Medium (DMEM) and Roswell Park Memorial Institute medium (RPMI 1640) supplemented with 10 % fetal bovine serum (FBS, Gibco), heat inactivated at 56 °C for 30 min. Exosome-deprived FBS (System Biosciences, Mountain View, CA) (*see* **Note 3**).

2. Human embryonic kidney 293T cells.

3. Lipofectamine 2000 (Invitrogen, Life Technologies).

4. *Spodoptera frugiperda* (Sf)9 cells.

5. SF900 II serum-free medium (Life Technology).

6. Cellfectin® Transfection Reagent (Life Technologies).

7. Sterile 125–500 mL polycarbonate Erlenmeyer flask (Corning Costar, Manassas, VA).

8. INNOVA refrigerated incubator shaker 4230 for Sf9 suspension culture.

2.3 Exosome Concentration, Purification, and Titration

1. Polyallomer ultracentrifuge tubes (*see* **Note 4**).
2. Iodixanol 60% solution (Axis Shield, Dundee, Scotland) (*see* **Note 5**).
3. Amplex Red kit (Molecular Probes, Life Technologies).

2.4 Exosome Characterization: Western Blot

1. Equipment and buffers for casting 10–12% SDS polyacrylamide gel electrophoresis (PAGE).
2. Recombinant (r)Nef protein. It can be obtained from NIBSC AIDS Reagent Program upon request or purchased from either EBI (Frederick, MD) or Intracel (Issaquah, WA).
3. Equipment and buffers for Western blot analysis.
4. Primary antibodies for Western blot analysis: anti-HIV-1 Nef ARP 444 from NISBC AIDS Reagent Program (*see* **Note 6**), anti-VSV-G from Immunology Consultant Laboratories (Newberg, OR), anti-TSG101 from Clontech (Palo Alto, CA), anti-ICAM-1 (Santa Cruz, Dallas, TX), and anti-CD63 (R&D System, Minneapolis, MN).
5. Secondary Abs for Western blot analysis: horseradish peroxidase (HRP)-conjugated anti-rabbit/mouse/sheep/human Abs.
6. Chemiluminescent detection reagents.

2.5 Exosome Characterization: FACS Analysis

1. Surfactant-free white aldehyde/sulfate latex beads (Invitrogen, Life Technology).
2. Kit for cell permeabilization Cytofix/Cytoperm (BD Bioscience, San Diego, CA).
3. Monoclonal antibodies (mAbs) to detect exosome-associated proteins: anti-Nef mAb clone 6.2 from NIH AIDS Research and Reference Reagent Program. Abs against envelope proteins and heterologous moiety of choice fused with Nef^{mut} suitable for FACS analysis (*see* **Note 7**); PE-conjugated anti-CD63 (R&D); FITC-conjugated cholera toxin subunit B (Sigma-Aldrich, St. Louis, MO).
4. FACSCalibur cytofluorimeter running Cell Quest software, or equivalent.

---

3 Methods

3.1 Vector Preparation

Here, we describe the methods for production, concentration, and titration of exosomes incorporating Nef^{mut} alone. The vector expressing Nef^{mut} is freely available upon request. To recover a vector expressing a Nef^{mut}-based fusion protein, amplify the Nef open reading frame and the polypeptide/protein sequence of interest separately by conventional PCR procedures. The final sequence codifying the fusion protein will be recovered by overlapping PCR procedures. In this regard, considering that the Nef moiety must be placed at the N-terminus of the fusion protein, design appropriate primers overlapping 3′ Nef and 5′ heterologous sequences. These primers should include a complementary sequence extending at least 10–15 nucleotides. On the basis of the experience we acquired with many Nef^{mut}-based fusion proteins we successfully constructed, no spacer amino acid sequences are needed between Nef^{mut} and the heterologous polypeptide/protein (*see* **Note 8**).

3.2 Recovery of Engineered Exosomes from Transiently Transfected Mammalian Cells

1. For 15 cm diameter dishes, seed 2×10^7 293T cells in DMEM 10% FBS without antibiotics the day before transfection.

2. The day of transfection, bring the volume of the medium to 12 mL. Add 3 mL of mix of transfection (i.e., Lipofectamine 2000 plus DNA) according to manufacturer's recommendations.

3. The day after, replace the medium. At this time, antibiotics may be included, but the use of exosome-depleted FBS is recommended. Pay special attention to leave the packaging cells attached.

4. The following day, harvest the supernatants. Additional supernatant harvestings may be done every 8–16 h for 2–3 days, according to the cell viability.

5. Clarify the supernatants by centrifugation at $1500 \times g$ for 30 min at 4 °C. At this time, supernatants can be stored at −80 °C.

3.3 Recovery of Cell Lines Stably Releasing Exosomes

In some cases, the availability of a cell line constitutively releasing engineering exosomes would be useful. We isolated a human cell line expressing Nef^{mut} inserted in the doxycycline-regulatable pLVX-TetOne-Puro lentiviral vector from Clontech-Takara (Mountain View, CA) (*see* **Note 9**). The experimental procedures for both LV production and cell transduction can be found in chapters of this volume as well as in previously published "Lentiviral gene engineering protocols" books of the MMB series.

3.4 Recovery of Engineered Exosome-Like Nanovesicles from Transiently Transfected Insect Cells

1. Seed $2.5–3 \times 10^7$ Sf9 cells in 150 cm² tissues culture flask from a suspension culture with a log phase of growth ($1–1.5 \times 10^6$ cells/mL) (*see* **Note 10**).

2. Incubate the cells at 27.5 °C until they adhere to the flask (about 2 h); replace the medium with 15 mL of fresh SF900 II w/o antibiotics (*see* **Note 11**).

3. Prepare the following solutions in Eppendorf tubes. Solution A: 60 µg DNA into final 500 µL of SF900 II w/o antibiotics. Solution B: 180 µL Cellfectin Reagent in 320 µL of SF900 II w/o antibiotics.

4. Combine the two solutions, mix gently, and incubate at RT for 30 min in a dark environment.

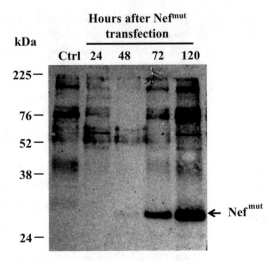

Fig. 1 Detection of Nef[mut] in exosome-like vesicles released by transfected Sf9 cells. These cells were transfected with the pBiEx-3 vector expressing Nef[mut]. Supernatants were harvested starting to 48 h after transfection, and exosome-like nanovesicles isolated through differential centrifugations. Equal amounts of exosome-like nanovesicles isolated from the supernatants harvested at the indicated times were loaded in a 10 % SDS-PAGE. Proteins were blotted, and filters revealed by a polyclonal anti-Nef Ab. In the ctrl lane, nanovesicles harvested from the supernatants of Sf9 cells 120 h after transfection with void pBiEx-3 vector were loaded. *Arrows* indicate the Nef [mut] migration. Molecular markers are given in kDa

5. Using a 1 mL sterile pipette, drop the DNA-Cellfectin mixture on the cells.

6. After max 16 h, replace the DNA containing medium with 30 mL of fresh medium and incubate the flask at 27.5 °C. Take particular care to avoid cell detachment.

7. For harvesting exosome-like nanovesicles, collect the medium from 2 days after transfection.

8. Centrifuge the supernatants at $1500 \times g$ for 30 min at 4 °C to remove both cells and cell debris. The cleared supernatants can be stored at −80 °C until processing, as described below.

9. By Western blot we detected increasing amounts of Nef[mut] in exosome-like vesicles purified from cell medium starting from 48 h post-transfection, with a peak at 5 days after transfection (Fig. 1).

3.5 Exosome Concentration

Although different commercial reagents useful to recover exosomes from cell supernatants are now available, we still consider differential centrifugations the gold standard method to concentrate and partially purify exosomes.

1. Load polyallomer SW 28 tubes with up to 30 mL of supernatant. Ultracentrifuge 30 min at $10,000 \times g$, 4 °C.

2. Harvest supernatants, filter 0.2 µM, and ultracentrifuge at 70,000 × g for 1 h.

3. Resuspend the pellet in 1× PBS, fill the tube with 30 mL of the buffer, and ultracentrifuge again at 70,000 × g for 1 h.

4. Decant the supernatants by inverting the tubes; eliminate possible residual drops with sterile paper.

5. Resuspend the pellet (which should not be visible) in 200–400 µL of 1× PBS.

6. Let stand the pellet at 4 °C overnight (*see* **Note 12**).

7. By gently scraping the bottom of the tube with a tip, harvest the resuspension volume, aliquot, and store at –80 °C.

3.6 Exosome Purification

1. To purify exosomes, pellets recovered by differential centrifugations can be subjected to 6–18% discontinuous iodixanol gradient. Pellets from 30–150 mL of supernatants can be effectively purified in 10 mL gradients which can be accommodated in Beckman SW 41 polyallomer tubes.

2. Put 1 mL of 30% iodixanol at the bottom of the tube. Then, gently stratify a total of ten fractions of 0.9 mL of iodixanol from 18% (bottom) to 6% in 1× PBS in 1.2% increments.

3. Stratify the exosome pellet on the top of the gradient. Ultracentrifuge at 200,000 × g for 1.5 h at 4 °C in an SW41 Ti rotor (Beckman).

4. Harvest 0.7 mL fractions starting from the top. Purified exosomes should concentrate in fractions 4–7.

We experienced that iodixanol present in the fractions does not significantly affect the outcomes of the most part of downstream applications (i.e., enzymatic titrations, Western blot analysis, cell assays). However, in the case exosome concentration needs to be increased and/or iodixanol has to be removed, the fractions can be further processed as follows:

1. Dilute half of fractions with two volumes of 0.9% sodium chloride.

2. Ultracentrifuge for 50 min at 392,000 × g in a TL-100 tabletop ultracentrifuge.

3. Resuspend the pellet with the same modalities here above described in case the recovery of untouched exosomes is desired. In case a molecular analysis of the exosomes is planned, the pellet can be immediately lysed and recovered by adding 50 µL of Tris–HCL pH 7.4 10 mM, NaCl 100 mM, EDTA 1 mM, and 0.1% Triton X-100.

3.7 Exosome Quantification: Acetylcholinesterase Assay

Determination of acetylcholinesterase (AchE) activity is a both rapid and convenient way to titrate exosomes. The enzyme acetylcholinesterase is specifically uploaded in exosomes [18], and the kit we routinely use, i.e., Amplex Red kit detects the activity in exosomes from both human and mouse cells. The AchE activity is measured as mU/mL, where 1 mU is defined as the amount of enzyme which hydrolyzes 1 pmole of acetylcholine to choline and acetate per minute at pH 8.0 at 37 °C. The title of a standard preparation of exosomes from 30 mL of supernatant of 293T transfected cells ranges 20–50 mU/mL upon 100-fold concentration (*see* **Note 13**).

3.8 Characterization of Exosome Preparations: Western Blot Analysis

This analysis is critical to determine the stability of the Nef^{mut}-based fusion product as well as its incorporation efficiency. The stability of the fusion product can be evaluated by conventional Western blot analysis on lysates from exosome-producing cells. In addition, Western blot analysis of the engineered exosomes as compared with exosomes incorporating Nef^{mut} alone will allow to establish a possible influence of the foreign product in the efficiency of incorporation in exosomes. Finally, the compared analysis with scaled amounts of recombinant Nef serves to evaluate the actual amounts of the fusion product uploaded in exosomes.

1. Load 0.2–1 mU of exosomes in three wells of 10–12% SDS-PAGE.

2. Blot the gel on filter, cut it in stripes, and reveal exosomes products through incubation with Abs detecting either Nef, the heterologous protein and, in case, the envelope protein. In addition, CD63, Alix, and Tsg101 can be considered appropriate exosome markers for Western blot-based molecular characterizations.

3. For the semi-quantitative analysis, load a unique 10–12% SDS-PAGE gel with serial dilutions of rNef (e.g., five wells containing from 100 to 6.25 ng) and additional five wells with serial dilutions of the exosome preparation.

4. Blot the gel on filter and incubate it with anti-Nef Abs and reveal.

5. Compare the signal intensities from both exosomes and rNef by quantitative densitometry.

3.9 Characterization of Exosome Preparations: FACS Analysis

Contents of engineered exosomes can be also detected by FACS analysis (*see* **Note 14**). In view of the exosome size which is near the detection threshold of most cytofluorimeters, exosomes should be preventively bound to aldehyde latex beads which interact with the lipids of nanovesicles (*see* **Note 15**). Exosome-coupled beads can be incubated with specific antibodies and analyzed by FACS. This method allows the detection of both membrane associated and intra-particle associated proteins.

1. Pretreat the required volume of surfactant-free white aldehyde/sulfate latex beads (i.e.,1 μL for up to 2 mU of exosomes) with an excess of exosome-depleted FBS at room temperature for 30 min.

2. Wash the beads once with 1× PBS, resuspend them in the buffer, and add the equivalent of 1 μL to exosome preparations. Bring the total volume to 50 μL in 1× PBS/5% exosome-depleted FBS.

3. Incubate at room temperature in a rotating plate from 2 h to overnight.

4. To detect exosome-associated envelope proteins, wash the beads once with 1 mL of 1× PBS and incubate the exosome-bead complexes with proper dilution of Abs in 50 μL of 1× PBS/5% exosome-depleted FBS. Always include the incubation with Abs against appropriate exosome markers, e.g., CD9 or CD63 tetraspanins.

5. Incubate at 4 °C for 1 h, wash, resuspend in 1× PBS-2% formaldehyde, and analyze by FACS.

6. In case a nonfluorescent Ab is used, the incubation with conjugated secondary Abs can be performed following the same protocol described for the primary one.

7. To detect both Nef and the fused foreign product, treat the exosome-beads complexes with Cytofix/Cytoperm solution according to manufacturer's recommendations.

8. For Nef detection, incubate with 1:30 dilution of the anti-Nef mAb clone 6.2 (NIH AIDS Research Reference Program). Specific Abs suitable for FACS analysis should be used for detecting the foreign protein.

4   Notes

1. We routinely use combinations of eukaryotic expression vectors regulated by the immediate-early CMV promoter without evident inhibitory interference. However, alternative promoters (e.g., PKG, e-IF2α) have been described working well in 293T cells.

2. In our pilot experiments, the Nef^{mut} open reading frame was subcloned into *BamH* I-*Acc* I sites of the pBiEx-3 vector (Novagen).

3. Although exosome-deprived FBS is commercially available, it can be easily prepared by ultracentrifuging heat-inactivated FBS $70,000 \times g$ at 4 °C for at least 2 h, and sterilizing with 0.45 μM pore diameter filter.

4. Do not use UltraClear tubes since the exosome pellet in these tubes is quite difficult to detach.

5. 20–60 % sucrose gradient is also effective, but in most instances, the use of pure exosomes in downstream cell assays requires sucrose elimination.

6. There are several good anti-Nef Abs for Western blot both in commerce and from NIH Research and Reference Reagent Program. Among the latter, we recommend also the polyclonal Abs #331 and #2949 and the monoclonal Abs #456 and #1535.

7. Although the foreign antigen incorporated in exosomes is expected to be part of a unique protein fused with Nef, we suggest to formally confirm the results using also Abs recognizing the heterologous moiety.

8. The longest protein we successfully accommodated as C-terminal fusion moiety of Nef^{mut} and incorporated in exosomes was HCV NS3 (i.e., 1890 nucleotides, 630 amino acids). However, often the exosome incorporation efficiency also depends on intrinsic features of the heterologous protein, such as intracellular localization, hydrophobicity, and interaction with cell membranes. As a general rule, highly hydrophobic amino acid domains which are expected to cross cell membranes should be deleted to avoid interference with Nef localization at the inner side of cell membranes.

9. We found the use of the pLVX-TetOne-Puro of particular convenience. Here, regulatory Tet-sequences, puromycine resistance, and transgene are accommodated in a single lentiviral construct. The unique shortcoming is the quite limited number of restriction sites available for cloning the desired open reading frame.

10. Sf9 cells are usually cultivated in suspension culture with serum-free medium (SF900 II) up to $2–4 \times 10^6$ cells /mL in polycarbonate flasks.

11. Sf9 cells can also be cultivated at a constant room temperature of 23–25 °C, either in a suspension culture using an opportune mild shaking instrument or in an adherent state on tissues culture flask. When Sf9 are cultivated at room temperature, their doubling time is longer. The temperature to manipulate and cultivate Sf9 must never exceed 28 °C, otherwise apoptosis would be induced. The flask working volumes are 20–50 mL for 75 cm^2 flask and 125–200 mL for 175 cm^2 flasks in incubator shaker at 27.5 °C, 60 rpm or faster depending on the instrument. The right rpm have to be fixed with the own shaker. Cell density and viability is checked every 24–48 h. Cells should be maintained at a density between 5×10^5 and 4×10^6 cells/mL.

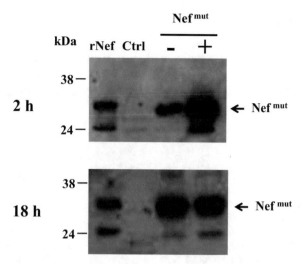

Fig. 2 Timing of exosome recovery after differential centrifugations. Quadruplicates of 10 mL of supernatants of 293T cells transfected with a Nef^{mut}-expression vector were processed by differential centrifugations, and pellets were resuspended in 300 μL of 1× PBS without (−) or with (+) 0.1 % Triton X-100. Resuspension volumes were then harvested after 2 or 18 h of incubation at 4 °C. Then, equal volumes of the exosome preparations were loaded in a 10 % SDS-PAGE. Proteins were blotted and filters revealed by a polyclonal anti-Nef Ab. As control, both 100 ng of recombinant HIV-1 Nef protein (rNef) and exosomes from mock-transfected cells (Ctrl) were loaded. **Arrows** indicate the Nef ^{mut} migration. Molecular markers are given in kDa

12. We experienced that the overnight incubation of exosome pellet with buffer increases significantly the exosome recovery (Fig. 2) without significant loss of their contents/functions.

13. The determination of the AchE enzymatic activity associated with exosomes is a rapid, simple, and quite specific assay. The most significant shortcoming we often experienced regards quite high blank values. This inconvenience can be minimized by complementing the reaction mix with the buffer of exosome dilution (e.g., PBS, 0.9 % sodium chloride, medium) rather than the dilution buffer provided by the kit.

14. For detecting exosome-associated proteins, the use of monoclonal rather than polyclonal Abs guarantees the best signal/background ratio. Also, two-steps labeling procedure using fluorochrome-conjugated secondary Abs could increase the sensitivity of the assay.

15. The small dimension of the beads implies that they can be detected at quite low values of both SSC/FSC parameters, i.e., similar to those used for detecting platelets.

Acknowledgments

This work was supported by a grant from "Ricerca Finalizzata" project n. RF-2010-2308334 from the Ministry of Health, Italy to M.F. We are also indebted to Pietro Arciero for the excellent technical support.

References

1. Gyorgy B, Szabo TG, Pasztoi M et al (2011) Membrane vesicles, current state-of-the-art: emerging role of extracellular vesicles. Cell Mol Life Sci 68:2667–2688

2. Usami Y, Popov S, Popova E et al (2009) The ESCRT pathway and HIV-1 budding. Biochem Soc Trans 37:181–184

3. de Gassart A, Geminard C, Fevrier B et al (2003) Lipid raft-associated protein sorting in exosomes. Blood 102:4336–4344

4. Fang Y, Wu N, Gan X et al (2007) Higher-order oligomerization targets plasma membrane proteins and HIV gag to exosomes. PLoS Biol 5:1267–1283

5. Lenassi M, Cagney G, Liao MF et al (2010) HIV Nef is secreted in exosomes and triggers apoptosis in bystander CD4+ T cells. Traffic 11:110–122

6. Muratori C, Cavallin LE, Kratzel K et al (2009) Massive secretion by T cells is caused by HIV Nef in infected cells and by Nef transfer to bystander cells. Cell Host Microbe 6:218–230

7. Chazal N, Gerlier D (2003) Virus entry, assembly, budding, and membrane rafts. Microbiol Mol Biol Rev 67:226–237

8. Simons K, Sampaio JL (2011) Membrane organization and lipid rafts. Cold Spring Harb Perspect Biol 3:a004697. doi:10.1101/cshperspect.a004697

9. Foster JL, Denial SJ, Temple BRS et al (2011) Mechanisms of HIV-1 Nef function and intracellular signaling. J Neuroimmune Pharmacol 6:230–246

10. Peretti S, Schiavoni I, Pugliese K et al (2005) Cell death induced by the herpes simplex virus-1 thymidine kinase delivered by human immunodeficiency virus-1-based virus-like particles. Mol Ther 12:1185–1196

11. Lattanzi L, Federico M (2012) A strategy of antigen incorporation into exosomes: comparing cross-presentation levels of antigens delivered by engineered exosomes and by lentiviral virus-like particles. Vaccine 30:7229–7237

12. Sistigu A, Bracci L, Valentini M et al (2011) Strong CD8(+) T cell antigenicity and immunogenicity of large foreign proteins incorporated in HIV-1 VLPs able to induce a Nef-dependent activation/maturation of dendritic cells. Vaccine 29:3465–3475

13. Hartman ZC, Wei JP, Glass OK et al (2011) Increasing vaccine potency through exosome antigen targeting. Vaccine 29:9361–9367

14. Sedlik C, Vigneron J, Torrieri-Dramard L (2014) Different immunogenicity but similar antitumor efficacy of two DNA vaccines coding for an antigen secreted in different membrane vesicle-associated forms. J Extracell Vesicles 3. doi:10.3402/jev.v3.24646

15. Xiu FM, Cai ZJ, Yang YS et al (2007) Surface anchorage of superantigen SEA promotes induction of specific antitumor immune response by tumor-derived exosomes. J Mol Med 85:511–521

16. Contreras-Gomez A, Sanchez-Miron A, Garcia-Camacho F (2014) Protein production using the baculovirus-insect cell expression system. Biotechnol Prog 30:1–18

17. Mena JA, Kamen AA (2011) Insect cell technology is a versatile and robust vaccine manufacturing platform. Expert Rev Vaccines 10:1063–1081

18. Rieu S, Geminard C, Rabesandratana H (2000) Exosomes released during reticulocyte maturation bind to fibronectin via integrin alpha 4 beta 1. Eur J Biochem 267:583–590

Chapter 19

Exosome-Mediated Targeted Delivery of miRNAs

Shin-ichiro Ohno and Masahiko Kuroda

Abstract

Many types of cells release phospholipid membrane vesicles that are thought to play key roles in cell–cell communication, antigen presentation, and the spread of infectious agents. These membrane vesicles, derived from the late endosomes, are called exosomes. Various proteins, messenger RNAs (mRNAs), and microRNAs (miRNAs) are carried by exosomes to cells in remote locations, like a message in a bottle. Because they can protect encapsulated small RNAs from ribonucleases (RNases) in body fluid, exosomes represent ideal carriers for nucleic acid drugs. In addition, because exosomes are constructed from self components, they are predicted to have low antigenicity and toxicity, extremely important properties for carriers used in drug delivery. This article describes a protocol for using exosomes as carriers for RNA drug delivery systems.

Key words Exosomes, Microvesicles, MicroRNA, Drug delivery system, Nucleic acid drugs

1 Introduction

MicroRNAs (miRNAs) are small (21–25 nucleotides) noncoding RNA molecules that bind to partially complementary mRNA sequences, resulting in target degradation or translation inhibition. A growing pool of evidence suggests that miRNA-related gain- or loss-of-function mutations can cause the development and/or progression of cancer [1]. For example, let-7a is thought to be a tumor suppressor that inhibits the malignant growth of cancer cells by reducing RAS and HMGA2 expression. Reduced expression levels of let-7 have been observed in colon, lung, ovary, and breast cancer cells [2]. Therefore, miRNA replacement therapies have emerged as promising treatment strategies for malignant neoplasms. Yet although miRNA-based modalities may eventually prove effective, their clinical application has been hampered by a lack of appropriate delivery systems.

Exosomes are small membrane vesicles (30–100 nm in diameter) that are secreted by a variety of cell types and tissues [3, 4] and can be isolated from the conditioned medium of a variety of cells or from body fluids using a sucrose gradient (1.13–1.19 g/ml) or

Maurizio Federico (ed.), *Lentiviral Vectors and Exosomes as Gene and Protein Delivery Tools*, Methods in Molecular Biology, vol. 1448, DOI 10.1007/978-1-4939-3753-0_19, © Springer Science+Business Media New York 2016

ultracentrifugation (100,000×*g* for 70 min) [5]. Exosomes are enriched in heat shock proteins (HSP70, HSP90), tetraspanin family molecules (CD9, CD63, CD81), and components of the ESCRT (endosomal sorting complex required for transport) machinery (e.g., Alix and TSG101) [4]. Of clinical interest, tumor cells have been shown to release exosomes containing miRNA [6] and miRNAs secreted from donor cells can be taken up and function in recipient cells [7]. These data indicate that exosomes are natural carriers of miRNA that could be exploited as an RNA drug delivery system. In this article, we present protocols for using exosomes as carriers for miRNA drug delivery [8].

Expectations for the clinical application of exosomes are increasing, necessitating further research and development of exosomes as a next-generation drug delivery system (DDS). On the other hand, attempts to apply exosomes as a DDS are still in their infancy, and the purification methods and analytical techniques are immature. We hope that the experimental techniques published in this paper will help researchers involved in exosome development in the future.

2   Materials

1. HEK293 cells (human embryonic kidney cell line), used as exosome-producing cells (*see* **Note 1**).

2. DMEM supplemented with 10% heat-inactivated fetal calf serum (FCS), penicillin, and streptomycin (*see* **Note 2**).

3. Ultracentrifuge (Optima L-70K) (Beckman Coulter) (*see* **Note 3**).

   Rotors (SW41Ti, SW28) (Beckman Coulter).

4. Ligand expression vectors (Fig. 1) (*see* **Note 4**).

5. Transfection reagent (*see* **Note 5**).

6. UltraClean Aldehyde/Sulfate Latex beads (Invitrogen).

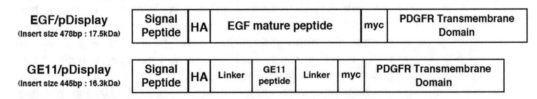

Fig. 1 Construction of a membrane-localized ligand to add a targeting function to exosomes. Diagrams of the modified epidermal growth factor (EGF) and GE11 proteins. Signal peptide, Igκ-chain leader sequence; HA, hemagglutinin epitope tag (YPYDVPDYA); Linker, (GGGGS) 3; Myc, Myc epitope (EEKLISEEDL); platelet-derived growth factor receptor (PDGFR) transmembrane domain, transmembrane domain from platelet-derived growth factor receptor. This figure was obtained from Ref. 8 with permission

7. 1 M glycine in phosphate-buffered saline (PBS).

8. 2% FCS in PBS.

9. Antibodies:

   Anti-HA (HA7) (Sigma-Aldrich).

   Anti-Myc antibody (Millipore).

   Anti-HLA-A/B/C (H-300) (Santa Cruz Biotechnology).

   Anti-CD81 antibody (BD Pharmingen).

10. RNAzol RT (Sigma-Aldrich).

11. TaqMan miRNA assays (Applied Biosystems).

12. Stratagene MX3000P thermal cycler (Agilent Technologies).

13. Flow cytometer: BD FACS Calibur (BD biosciences).

14. Dye for exosome.

    PKH67 with Diluent C (Sigma-Aldrich); for in vitro experiment.

    XenoLight DiR (Perkin Elmer).

15. Protein Assay Rapid Kit (Wako Pure Chemicals).

16. Confocal fluorescence microscopy (Leica).

17. IVIS Lumina (Perkin Elmer).

3   Methods

3.1   Selection of Exosome-Producing Cells and Targeting

Secretion of exosomes by cells is a common physiological phenomenon. However, the characteristics of exosomes, including their size, amount secreted, and the expression of molecules on their membranes (included proteins and nucleic acids), differ between cell types. Thus, depending on the therapeutic target and purpose of the experiment, it is necessary to select suitable exosome-producing cells. On the other hand, because the molecules that constitute exosomes are diverse, it is not feasible to predict all of their effects and side effects. Therefore, exosomes have properties distinct from those of single biological products, such as purified antibodies, and are in some ways more similar to cell transplantation therapy (e.g., immunotherapy). The main problem with exosomes is immunogenicity, which can be addressed using autologous cells for exosome production. Immune cells or induced pluripotent stem cell (iPS) cells that can be grown in vitro are a potential source of safe exosomes. In particular, dendritic cells (DCs) have a high exosome production capacity.

When exosomes are administered systemically into mice via the tail vein, most exosomes are integrated into the liver. This is a consequence of the purifying effect of the reticuloendothelial system of the liver and has been observed in many DDSs including exosomes. If the target is not the liver, it is necessary to devise a method for efficiently delivering the exosomes to target cells. For example, in order to efficiently deliver exosomes to breast cancer cells, we developed exosomes that target EGFR. In particular, we focused on EGF and an artificial ligand (GE11 peptide) as EGFR ligands and prepared exosomes that express these molecules on their membrane surface [8].

3.2 Preparation of Exosomes

1. Transfect the ligand-expressing vectors (Fig. 1) into HEK293 cells (exosome-producing cells).

2. After 2 days, select cells stably expressing the ligand by G418.

3. Transfect miRNA drugs (e.g., let-7a) to the ligand-expressing cell lines at a concentration of 100 nM.

4. After 2 days, collect the culture supernatant.

5. To remove dead and floating cells, centrifuge the supernatant at $2000 \times g$ for 20 min at 4 °C and collect the supernatant.

6. To remove cell debris, centrifuge the resultant supernatant at $10,000 \times g$ for 30 min at 4 °C and collect the supernatant.

7. To precipitate the exosome fraction, centrifuge the resultant supernatant at $100,000–120,000 \times g$ for 70 min at 4 °C and discard the supernatant.

8. Wash the exosomes fraction with PBS and re-centrifuge at $100,000–120,000 \times g$ for 70 min at 4 °C and discard the supernatant.

9. Suspend the pellet in 100 μl PBS and store the exosome fraction at 4 °C.

10. Measure the protein concentration using the Protein Assay Rapid Kit. In the case of HEK293, about 70 μg of exosomes can be obtained from 100 ml culture supernatant.

3.3 Analysis of Exosomes

Immunoblots of protein extracts (Fig. 2, left) and real-time PCR from RNA extracts allow relatively straightforward of exosome components, because it is possible to obtain and analyze these extracts under the same conditions used for cells. For the internal control, it is necessary to consider whether GAPDH and β-actin are suitable. We used HLA as an internal control for immunoblotting and let-7a as an internal control for miRNA expression analysis.

Several methods may be used to confirm the quality of the purified exosomes. One option is electron microscopy. Either transmission electron microscopy (TEM) or scanning electron microscopy (SEM) can be used to verify that the exosomes are spherical and have a diameter of 30–100 nm. Although exosomes were previously considered to have a cup shape (i.e., a dented ball), the current mainstream view is that they are spherical. Also, by using immuno-electron microscopy in TEM, antigen expression

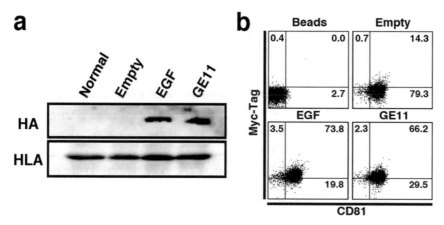

Fig. 2 Analysis of exosomes by immunoblotting and flow cytometry. (**a**) Western blots of HA-tagged constructs in exosomes obtained from culture supernatants of HEK293 cells that had been transfected with pDisplay encoding EGF or GE11. The quality of each exosome preparation was confirmed by incubation with antihuman leukocyte antigen (HLA) antibodies. (**b**) For flow cytometry, exosomes from transfected HEK293 cells were incubated with latex beads and stained with anti-Myc tag antibodies. Tetraspanin CD81 was used as a positive control for the exosomes. This figure was obtained from Ref. 8 with permission

can also be detected. By simultaneously detecting exosome markers such as CD63, Alix, and TSG101, it is possible to improve the accuracy of exosome detection. Furthermore, in recent years, beautiful images of spherical exosomes have been obtained by cryo-SEM [9]. For measurements of the size and concentration of exosomes, particulate-measuring devices such as qNano and NanoSight are used [10].

Another approach to identify exosomes involves analyzing the expression of exosome markers. Completely exosome-specific markers do not exist, but exosomes do contain multiple antigens. Representative examples are tetraspanins such as CD81, CD63, and CD9 and proteins involved in vesicle formation such as Alix and TSG101 [4]. Membrane antigens can also be detected by flow cytometry rather than immunoblotting. The size of exosomes, which falls below the detection limit of most of flow cytometers, makes it difficult to analyze individual exosomes. Therefore, latex beads are used to adsorb exosomes. This procedure allows the staining of the desired antigen whose analysis can be then performed using a flow cytometer.

3.4 Analysis of Exosomes by Flow Cytometry

Here we present a protocol, modified from that of Alvarez-Erviti et al. [11].

1. Wash an UltraClean Aldehyde/Sulfate Latex beads, 200 μl (8 mg) twice with 1 ml PBS, and resuspend in 200 μl PBS.

2. Mix the purified exosomes (8 μg) with the 12.5 μl washed beads (adjusted to 100 μl with PBS) and then incubate with slow stirring in a rotator at room temperature for 2 h.

3. Add 11 µl 1 M glycine to the bead/exosome mixture and incubate with slow stirring in a rotator at room temperature for 30 min.

4. Wash three times with 1 ml 2 % FCS in PBS.

5. Resuspend the pellet in 50 µl 2 % FCS in PBS.

6. Incubate the beads/exosomes with appropriate amount of fluorescently labeled antibody for 20 min at room temperature.

7. The pDisplay construct can be detected with an anti-Myc antibody. In addition, anti-CD81 antibody is available as a positive control. The fluorescently labeled isotype control antibodies are used as negative control.

8. Wash with 1 ml 2 % FCS in PBS and then resuspend in 300 µl 2 % FCS in PBS.

9. Perform flow cytometry analysis (Fig. 2 right).

3.5 Tracking of Exosomes

To confirm that exosomes accumulate in the target organ, it is necessary to label them. PKH67, a fluorescent dye that is stably integrated into the lipid region of the cell membrane, can be used to stain exosomes composed of lipid bilayer membranes. In in vitro experiments, it is possible to observe uptake into cells by confocal fluorescence microscopy.

Here we present a protocol to fluorescently label exosomes modified from Lässer et al. [12]:

1. Add PKH67 (0.4 µl) in 200 µl Diluent C to 10 µg exosomes in 200 µl PBS. PBS alone, without exosome, is used as a negative control.

2. Incubate the mixture for 2 min at room temperature.

3. Wash with 10 ml PBS and ultracentrifuge at $120,000 \times g$ at 4 °C for 70 min.

4. Discard supernatant and resuspend the pellet, containing fluorescently stained exosomes, in 100 µl PBS.

5. For an uptake assay of PKH67-labeled exosome, incubate 1 µg of PKH67-labeled exosomes with 10^5 breast cancer cells in 24 well cell culture plate at 37 °C or 4 °C for 4 h. The uptake of PKH67-labeled exosomes is analyzed using flow cytometry and confocal fluorescence microscopy (Fig. 3).

On the other hand, when administered in vivo, exosomes can be stained using XenoLight DiR as the fluorescent dye. Because it fluoresces in the near-infrared, the emissions of this dye have high tissue permeability. Behavior of exosomes after administration can be observed using an in vivo imaging system (IVIS). A strong signal can be observed under anesthesia without dissection, and it is possible to increase sensitivity by extracting an organ, as in Fig. 4.

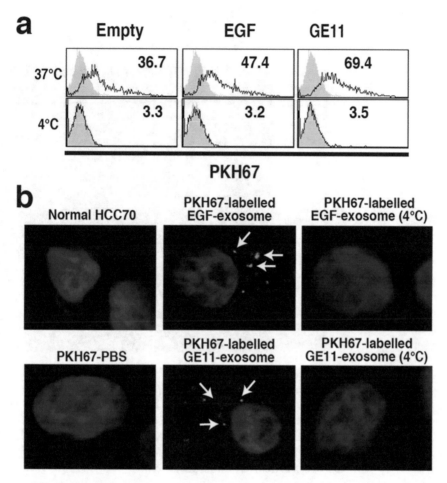

Fig. 3 Uptake of ligand-targeted exosomes by breast cancer cell lines. (**a**) Uptake of fluorescently labeled exosomes by the breast cancer cell lines was detected using flow cytometry. PKH67-labeled exosomes were incubated with the breast cancer cell lines at 37 °C or 4 °C for 4 h. The degree of uptake was relatively low at 4 °C. (**b**) Intracellular PKH67-labeled exosomes were detected in HCC70 cells (*arrows*) using confocal fluorescence microscopy. This figure was obtained from Ref. 8 with permission

For the fluorescence staining of exosomes using XenoLight DiR:

1. Dilute XenoLight DiR to 300 μM in Diluent C (*see* **Note 6**).

2. Add diluted XenoLight DiR to 10 μg exosomes in 1 ml PBS at a final concentration of 2 μM.

3. Incubate at room temperature for 30 min.

4. Wash with 10 ml PBS and ultracentrifuge at 120,000 × *g* for 70 min.

5. Resuspend the pellet, containing fluorescently stained exosomes, in 100 μl PBS.

6. Administer 4 μg of exosomes systemically via the tail vein and perform IVIS analysis and dissection after 24 h.

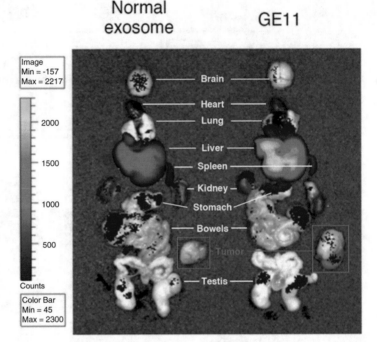

Fig. 4 Analysis of fluorescently labeled exosomes after systemic administration. Exosomes labeled with XenoLight DiR (near-infrared) were intravenously injected (4 μg of purified exosomes) into mice bearing transplanted HCC70 cells. Brain, heart, spleen, liver, lung, kidney, small intestine, colon, and tumor tissues were harvested 24 h postinjection for ex vivo imaging. The migration of fluorescently labeled exosomes was detected with an in vivo imaging system (IVIS). This figure was obtained from Ref. 8 with permission

4   Notes

1. Because it is possible that exosomes derived from cancers contain oncogene products, we used HEK293 cells to produce exosomes. However, HEK293 cells produce very low levels of exosomes, and it is also necessary to be consider the potential incorporation of gene products from the introduced adenovirus.

2. Because FCS contains exosomes derived from cattle, we deplete the exosome fraction by ultracentrifugation. It is also possible that serum-free medium such as Knockout DMEM could be used, although we have no direct experience with this reagent. Also, if a decrease in exosomes yield is a concern, medium without serum can be used.

3. There are several methods for purifying exosomes: ultracentrifugation, sucrose gradients, ultrafiltration through a membrane, and the use of commercially available co-precipitants.

Ultracentrifugation, an inexpensive method with a relatively high capacity, is used in most cases.

4. In order to add a targeting function, we express a ligand on the membrane of the exosomes. To this end, we construct a chimeric molecule consisting of the ligand and a cell membrane localization domain that binds to the target cell. The expression of chimeric molecules is confirmed by Western blot and flow cytometry. We focused on epithelial growth factor (EGF) and an artificial ligand (GE11 peptide) as epithelial growth factor receptor (EGFR) ligands and prepared exosomes expressing these molecules on their surfaces using the pDisplay vector (Life Technologies), which adds the cell membrane localization domain of PDGFR and a peptide tag (HA, Myc) to the ligand (Fig. 1). In addition, to express targeting peptide on the exosomal membrane, the group of Alvarez-Erviti used modified Lamp2b, a protein found abundantly in exosomal membranes [11]. This method is also considered to be effective.

5. Techniques for encapsulating nucleic acid drugs into the exosomes can be divided into two broad categories. To directly introduce the RNAs, exosomes can be electroporated [13]. Alternatively, to encapsulate the nucleic acids during the formation stage, the exosomes can be obtained from cells expressing a high level of the desired RNAs. We used the Lipofectamine RNAi MAX transfection reagent (Life Technologies) to introduce the tumor-suppressive miRNA let-7a into exosome-producing cells, which then produced this miRNA at high concentrations.

6. Be aware that the incubation with exceeding amounts of dye decreases the signal.

References

1. Calin GA, Croce CM (2006) MicroRNA signatures in human cancers. Nat Rev Cancer 6(11):857–866

2. Barh D, Malhotra R, Ravi B et al (2010) MicroRNA let-7: an emerging next-generation cancer therapeutic. Curr Oncol 17(1):70–80

3. Lotvall J, Valadi H (2007) Cell to cell signalling via exosomes through esRNA. Cell Adh Migr 1(3):156–158

4. Théry C, Ostrowski M, Segura E (2009) Membrane vesicles as conveyors of immune responses. Nat Rev Immunol 9(8):581–593

5. Théry C, Amigorena S, Raposo G, et al (2006) Isolation and characterization of exosomes from cell culture supernatants and biological fluids. Curr Protoc Cell Biol Chapter 3:Unit 3.22

6. Skog J, Würdinger T, van Rijn S et al (2008) Glioblastoma microvesicles transport RNA and proteins that promote tumour growth and provide diagnostic biomarkers. Nat Cell Biol 10(12):1470–1476

7. Pegtel DM, Cosmopoulos K, Thorley-Lawson DA et al (2010) Functional delivery of viral miRNAs via exosomes. Proc Natl Acad Sci U S A 107(14):6328–6333

8. Ohno S, Takanashi M, Sudo K et al (2013) Systemically injected exosomes targeted to EGFR deliver antitumor microRNA to breast cancer cells. Mol Ther 21(1):185–191

9. Gallart-Palau X, Serra A, Wong AS et al (2015) Extracellular vesicles are rapidly purified from human plasma by PRotein Organic Solvent PRecipitation (PROSPR). Sci Rep 5:14664

10. Mehdiani A, Maier A, Pinto A et al (2015) An innovative method for exosome quantification and size measurement. J Vis Exp 95:50974

11. Alvarez-Erviti L, Seow Y, Yin H et al (2011) Delivery of siRNA to the mouse brain by systemic injection of targeted exosomes. Nat Biotechnol 29(4):341–345

12. Lässer C, Alikhani VS, Ekström K et al (2011) Human saliva, plasma and breast milk exosomes contain RNA: uptake by macrophages. J Transl Med 9:9

13. Kooijmans SA, Stremersch S, Braeckmans K et al (2013) Electroporation-induced siRNA precipitation obscures the efficiency of siRNA loading into extracellular vesicles. J Control Release 172(1):229–238

INDEX

Maurizio Federico (ed.), *Lentiviral Vectors and Exosomes as Gene and Protein Delivery Tools*, Methods in Molecular Biology,
vol. 1448, DOI 10.1007/978-1-4939-3753-0, © Springer Science+Business Media New York 2016

Printed in the United States
By Bookmasters